A Note from the Kaplan Director of European Operations

Welcome to the first edition of Kaplan Test Prep and Admissions' BMAT preparation book! We want you to perform at your very best on test day, and that is what this book will help you do.

Kaplan Test Prep and Admissions is the world leader in test preparation, and our books, software, courses and tutoring services are second to none. Kaplan was founded in the U.S. in 1938, and in the UK we have helped thousands of students do better on university admissions tests since 1994.

Take full advantage of all the strategies, practice questions, review materials, and online practice available through buying this book, to make sure that test day presents no surprises and is as stress-free as possible for you.

Kaplan's BMAT online companion is accessible through **kaptest.com/BMATbooksonline**. Here you'll find additional practice questions and more writing practice, including sample essay responses.

If after working through this book, you would like further help with your BMAT preparation, Kaplan Test Prep and Admissions also offers specialised preparation courses and tutoring at its London Centre and at secondary schools across the UK. See our web site or contact us at the address below for more information.

Entry into the UK's top medical schools is becoming ever more competitive. The number and quality of applicants is increasing every year. As a result, a number of the more selective medical schools now require applicants to take the BioMedical Admissions Test (BMAT) to help them distinguish between highly-qualified candidates and assess whether they have the skills needed to do well in medical programmes.

During a successful career in medicine you will encounter many challenges, and that is probably one of the reasons you were attracted to a medical career in the first place. View the BMAT as one of these challenges on a path toward a successful future career, as well an opportunity for you to show medical schools that you are committed and well-suited to a career in medicine. We are pleased to be able to work with you on achieving this goal.

Good luck on test day!

Kind regards,

Louise Cook
Director of European Operations
Kaplan Test Prep and Admissions

London Centre
3-5 Charing Cross Road
London WC2H 0HA
Tel: 020 7930 3130
Fax: 020 7930 8009
london_centre@kaplan.com
www.kaptest.com/uk

BMAT®
Biomedical
Admissions Test

by the Staff of Kaplan Test Prep and Admissions

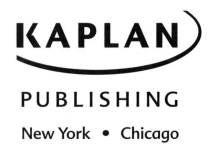

PUBLISHING

New York • Chicago

This publication is designed to provide accurate and authoritative information in regard to the subject matter covered. It is sold with the understanding that the publisher is not engaged in rendering legal, accounting, or other professional service. If legal advice or other expert assistance is required, the services of a competent professional should be sought.

Editorial Director: Jennifer Farthing
Senior Editor: Tonya Lobato
Production Artist: Dave Chipps
Cover Designer: Carly Schnur

© 2006 by Kaplan, Inc.

Published by Kaplan Publishing, a division of Kaplan, Inc.
888 Seventh Ave.
New York, NY 10106

Printed in the United States of America

June 2006
10 9 8 7 6 5 4 3 2

ISBN-13: 978-1-4195-4170-4
ISBN-10:   1-4195-4170-6

Kaplan Publishing books are available at special quantity discounts to use for sales promotions, employee premiums, or educational purposes. Please call our Special Sales Department to order or for more information at 800-621-9621, ext. 4444, e-mail kaplanpubsales@kaplan.com, or write to Kaplan Publishing, 30 South Wacker Drive, Suite 2500, Chicago, IL 60606-7481.

Table of Contents

AVAILABLE ONLINE

Online Companion

The best preparation for a standardized test is practice in the test format. That's why we've provided even more practice in your online companion which can be accessed at kaptest.com/BMATbooksonline. Look there for additional reading passages and questions and more essay practice with a sample response.

Updates and Corrections

The material in this book is up-to-date at the time of publication. However, the LNAT Consortium Ltd may have instituted changes in the test after this book was published. Be sure to carefully read the materials you receive when you register for the test. If there are any important late-breaking developments—or any changes or corrections to the Kaplan test preparation materials in this book—we will post that information at kaptest.com/publishing.

Feedback and Comments

If you have comments or suggestions about this book, we invite you to fill out our online survey form at kaplansurveys.com/books. Your feedback is extremely helpful as we continue to develop high-quality resources to meet your needs.

PART I

BMAT Basics

Chapter 1: **Introduction to the BMAT**

While laughter may be the best medicine for the soul, *preparation* is the best "medicine" for an exam. Because you aspire to be a medical professional, you'll need to take the BMAT, a requirement for admission to many biomedical degree programmes. It's an important test, one that can have a significant impact on your future. This book has everything you need to get ready for the exam and succeed on test day.

A BMAT OVERVIEW

The BMAT – BioMedical Admissions Test – is a standardised test designed to help universities select the most qualified candidates for biomedical classes and programmes more effectively. While most standardised tests aim to measure either aptitude or knowledge (usually the latter), the BMAT is designed to do both, with an emphasis on your abilities and skills.

The two-hour exam consists of three sections:

- Section I: Aptitude and Skills (60 minutes)
- Section II: Scientific Knowledge and Applications (30 minutes)
- Section III: Writing Task (30 minutes)

The test takes place just once a year and is administered by Cambridge Assessment, which also researches and develops the exam. It's an old-fashioned pen-and-paper test, and with the exception of the essay portion of the exam, most of the questions are multiple-choice. A few questions will ask you to make calculations or respond in a short answer.

It's important to note that the BMAT *does not* assess your qualification to practise medicine. That is something your university will do on an ongoing basis as you work toward your degree. Instead, the BMAT aims to measure your *potential* to do well in a rigourous undergraduate programme. Test items focus on assessing generic but essential academic skills such as critical thinking and basic scientific knowledge, not specialised knowledge or skills.

Why Take the BMAT?

Many universities require the BMAT for certain pre-med classes and programmes. If you wish to enroll in any of these programmes or classes, you must take the BMAT.

While we know you'd rather not take *another* test if you don't have to, we also know that with preparation, you can make the BMAT work to your advantage. Because the BMAT is so different from other assessment tools that universities use to assess candidates, it gives you the opportunity to distinguish yourself from other applicants.

Institutions requiring the BMAT for courses and degree programmes include:

- University of Bristol Veterinary School
- University of Cambridge Medical & Veterinary Schools
- University of Oxford Medical School
- Royal Veterinary College
- Imperial College London
- University of Manchester
- University College London

The official BMAT website, **bmat.ucles-red.cam.ac.uk**, offers a complete list of the specific universities and courses that require the BMAT.

Why *Make* the BMAT?

Because medical programmes are so competitive, and because so many qualified candidates apply, many universities felt the need for another tool to help them determine which candidates are the *most* qualified. That's why Cambridge Assessment created the BMAT. Because the BMAT is a standardised test, universities can see how you compare to other applicants. And that's good news for you: because you're taking the time to prepare for the exam, you're more likely to do your best on the test.

WHAT TO EXPECT ON THE BMAT

As we noted, the BMAT aims to measure both aptitude and knowledge – what you know and, more importantly, how you think and learn. Generic skills tested throughout the exam include the ability to:

- read and understand formal written English
- follow written directions
- work efficiently and accurately under time pressure
- make logical generalisations and inferences based on textual information and quantitative data
- use critical thinking in approaching problems and texts
- recognise elements of effective arguments and logical conclusions
- use a scientific (evidence-based) approach to evaluating problems

Specifically, the test breaks down as follows:

Section I: Aptitude and Skills

Time: 60 minutes

Format: Multiple-choice and a few short answer

Goal: To test generic skills needed for successful undergraduate study

A full half of the BMAT, this first section is devoted to assessing your aptitudes and skills, especially problem-solving. You can see the BMAT's emphasis on strategies you will use regularly in undergraduate courses, particularly in science and mathematics classes.

Question Types
Problem Solving

Approximately 30 minutes

Worth 13 marks

Questions will ask you to solve problems using simple numerical and algebraic operations. You'll need to:
- determine what information is relevant (3-7 marks)
- recognise analogous cases (3-7 marks)
- determine appropriate procedures to apply (3-7 marks)

Understanding Argument

Approximately 15 minutes

Worth 10 marks

Questions will present a series of arguments for you to evaluate. You'll need to:
- identify elements of argument: reasons, assumptions, and conclusions
- recognise flaws in logic
- draw logical conclusions

Data Analysis & Inference

Approximately 15 minutes

Worth 12 marks

Questions test your ability to understand and draw conclusions from information presented in different forms. You'll need to:
- analyse and interpret verbal, statistical, and graphical data
- use inductive and deductive reasoning to draw appropriate conclusions from the information presented

Please note that you may not use a calculator on this or any other section of the exam.

You'll find a detailed discussion of Section I, along with sample and practice questions, in Chapters 3, 4, 5, and 6.

Section II: Scientific Knowledge and Applications

Time: 30 minutes

Format: Multiple-choice and a few short answer

Goal: To measure core knowledge in four disciplines – biology, chemistry, physics and mathematics – and the ability to apply that knowledge.

You haven't begun your university-level biomedical courses, so you won't be expected to have specialised scientific or mathematical knowledge. The questions in this section will only cover material normally included in non-specialist school science and mathematics curricula – ideas and information you've already studied and hopefully remember well.

Question Types
Biology
Approximately 8 minutes
Worth 6-8 marks

Chemistry
Approximately 8 minutes
Worth 6-8 marks

Physics
Approximately 8 minutes
Worth 6-8 marks

Mathematics
Approximately 6 minutes
Worth 5-7 marks

Sections IV to VII inclusive of this book are devoted to reviewing important science and mathematics concepts. Studying these chapters will help you refresh your memory of topics you studied in school and that may show up on the BMAT. Each chapter opens with a list of the primary topics covered in that chapter to help you find information you need quickly and easily.

Section III: Writing Task

Time: 30 minutes

Format: 1-page essay

Goal: To assess your ability to develop ideas and communicate them clearly and effectively in writing.

You may spend most of your college days studying science and mathematics, but throughout your academic and professional careers, you'll need to be able to express yourself effectively in writing. In fact, communication skills are so important that a copy of your essay will be sent along with your BMAT scores to each university to which you apply. It may even come up as a topic of discussion during your interview.

Question Types

For the essay, you'll choose **one** of three possible topics. Each will present a short proposition, and in your response you may be asked to:

- explain the implications of the proposal
- address counter-arguments
- propose a resolution

Please note that you may not use a dictionary, spell checker, or grammar checker for this or any section of the BMAT.

REGISTERING FOR THE BMAT

If you are currently at school, ask your Examinations Officer if your school will administer the BMAT. If not, you'll have to take the exam at an Open Centre. You can check the BMAT website (see "How Do I Register?") to find the Open Centre nearest you. Or, if you prefer, you can call the BMAT Support Desk at 01223 553366 or email the BMAT Support Team at bmatinfo@cambridgeasessment.org.uk.

BMAT CONTACT INFORMATION

Website: bmat.ucles-red.cam.ac.uk

Phone: 01223 553366

Email: bmatinfo@cambridgeassessment.org.uk

The Examinations Officer at your school or the BMAT contact at an Open Centre will register you for the BMAT via the BMAT Entries Extranet. Once your entry has been processed, your centre or school will receive a 5-digit BMAT candidate number for your entry. *Don't lose this number!* It's your unique BMAT ID, and you'll need it on test day and whenever you enquire about your scores.

The 2006 BMAT will take place on Wednesday, 1st November. You must register for the exam **no later than Friday, 29th September**. Late applicants with exceptional circumstances *may* be accepted up until Thursday, 12th October and will be charged a late fee. If you absolutely cannot sit the exam on the given test date, speak to your Examinations Officer or Open Centre contact about the possibility of making other arrangements.

The entry fee for the BMAT is £26.00 if you take the test in the UK, £48.50 if you take it internationally. Please note that some testing centres also charge a nominal administration fee for use of their facilities.

Registration deadline: Friday, 29th September.

Test date: Wednesday, 1st November.

Fees: £26.00 in the UK, £48.50 internationally. **Testing centre fees may also apply.**

At registration, be sure to indicate if you need any special testing arrangements. If English is not your native language and you need a multilingual dictionary, this must also be specified at the time of registration.

GETTING AND UNDERSTANDING YOUR RESULTS

Of course you'll be anxious to get your BMAT results, but they won't come to you right away. In fact, they won't come to you at all; you'll have to go and get them. Your test results and essay are sent first to the universities to which you are applying and then, on 30th November 2006, to your test centre. You must then contact your test centre directly to get your results.

Your scores for Sections 1 and 2 will range from 1 (low) to 9 (high) to one decimal point (e.g., 6.7). While you may yearn for a 9, don't be surprised if you end up with a much lower score. The test is designed so that even the very best students rarely score higher than 7. Most students score between 4 and 5.5, creating typical "bell curve" results. Keep in mind that if you score on the upper half of the curve with a 6, you've still distinguished yourself from more than half of the applicants.

The Writing Task is scored on a 3-point scale running from 0 (lowest) to 15 (highest). Essays are graded holistically; readers will be assessing the *overall* quality and effectiveness of your writing, taking into account your argument, organisation, grammar and style.

Your essay will be marked by two separate readers. If their marks are the same or adjacent on the scale (e.g., two 9s or a 9 and 12), your writing score will be the average of those two marks. If the scores are not adjacent, a third reader will mark your essay to determine your score.

You'll find a detailed discussion of the Writing Task scoring rubric in Part VIII on page 390.

SAMPLE BMAT SCORES

Section 1: 6.1

Section 2: 5.8

Section 3: 13.5 (average of Reader 1 score 12 and Reader 2 score 15)

PREPARING FOR THE EXAM

Your job is to do your best on the BMAT. Our job is to help you do that by telling you everything you need to know to earn your best score. We'll show you exactly what to expect on the exam so you can review content, practise skills and test-taking strategies and minimise test anxiety.

We begin by presenting you with test-preparation and test-taking strategies, including strategies specific to the BMAT as well as general stress management. A diagnostic test follows. Be sure to take it before you begin the next chapter; it will introduce you to the kinds of questions you'll see on the BMAT and help you determine which sections to focus on as you work through this book.

The next chapters of the book cover each section of the exam in detail, describing exactly what kinds of questions to expect and how you can dramatically improve your chances of answering those questions correctly. Parts IV through VII offer review material that you can use as a reference for reinforcing your understanding of key science and maths concepts that you may encounter in Section II of the test. You'll have many opportunities to apply what you learn through the practice questions in each chapter. Make sure you read the answers and explanations for all practice questions throughout these chapters. Then take the practice test at the end. See how you can expect to measure up on the real BMAT and if there are any areas in which you need further practice or study.

Additional Practice Online

Don't forget to check out the additional online resources, accessible through **kaptest.com/BMATbooksonline**. Here you'll find more test item questions, review material and sample essays to help ensure your success on the BMAT.

Congratulations. Your journey towards a medical degree has begun!

Chapter 2: **BMAT Preparation Strategies**

You know from experience that there's a strong correlation between how much you prepare and how well you do on an exam. The BMAT, of course, is no exception. And because it's a somewhat unusual test for a very competitive and limited pool of candidates, it's especially important to prepare effectively.

The three sections in this chapter offer a well-rounded approach to preparing for the BMAT. You'll find ten indispensable BMAT strategies, essential stress management techniques, and practical guidelines for the days leading up to the exam. Read this chapter now and come back to it again and again until you're sure you know the BMAT strategies inside and out. Refer to the Stress Management section any time you feel yourself starting to get overwhelmed. And use the advice in the Countdown section to get you into the test centre feeling confident and ready to do your absolute best on the exam.

TOP 10 BMAT STRATEGIES

Here are our top ten strategies to get you a top score on the BMAT.

- Be prepared.
- Stay calm.
- Be confident.
- Have the right attitude.
- Predict the right answer.
- Move around as needed.
- Use the process of elimination.
- Use the answers and explanations.
- Pace yourself.
- Write neatly.

1. Be prepared.

Do we already sound like a broken record? Well, sorry, but there's simply no substitute for preparation. Know what to expect on the exam: the types of questions that will be asked, the kinds of skills you'll need to use, the content you'll be expected to know. Learn that content if you don't know it already; practise the kinds of questions you'll face on test day. Carefully review your performance on practice questions so you can work towards improving your score.

Knowing what to expect enables you to employ many of the other strategies on our list effectively. It eases test anxiety so you can stay calm; it gives you confidence so that you can answer questions quickly and accurately; and it gives you the knowledge you need to pace yourself effectively on the exam. Practice helps you to predict the right answers better and eliminate incorrect ones; and the more you know about the exam, the easier it is to have the right attitude.

2. Stay calm.

Any standardised test demands time-management skills, and the BMAT is no exception. You need both speed and accuracy to complete each section on time.

It may help to know that test developers put you under such pressure for a reason. Medical school is a frenzied experience for most students. To meet the requirements of a rigorous work schedule, students must learn to prioritise and budget their time or else fall hopelessly behind. Your performance on a timed exam serves as one indicator of how well you may perform as a medical student. It also suggests whether or not you've got that *sine qua non* of the successful physician: grace under pressure.

Thus it's imperative that you remain calm and composed while working through each section of the BMAT. You can't allow yourself to become so rattled by a difficult question that it affects your performance in the rest of the test. Remember, the BMAT is designed to be challenging, and you're bound to come across some rather difficult questions. But remember, too, that you won't be the only one having trouble with that question. And don't forget that the test results are curved to take the difficult material into account.

Struggling with a couple of difficult questions won't ruin your score. Getting upset about it and letting it throw you off track *will*. Keep calm during the exam (see our stress management strategies for tips on keeping stress under control).

3. Be confident.

Confidence feeds on itself, and, unfortunately, so does self-doubt. Confidence in your ability to do well on the BMAT leads to quick, sure answers and a sense of well-being that translates into more points. If you lack confidence, you may end up reading questions and answer choices two, three or four times until you get confused and off-track, not to mention behind in time. This creates a downward spiral, causing anxiety and a tendency to rush, which leads to incorrect answers and haphazard guessing. Worse, it could cause you to simply shut down.

But that won't happen to you, because you're taking the time to prepare thoroughly for the BMAT, and that puts *you* in control. Armed with test-taking strategies and a detailed understanding of each section, buoyed by plenty of practice, you'll be ready to face the BMAT with supreme confidence—and that's the one sure way to do your best on test day.

If self-doubt does strike you on test day, simply take a moment to reflect upon how well you've prepared. Think of the specific things you did to get ready for this test. Remember how much you know about each section and the test-taking strategies you've internalised through practice. Focus on what you *can* do, what you *do* know, not on what you think you can't do or don't know. Keep the positive energy strong.

4. Have the right attitude.

Your attitude towards an event has a significant impact on how you experience that event. If you dread going, for example, you're more likely to have an awful time than if you are eagerly looking forward to it. The BMAT is that kind of event. You can be calm and confident, but if you approach the exam with the wrong attitude, those two hours are going to be torture, and you're not going to earn your best score.

You need to approach the BMAT with the right attitude – and in this case, *right* means *positive*. Remember that you're taking the BMAT for a good reason. You want to be a doctor – and not just any doctor, but a *great* doctor. The BMAT is not an obstacle to that goal but a stepping stone – a tool to help you get where you need to go.

The right attitude also means keeping things in perspective. Yes, the BMAT is an important exam, but it is by no means the only tool universities use to determine whether or not to accept you into their programme, and a poor performance isn't going to prevent you from following your dream and earning a medical degree. So prepare diligently, but don't put too much pressure on yourself. And remember, if you're prepared, the BMAT can actually help you by distinguishing you from the other candidates.

5. Predict the right answer.

It's important to know that on standardised tests, test-makers *try* to trick you. They intentionally include answer choices that look correct, but aren't. But we have a way to avoid falling for these distractors: predicting the right answer.

Read the question, but don't look at the answer choices until you think of what the answer should be. How would *you* answer the question? What kind of answer does the question call for? *Then* look for that answer among the choices. Now you're looking for a particular kind of answer, so you're more likely to quickly identify the correct choice. You're also less likely to rush and make sloppy errors.

6. Move around as needed.

With an occasional exception, all questions on the BMAT are worth one point—which means you need to answer as many questions correctly as quickly as possible to maximise your score. Thus one of the most valuable strategies for the BMAT is to learn to recognise and deal first with the questions that are easier and more familiar to you. That means temporarily skipping those that seem difficult and time consuming. The questions you know right off the bat count the same as those that you struggle over for several minutes, so answer all the ones you know as quickly as you can—then come back to the more difficult questions at the end. You're guaranteed to earn more points than if you go in order and get bogged down by questions that stump you.

We know that skipping a difficult question is easier said than done; we all have the natural instinct to plough through test sections in order. But it just doesn't pay off on the BMAT—or on any timed exam, for that matter. In fact, this is one of the single most important strategies for a timed exam. On the BMAT, it's not just getting the questions right that matters—it's getting the most number of questions right in the shortest amount of time that ensures success.

As you work through the exam, then, determine as quickly as possible which category a question falls into:

1. Green light: You're good at this kind of question—it's your strength. You usually get it right. In fact, you may even instantly know the answer.

2. Amber light: You're okay at this kind of question; it may not be so easy, but you can do it, maybe taking a little more time.

3. Red light: This kind of question is your weakness on the exam; you tend to get them wrong because you haven't mastered either the skills involved or the content.

If a question ranks 1 or 2, do it immediately. If it's a 3, leave it. Come back to it later after you've racked up points from quickly completing all the 1s and 2s.

BE GRID SMART

What's one of the worst things that can happen during a timed exam? Moments before the bell rings, you realise you put all the answers in the wrong grids on your answer sheet.

It sounds so simple, but it's extremely important: Do not make mistakes filling out your answer grid! Here are some tips to help prevent this from happening to you:

1. Always circle questions you skip. That way these questions will be easy to find when you're ready to come back to them. Also, if you accidentally skip an oval on the grid, you can easily check your grid against your test booklet to see where you went wrong.

2. Always circle the answer you choose in your test booklet. This will make it easier to check your answers on the grid.

3. Grid answers in chunks. Don't mark your answers to the grid after every question. After you've answered four or five questions, then transfer the answers. You'll save time and have less chance of making an error on your answer sheet. Just make sure you're not left at the end with ungridded answers!

4. Save time at the end for a final grid check. Make sure you have enough time at the end of every section for a quick check of your grid and to make sure you've got an answer filled in for each question. Remember that a blank grid has no chance of earning a point, but a guess does.

---

7. Use the process of elimination.

There are two ways to answer a multiple-choice question correctly: you either know the *right* answer, or you know all the *wrong* answers.

Each multiple-choice question on the BMAT offers you five choices. That means one is correct and four are incorrect. Some you will recognise as incorrect immediately; others after a little thought. By eliminating those incorrect answers, you either get to the correct response or significantly increase your chances of guessing the correct answer.

Remember, most of the BMAT is multiple-choice, which means you have a 20% chance of answering the question correctly even with a blind guess. Eliminate one choice, and you increase your chances to 25%; eliminate two, it's 33%; eliminate three, and you've got a 50-50 chance of getting the answer right.

As you eliminate incorrect answers, be on the lookout for wrong-answer traps – those answers that *look* right but are in effect a distortion of the correct answer. Be sure to read each answer choice carefully and make sure it answers the question accurately. Don't rely on knowledge you may have outside the scope of the question prompt; answer only what the question asks.

SHOULD YOU GUESS? YES!

If you can't answer a question or can't get to it before time runs out, by all means, guess! Fill in an answer – any answer – on the answer sheet. There's no penalty if you're wrong, but you score a point if you're right. (And if you've eliminated any answer choices, you've significantly increased your chances of guessing correctly.)

---

8. Use the answers and explanations.

Tests like the BMAT tend to stick to certain types of questions with predictable formats and patterns. We provide you with detailed explanations for *why* right answers are right and wrong answers are wrong. Read these explanations carefully – even if you get the answer right. Why? Because then you will be able to recognise these formats and patterns, making it more likely that you can quickly identify the correct answer. It'll help you recognise distractors and common wrong answer types found on standardised tests like the BMAT.

Of course, if you get a question wrong, you need to know why. Do you need to review content? Do you need to practise a particular skill? Or were you fooled by a distractor? Isolate the weakness—content, skill or test-taking strategy—so you can turn it into a strength before Test Day.

Here's another tip: For incorrect answers, work out why your answer isn't right *before* you look at the explanation. Think it through on your own before we explain it to you. This will reinforce your knowledge and skills and help prevent you from making the same kind of mistake next time.

As you prepare, don't get frustrated by your mistakes. Remember that every mistake you make during practice is an opportunity to improve your score on Test Day.

9. Pace yourself.

You know the saying: Timing is everything. This is especially true for standardised tests like the BMAT. The last thing you want to happen is to run out of time before you've finished a section. So it's essential that you pace yourself: work quickly and steadily, keeping in mind the general guidelines for how long to spend on any individual question or passage (see the table below). *Practise* your timing and memorise how long you have to do each question so you know when you're exceeding the time limit and should start to move on or move faster.

Remember, don't spend a wildly disproportionate amount of time on any one question or group of questions. (See strategy 6: skip a question and move on if you think it's going to take too much time.) Also, allow yourself 30 seconds or so at the end of each section to fill in answers for any questions you weren't able to get to.

Section I: Aptitude and Skills

	Approximate number of questions	Approximate time per section	Approximate time per question
Understanding argument	6	10	1.5-2 minutes
Problem solving	13	24	1.5-2 minutes
Data analysis	12	18	1.5 minutes
Inference (reading comprehension)	4	8	4 minutes for the passage, 1 minute per question
Total:	35	60	

Section II:

	Approximate number of questions	Approximate time per section	Approximate time per question
Biology	6-8	8	1 minute
Chemistry	6-8	8	1 minute
Physics	6-8	8	1 minute
Mathematics	5-7	6	1 minute
Total:	27	30	

Section III: Writing Task

On a timed writing exam, your time should roughly be divided ¼, ½, ¼ among brainstorming/outlining, writing, and revising/editing, respectively. Thus spend your 30 minutes as follows:

- 5 minutes brainstorming/outlining
- 10 minutes writing
- 5 minutes revising/editing

More about this in Part VIII.

A word of caution: while you need to keep track of time and should follow the guidelines in the chart above, don't obsess to the point of distraction. If you're checking your watch before and after each question, you're focusing too much on time and not enough on answering the questions correctly.

TAKE FIVE!

Well, okay, you don't have the luxury of a five-minute break during the exam. But you should take a quick break if you need to, even if it's in the middle of the test. The minute or so you take to regroup can give you the concentration and energy you need to keep performing your best on the exam. On the contrary, if you just keep ploughing through, you might get more frustrated and unfocused and answer more questions incorrectly. So: if you find yourself losing focus or getting frustrated, stop, close your eyes and take two or three deep breaths. Stretch your fingers, arms, neck and shoulders. Then, sufficiently renewed, get back to work!

10. Write neatly.

It may seem silly for handwriting to count in this day and age, but on this exam, like it or not, penmanship matters. You could write a truly magnificent essay, but it will all be for nothing if your readers can't understand what you've written. The challenge, of course, is that you need to write quickly *and* neatly.

On this pen-and-paper test, illegible writing is simply out of the question. You don't want your hard work to be for nothing because your handwriting is just too garbled to be understood. But even untidy-but-still-legible handwriting should be avoided. Your readers will probably be pretty good at deciphering sloppy text, but you don't want to make them struggle. If they have to work to decipher what you've written, however much they might like your essay in the end, they may subconsciously believe you deserve a lower score. This may be due in part to the fact that poor handwriting suggests a lack of control. Whether that's true or not doesn't matter; the fact is that it's often perceived that way and could be reflected in your score.

Your best bet? *Practise, practise, practise.* Do as many practice essays as you can under timed conditions to get used to writing quickly and neatly. Evaluate your handwriting after each session. Ask others to read it and tell you if they have any difficulties.

If you are a particularly untidy writer, take heart. While focusing on neater writing may be a challenge, it can help you by forcing you to slow down a little—which may help you craft your sentences and choose your words a little more carefully.

STRESS MANAGEMENT

You know it when you feel it, but what exactly *is* stress? Before we tell you how to manage it, let's take a moment to define it.

Some define stress as the tension we feel when the way our life is is different from the way we want it to be. For example, we need to be somewhere at 9:00, but we're stuck in traffic, and it's already 9:15. The way it is isn't the way we want it to be—so we feel stress. Here's a more scientific definition: stress is the psychological and physiological response we have when we perceive we cannot cope with the demands placed upon us.

That feeling of being unable to cope causes a physical reaction—our sympathetic nervous system prepares the body for flight-or-fight mode, tensing the muscles, increasing heart rate and blood pressure and causing us to sweat. Thus stress is both a physical and emotional reaction to a situation.

Of course, a little stress can be a good thing. That fight-or-flight response can give you an edge that may make you more productive on the exam. The key is to keep your stress at that productive level. Only you know how much nervous tension is good for you. Use our top five stress management strategies to keep your stress under control and do your best on the exam.

Kaplan's Top Five Strategies to Beat Stress

1. **Identify and address your sources of stress.** Determine exactly what is causing your stress. Be as specific as possible. To say you're "stressed about the BMAT" is too general. Are you worried that you won't score highly enough to be accepted to your first choice university? Are you stressed because you can't seem to find the time to study? Are you afraid that you will freeze up on test day? Are you worried that you'll disappoint your parents with your score? When you identify your specific sources of BMAT-related stress, write them down in the spaces below.

_____

_____

_____

_____

_____

_____

_____

Now determine whether each stressor already exists or is just a possibility. Next to each stressor on your list above, put E (exists) or P (possibility).

Example:

Stressor: Can't find the time to study - E

Stressor: Afraid of writing a terrible essay - P

The existing stressors are, of course, real and tangible situations. Your next step is to address them – decide what you're going to do about them to relieve your stress. You may not be able to change the situation, but you *can* find a solution. For example, if writing is not one of your strengths, having to write an essay on the BMAT may be a real stressor. The solution? Practise and prepare, and spend extra time on Part VIII.

As for those stressors that remain future possibilities, remember this: most of the things people worry about *never happen*. Be realistic – how likely is it that what you're worrying about will happen? – and think positively. And then take action. What can you do now to make sure that what you're worrying about doesn't happen? Prepare, practise test-taking strategies, become so comfortable with the exam that your fears will be unwarranted.

2. **Visualise success.** Have you ever imagined a situation beforehand, and it turned out just the way you'd pictured it?

Visualisation is such a powerful tool that we can to a large degree "create" our day – or at least the tenor of it. And it's remarkably easy: simply imagine yourself doing what you would like to do the way you'd like to do it. In your mind's eye, picture yourself doing really well on the exam. Take the time to really imagine the scene: your eyes moving calmly over the question, your smile as you quickly identify the correct answer, the way you'll feel as you finish the section ahead of time after answering each question correctly. Picture yourself celebrating after you've called the test centre to get your results.

Visualisation works largely because it gives you the confidence to make something happen the way that you imagine it happening. It creates subtle but important changes in your subconscious, neutralising fear, self-doubt and other negative emotions. It generates a positive mental attitude that puts *you* in control.

Practise it!

3. **Exercise.**

Running, walking, biking, football, yoga – whatever your preference, physical exercise is a very effective way to stimulate both your mind and body and to improve your ability to think and concentrate. It's also a powerful way to relieve stress.

Unfortunately, many students fall out of the habit of regular exercise when they're preparing for an exam. And many other students are simply in a sedentary routine. If either case is true for you, you need to get physical!

After all, a big test is a bit like a race. Finishing the race strongly is just as important as being quick early on. If you can't sustain your energy level in the last section of the exam, you could blow it. Along with a good diet and adequate sleep, exercise is an important part of keeping yourself in fighting shape and thinking clearly for the long haul.

There's another thing that happens when students don't make exercise an integral part of their test preparation. Like any organism in nature, you operate at your best if all your energy systems are in balance. Studying uses a lot of energy, but it's all mental. Take a five to ten minute break for every hour of study and do something active to restore the balance. When you come back to your work, you'll feel more energised and be better able to retain what you learn and practise.

One warning, however. It's not a good idea to exercise vigorously right before you go to bed – you may find it very difficult to go to sleep if you do. For the same reason, it's also not a good idea to study right up to bedtime. Make time for a "buffer period" before you go to bed to do something relaxing – take a long hot shower, knit, read for pleasure, do some deep breathing. You'll find it much easier to nod off and sleep restfully.

4. **Feed your body right.**

Outside circumstances – for example, the fact that you have to take the BMAT – may be beyond your control, but one thing that *is* in your control is what you put in your body. How you feed yourself can help alleviate stress or exacerbate it. As you prepare for the BMAT, and especially in the final days right before and day of the exam, *eat well*. Your body needs proper nutrition to function at its best, and a steady diet of cakes and tea does not qualify as "proper nutrition".

While you may be eager for that caffeine or sugar buzz, caffeinated and high-sugar foods and beverages usually only offer empty calories and temporary energy surges that lead to a crash an hour or so later. Your blood sugar needs to be on an even keel, not a rollercoaster ride.

Now's probably not the best time for a major diet overhaul, but it is in your best interests (now and even after the test) to avoid foods in the following categories:

high-sugar foods such as sweets, biscuits, cakes and fizzy drinks. These send a surge of sugar into your bloodstream, giving you a temporary burst of energy. But it's very temporary, and when the rush subsides, you're likely to feel even *more* tired. If you have a sweet tooth, try fresh or dried fruits or yogurt.

empty calorie foods such as crisps or pretzels. Your body needs more nutrients to be energised. Try munching on carrot sticks, nuts, or whole grain breads or cereals instead.

excessive caffeine. If you're used to one or two cups of coffee a day, fine; moving up to three may even be okay if you're highly tolerant. But too much caffeine is likely to make you jittery and unable to focus. It can also interfere with sleep. Avoid caffeinated beverages after lunchtime so you can get a good night's rest. Instead of fizzy drinks or coffee, try fresh fruit juices or green tea (which calms *and* is full of immune system-boosting antioxidants).

5. Get enough rest.

You know that it can be very difficult to think clearly when you're tired. As much as you may want to cut out sleep time to get more studying done, *don't*. Make sleep a priority throughout your test-preparation process and especially in the days right before the exam. You don't want to walk into your test centre exhausted; you want to walk in there refreshed and ready to do your best in the exam.

If you have trouble relaxing and getting to sleep at night, try deep breathing, muscle relaxation or visualisation exercises. The deep breathing relaxes your body and calms your mind. By tightening and then relaxing each muscle in your body, in succession, you will release tensions and relax the body so it can sleep. And visualisation will often chase away the self-doubt and worry that may be keeping you up at night.

COUNTDOWN TO THE BMAT

Today, your countdown to the BMAT begins. Here are some guidelines to help you make the most of your time between now and test day.

Now: create a study plan. Whether the BMAT is months or only a few weeks away, you need to plan your preparation time wisely. Create a study plan that will enable you to prepare at a manageable pace. Schedule your diagnostic test and then allocate specific days or weeks to each section.

Every day between now and test day: visualise success.

Three days before: take a full-length practice test under timed conditions. Use the techniques and strategies you've learned in this book. Approach the test strategically, actively and confidently. Assess your performance. Visualise success.

Two days before: go over the results of your practice test. Don't worry too much about your score, or about whether you got a specific question right or wrong. After all, the practice test doesn't count, and you might do much better on the actual exam. But do examine your performance on specific questions with an eye to how you might get through each one better and faster on the test to come. Visualise success.

The night before: do not study. Repeat: do not study. Do not take a practice exam or do practice questions. Instead, relax. Prepare a "BMAT kit" containing the following items:

- a watch
- a few pencils with rubbers
- photo ID card
- your BMAT ID number
- a healthy snack (There'll be breaks between the sections and you may be hungry during the exam, especially if you were nervous and couldn't eat much breakfast.)
- a bottle of water (especially if you tend to get a dry mouth when you're nervous).

Know exactly where you're going, exactly how you're going to get there and exactly how long it takes to get there. Do a test run so you know what to expect. Do not study; spend your time visualising instead. Set your alarm a few minutes early and ask someone to make sure you're up, just in case. Get a good night's rest.

On test day: think positively. Eat a substantial breakfast, but not anything too heavy or greasy. Get to the test centre early. Do your best in the exam!

| PART II |

Diagnostic Test

Diagnostic Test

This quick 20-question diagnostic is designed to help you gauge how well prepared you are for the BMAT and to help you identify areas in which you should spend more time reviewing. The test includes questions similar to those you might find on the Aptitude and Skills section and the Scientific Knowledge and Applications section of the BMAT.

Complete answers and explanations follow the test. After determining how many questions you answered correctly and incorrectly, use the correlation chart at the end of the test to determine which sections of the book you should spend the most time reviewing.

Time: 20 minutes

Directions: Mark your answers on the answer sheet provided.

1. Gametes have a single copy of the genome, and diploid cells have two copies of the genome. All human cells are diploid, with the exception of the gametes. Which **two** of the following must be true?

   (A) Gametes never have two copies of the genome.
   (B) Diploid cells are always human.
   (C) Genomes can only be copied once or twice.
   (D) All cells are diploid except for gametes.
   (E) Human cells never have three copies of the genome.

2. At University X, the faculty-to-student ratio is 1:9. If two-thirds of the students are female and one-quarter of the faculty is female, what fraction of the combined students and faculty are female? (Reduce your answer to its lowest form.)

3. In a certain game, each player scores either 2 points or 5 points. If n players score 2 points and m players score 5 points, and the total number of points scored is 50, what is the least possible positive difference between n and m?

   (A) 1
   (B) 3
   (C) 5
   (D) 7

MEGACORP, INC. REVENUE AND PROFIT DISTRIBUTION
FOR FOOD- AND NON-FOOD RELATED OPERATIONS, 1999–2004

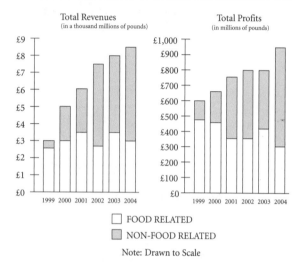

Total Revenues
(in a thousand millions of pounds)

Total Profits
(in millions of pounds)

☐ FOOD RELATED
☐ NON-FOOD RELATED

Note: Drawn to Scale

PERCENTAGE OF REVENUES FROM FOOD-RELATED
OPERATIONS IN 2004 BY CATEGORY

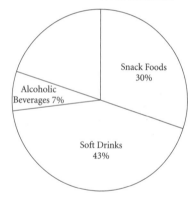

4. Approximately how much did total revenues increase from 1999 to 2002?

_____

5. For the year in which profits from food-related operations increased over the previous year, *total revenues* were approximately

   (A) £3.5 billion
   (B) £4.5 billion
   (C) £5.7 billion
   (D) £6.0 billion
   (E) £8.0 billion

6. Which of the following statements must be true based on the information given?

   1) In 2003, the percentage of total profits compared to total revenues was less than the percentage of revenues from frozen foods in 2004.

   2) The exact value of total revenues from food-related operations affects the value of total revenue from non-food related operations.

   3) You can calculate the revenues from non-food related operations by category.

   (A) 1 only
   (B) 2 only
   (C) 1 and 2 only
   (D) 2 and 3 only
   (E) 1 and 3 only

7. In 2004, approximately how many millions of pounds were revenues from frozen food operations?

   (A) 1,700
   (B) 1,100
   (C) 900
   (D) 600

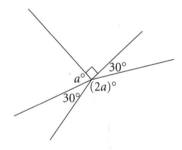

Note: Figure not drawn to scale.

8. In the figure above, what is the value of *a*?

   (A) 55
   (B) 60
   (C) 65
   (D) 70

GO ON TO THE NEXT PAGE

9. Jan types at an average rate of 12 pages per hour. At that rate, how long will it take Jan to type 100 pages?

_____

10. If a poor harvest season in a major corn-producing state results in higher prices for a bushel of corn, corn prices in other states will rise as well, whether or not those states are net importers of corn.

Which **one** of the following is an underlying assumption of the above argument?

(A) Poor harvesting seasons come at predictable regular intervals.

(B) Higher prices for corn tend to lead to increased prices for livestock, which rely on corn feed.

(C) The corn market in any state is part of the national corn market even if most of the corn consumed in the state is produced in the state.

(D) National corn supply disruptions have little, if any, effect on the price of local corn.

(E) States engage in price fixing of produce.

11. Which of the following best describes what happens when an electron in an oxygen atom jumps from a higher energy level to a lower energy level?

(A) A photon is emitted with its energy determined by the higher level.

(B) A photon is emitted with its energy determined by the difference between the levels.

(C) A photon is absorbed with its energy determined by the higher level.

(D) A photon is absorbed with its energy determined by the difference between the levels.

(E) A photon is absorbed with its energy determined by the lower level.

12. Which element forms a binary compound with hydrogen that is a strong acid?

(A) Mg

(B) Si

(C) P

(D) S

(E) Cl

13. Which of the following pairs of substances will react to produce H_2 (g)?

(A) HCl (aq) and $NaHCO_3$ (aq)

(B) HCl (aq) and Cu (s)

(C) HNO_3 (aq) and Cu (s)

(D) H_2O (l) and Na (s)

(E) NaOH (aq) and NH_4Cl (aq)

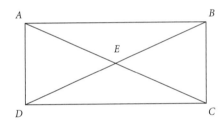

14. In the figure above, ABCD is a rectangle. If the area of $\triangle AEB$ is 8, what is the area of $\triangle ACD$?

(A) 8

(B) 12

(C) 16

(D) 24

(E) 32

15. If $4\sqrt{2}x - 2 = 16$, then $x =$

_____

GO ON TO THE NEXT PAGE

KAPLAN

16. A 6-digit code is required to secure a safe at a laboratory. The first, third and fourth digits cannot be multiples of 3. The last two digits cannot be even numbers, and the second digit must be an even number. The third number cannot be a prime number and no digit can be used more than once.

    Which **one** of the following correctly shows a possible order of the digits of the code?

    (A) 4, 6, 8, 5, 0, 1
    (B) 5, 6, 2, 7, 3, 9
    (C) 1, 2, 0, 6, 3, 9
    (D) 1, 0, 8, 2, 7, 5

17. If attendance at a school had increased by 30% over last year, this year's attendance would have been 10,972. Actually the attendance decreased by 35% from last year. What is this year's attendance?

    (A) 5,126
    (B) 5,206
    (C) 5,486
    (D) 6,136
    (E) 6,300

18. We gave working parents the opportunity to use a trial membership to our new Flash Fitness Centres. More than 85% found this convenient new workout to be very effective. If you're a parent who is pressed for time, Flash Fitness is the quick solution!

    Which **one** of the following is the best statement of the flaw in the above argument?

    (A) Working parents are not necessarily representative of the general population.
    (B) Other fitness centres are just as convenient and effective as Flash Fitness.
    (C) The fact that working parents found Flash Fitness effective does not mean that it was quick.
    (D) "Effective" is a subjective term and makes no representation as to a measurable degree of success.
    (E) Most people do not consider convenience as an important factor when choosing a fitness centre.

19. Studies show that people who write down their goals are more likely to achieve those goals. If I write my goals down, I will be a success.

    Which **one** of the following is an underlying assumption of the above argument?

    (A) The studies were conducted by reliable sources.
    (B) People who write well are more likely to succeed.
    (C) Goals must be realistic if they are to be achieved.
    (D) Writing down your goals is the most important factor in achieving them.
    (E) Being clear about your goals makes it easier to achieve them.

GO ON TO THE NEXT PAGE ⟩

KAPLAN

20. Which of the following is a correct association?

  (A) mitochondria: transport of materials from the nucleus to the cytoplasm

  (B) Golgi apparatus: modification and glycosylation of proteins

  (C) endoplasmic reticulum: selective barrier for the cell

  (D) ribosomes: digestive enzymes most active at acidic pH

  (E) lysosomes: membrane-bound organelles that convert fat into sugars

ANSWERS AND EXPLANATIONS

1. A, E

Choice **(A)** is true because the first statement clearly mentions that gametes have a single copy of the genome. Therefore, it must be true that gametes never have two copies of the genome. Choice **(E)** is true because the second statement reads, "All human cells are diploid, with the exception of the gametes". This is another way of saying that human cells have only one copy of the genome or two copies of the genome, but never three copies of the genome. Choices **(B)**, **(C)** and **(D)** might be true, but they might not be true.

2. $\frac{5}{8}$

Pick a number for the smallest given quantity described in the question—the number of female faculty: if there is 1 female member of the faculty, then the total number of faculty is 4 times 1, or 4. There are 9 times as many students, or 36 students. $\frac{1}{3}$ of 36 students are female, so there are 24 female students. Therefore, the total number of females is 1 + 24, or 25, and the total number of students and faculty is 36 + 4, or 40. That makes the fraction $\frac{25}{40}$ or $\frac{5}{8}$.

3. B

The quickest solution is to pick numbers for n and m. Since $n = 1$ and $m = 1$ would amount to 7 points, and since we want to minimise the difference between n and m, and since $50 \div 7$ is just a bit more than 7, start with values near 7. The key is to discover what values for n, when

multiplied by 2 points, will leave a multiple of 5 as the remaining points. The solution turns out to be 5 for n (10 points), which allows 8 for m (40 points). That is a total of 50 points, and the positive difference between the two values is only 3. If you investigate further, you find that it is impossible for there to be a difference of only 1 (choice **(A)**).

4. £4.5 billion

This question asks about total revenues, so you should refer to the left bar graph. The most difficult part of the question is making certain you correctly extract information from the appropriate bars, in this case for 1999 and 2002. Total revenues for 1999 appear to be £3 million and for 2002 they appear to be about £7.5 million (if you are ever having trouble pinpointing a quantity on a bar graph, place the edge of a piece of paper along the top of the bar to read the scale better). So the increase is roughly £7.5 billion − £3 million = £4.5 billion.

5. E

The wording is somewhat tricky here, and you have to refer to both bar graphs. Firstly, you have to refer to the right bar graph to find the lone year in which food-related profits increased over the previous year—the only year in which the unshaded portion of the bar goes up is 2003. Now that you have found that specific year, you must refer to the left bar graph to determine the total *revenues* for that year, which appear to be about £8.0 billion.

6. A

If you test the statements one by one, you can deduce the correct answer.

Statement 1 is true because in 2003 the percentage of total profits was 10% $\left(\frac{800 \text{ million}}{8,000 \text{ million}} = \frac{1}{10} = 10\% \right)$ and in 2004, the percentage of revenues from frozen foods was 20%. Because 10% is less than 20%, statement 1 is true. Statement 2 is not true because there is no data in either chart to suggest that the value of total revenues from food-related operations affects the value from non-food related operations.

Statement 3 is not true because you are not given the categories for non-food related operations. If you were reading too quickly, you may have mistaken this statement for food-related categories. If that were the case, statement 3 would be true.

Because only statement 1 must be true, choice **(A)** is correct.

7. D

Here is a question that refers to the pie chart. You are asked about revenues from frozen food operations, and the pie chart informs you that frozen foods represent 20% of all food-related revenues for 2004. To convert this into an amount you need to locate the amount of food-related revenues for 2004, so once again refer to the left bar graph where you will find the food-related revenues in 2004 were about £3,000 million. 20% of £3,000 million is £600 million.

8. D

The number of degrees around a point is 360. Therefore:

$$90 + 30 + 2a + 30 + a = 360$$
$$150 + 3a = 360$$
$$3a = 210$$
$$a = 70$$

9. y

Set up a proportion:

$$\frac{12 \text{ pages}}{1 \text{ hour}} = \frac{100 \text{ pages}}{x \text{ hours}}$$
$$12x = 100$$
$$x = \frac{100}{12} = 8\frac{1}{3}$$

One-third of an hour is $\frac{1}{3}$ of 60 minutes, or 20 minutes. So $8\frac{1}{3}$ hours is 8 hours and 20 minutes.

10. C

The stimulus says that if the price of corn rises in a major corn-producing state because of a poor harvest, the price of corn will increase in other states, whether those states import or grow most of their corn. In other words, the price of corn must somehow be standardised. This implies that all states are part of a national corn market (choice (C)). (A) is out of scope; the passage focuses on corn prices, not bad harvests or their frequency. (B), too, is out of

scope, since livestock isn't part of the argument. It might be tempting because it certainly could be true, but it is out of scope and doesn't have to be true based on the stimulus. (D) actually contradicts the argument, which states that the price of all corn – local and imported – is affected by a bad harvest in one state. And (E) is a distortion. The evidence is linked to the conclusion by the assumption of a national corn market, not a price-fixing conspiracy among the states.

11. B

When an electron jumps to a lower energy level in an atom, it emits a photon. The photon energy equals the difference in energy between the two energy levels.

12. E

The binary compound of Cl and H is HCl, which forms hydrochloric acid in aqueous solution.

13. D

The alkali metals react with water to produce H_2 (g) and OH^- ions. The substances in (A) would react to produce CO_2 (g); (B) would give no reaction (though HCl does react with active metals such as Mg and Zn to produce H_2); (C) would react to produce NO gas, which would be converted to brown NO_2 on contact with air; (E) would produce NH_3 (aq) and NaCl (aq).

14. C

CDE has the same area as $\triangle$AEB; they're congruent triangles. But we want the area of $\triangle$ACD, which means that we need to know $\triangle$ADE's area as well. So we want to find a relationship between $\triangle$ADE's area and $\triangle$CDE's area. Let's make AD the base of $\triangle$ADE. Its height, a line drawn perpendicularly from E (the rectangle's midpoint, where its diagonals meet) to AD is just one-half the length of side DC. So the area of $\triangle$ADE is $\frac{1}{2} \times AD \times \frac{DC}{2} = \frac{1}{4} \times AD \times DC$. Applying similar reasoning, let DC be the base of $\triangle$CDE. Its height is then a line drawn perpendicularly from E to DC, which is one-half the length of side AD. So $\triangle$CDE's area is:

$$2 \times DC \times\times DC \times AD.$$

The two triangles are equal in area; each has an area of 8. Therefore, the area of $\triangle$ACD is

$$8 + 8 = 16. \text{ (C) is correct.}$$

15. $\dfrac{81}{8}$

$$4\sqrt{2x} - 2 = 16$$
$$4\sqrt{2x} = 18$$
$$\sqrt{2x} = \dfrac{18}{4}$$
$$\left(\sqrt{2x}\right)^2 = \left(\dfrac{18}{4}\right)^2$$
$$2x = \dfrac{18 \times 18}{4 \times 4 \times 2} = \dfrac{9 \times 9}{2 \times 2 \times 2} = \dfrac{81}{8}$$

16. D

Apply each answer choice systematically to the rules.

A   4, 6, 8, 5, **0**, 1

This is incorrect. There can be no even number in the fifth position. Remember, zero is an even number.

B   5, 6, **2**, 7, 3, 9

This is incorrect. There can be no prime number in the third position. Two is a prime number.

C   1, 2, 0, **6**, 3, 9

This is incorrect. There can be no multiple of 3 in the fourth position. Six is a multiple of 3

D   1, 0, 8, 2, 7, 5

This is correct.

17. C

In questions involving percent increase or percent decrease, it is often helpful to ask yourself,

"What percent of the original whole is the new whole?" This is easy to calculate: just add (or subtract) the percent increase (or decrease) to (or from) 100%. Here, a 30% increase over the previous year's attendance would make this year's attendance 10,972. In other words, if A represents the previous year's attendance, 100% of A + 30% of A = 10,972 or 130% of A = 10,972. Solve for A here, and then from that find this year's actual attendance. However, there is a faster way to solve this question. The actual attendance decreased 35% from the previous year's attendance, so it can be represented as (100% of A) − (35% of A), or 65% of A. Note that 65% of A is just one-half of 130% of A. Therefore, if 130% of A = 10,972, then 65% of A = $\dfrac{1}{2}$ of 10,972, or 5,486, making **(C)** the answer.

18. C

The conclusion is that for parents who are pressed for time, Flash Fitness is the "quick solution". The evidence, however, doesn't have anything to do with being quick; it tells us that working parents "found this convenient new workout to be very *effective*". As stated in (C), there's no evidence that Flash Fitness is "quick". Note that none of the wrong choices address quickness, which is the new element introduced in the conclusion. (A) may be true, but it's not a serious criticism of the advert since time-pressed parents are the target audience (and so we really don't care whether the rest of the world would like the programme). The information in (B) is irrelevant. The advert makes no claim that Flash Fitness is more effective or convenient than other fitness centres, only that it is an effective and convenient centre. (D) may be true, but it's not important, because the conclusion of the argument is that the programme is a "quick" solution—we're not trying to prove its effectiveness. (E) is also irrelevant. While it may be true that some people are not concerned with convenience when choosing a fitness centre, this advert attempts to appeal to those who do have that concern.

19. D

The author makes the leap from the results of the study (people who write down their goals are more likely to achieve them) to his own future. The missing link must connect the study to the likelihood of the author indeed becoming a success. The only way this is possible is with the assumption that simply writing down one's goals is the most important factor in actually achieving them (D). Otherwise, the argument falls apart. (A) is irrelevant; we hope the studies were conducted by reliable sources, but the issue remains a matter of how the author can come to the conclusion that he does about his own success. (B) is a distortion; it's not a matter of writing *well* but of articulating one's goals. (C) may be true, but it is outside the scope of the argument. We do not know if the studies in any way address whether or not the goals are realistic, nor do we know whether the author's goals are or are not realistic. (E) may be tempting, but it does not answer the question – that is, it does not connect the evidence to the conclusion. Rather, it clarifies the evidence by explaining why people who write their goals are more likely to achieve them.

20. B

The Golgi apparatus consists of a stack of membrane-enclosed sacs. The Golgi receives vesicles and their contents from the smooth ER, modifies them (as in glycosylation), repackages them into vesicles, and distributes them. In (A), mitochondria are involved in cellular respiration, and in (C), the ER transports polypeptides around the cell and to the Golgi apparatus for packaging. The ribosome (D) is the site of protein synthesis, while lysosomes (E) are membrane-bound organelles that contain digestive enzymes and typically have a low pH.

DIAGNOSTIC TEST CORRELATION CHART

Question	Topic
1	Aptitude and Skills: Problem Solving
2	Aptitude and Skills: Problem Solving
3	Aptitude and Skills: Problem Solving
4	Aptitude and Skills: Data Analysis & Inference
5	Aptitude and Skills: Data Analysis & Inference
6	Aptitude and Skills: Data Analysis & Inference
7	Aptitude and Skills: Data Analysis & Inference
8	Mathematics
9	Mathematics
10	Aptitude and Skills: Understanding Argument
11	Physics
12	Chemistry
13	Chemistry
14	Mathematics
15	Mathematics
16	Aptitude and Skills: Problem Solving
17	Aptitude and Skills: Problem Solving
18	Aptitude and Skills: Understanding Argument
19	Aptitude and Skills: Understanding Argument
20	Biology

How to Approach the Aptitude and Skills Section

Chapter 3: **Problem Solving**

This chapter reviews the essentials for mastering Problem Solving questions on the Biomedical Admissions Test. Question format and structure, as well as basic principles and strategies are offered here. Be sure to answer all the practice questions found in this chapter to ensure you have understood the material covered.

QUESTION FORMAT AND STRUCTURE

Problem Solving questions are better described as word problems primarily requiring the use of maths and logic skills. The thirteen questions are designed to test your ability to translate and compute information using arithmetic methods and reasoning. Problem Solving questions also test your skill at recognising information that is relevant and omitting information that is not; identifying and reasoning with similar problems or situations; and understanding and executing the calculations needed to solve a problem. Bear in mind that although some numerical information is tested, the use of a calculator is NOT permitted.

Problem Solving Skill	Number of Questions	Time Allowed
Select relevant information	3–7	—
Recognise analogous cases	3–7	—
Determine and apply appropriate procedures	3–7	—
	TOTAL: 13 (approximate)	TOTAL: 30 minutes

An important thing to note about Problem Solving questions is that they are not found in a distinct section of the BMAT. In other words, while completing the 35 questions in the Aptitude and Skills section of the BMAT, these questions are interspersed with Understanding Argument questions and Data Analysis & Inference questions. For this reason, there are no specific directions for these questions.

POINT VALUE

On the BMAT, all Problem Solving questions are valued at one point each. There is no penalty for incorrect answers, so you should complete every question in the Aptitude and Skills section.

Multiple-Choice and Short Answer Questions

There are two ways that Problem Solving questions are presented. The first is multiple-choice format. In this format, the question is followed by possible answer choices. Some questions have five answer choices (A–E), while others have only four answer choices (A–D). Although uncommon, it is possible to have only three answer choices (A–C). For this question format, you have to select a correct answer, or two correct answers, from among the possibilities listed. When answering these questions it is strongly advised to use the process of elimination, which is covered in the Top 10 Strategies for Success with Problem Solving Questions.

Short answer questions are quite different. This format presents information followed by a question. There are no answer choices provided. You are responsible for generating and submitting the correct answer to the question. Short answer questions are almost exclusively maths questions, so be very careful in your calculations. You should always review your solutions as you will not be able to compare your answer with a provided answer choice. Even though your chances of guessing the correct answer are low, you should never leave a short answer question blank. If you are completely unsure of how to solve a short answer question, do not waste time trying to find the correct answer. Write down a reasonable answer and move on.

Problem Solving–Maths

Problem Solving questions can be divided into two categories: Maths and Logic. Although maths is tested specifically in the Scientific Knowledge and Applications section of the BMAT, there are some word-based maths problems among the Problem Solving questions. For this category of Problem Solving question, you will have to extract the relevant numerical information and apply the appropriate methods to arrive at the answer. Here is an example of a word problem:

> In a certain laboratory, chemicals are identified by a colour-coding system. There are 20 different chemicals. Each one is coded with either a single colour or a unique two-colour pair. If the order of colours in the pairs does not matter, what is the minimum number of different colours needed to code all 20 chemicals with either a single colour or a unique pair of colours?
>
> (A) 5
> (B) 6
> (C) 7
> (D) 20
> (E) 40

The answer is (B).

It is reasonable to assume that of the approximately thirteen Problem Solving questions, a majority of them will be based on maths.

When answering Problem Solving maths questions, you must know how to translate the words you are reading into maths you can solve. Here is a table of some common translations.

English	Maths
equals is, was, will be has costs adds up to is the same as	=
times of multiplied by product of twice, double, triple, half	×
per out of divided by each ratio of __ to __	÷
and plus added to sum combined total	+
minus subtracted from less than decreased by difference between	−
what how much how many a number	x, n (variable)

Remember: If you are completely baffled by a word problem, look for some of the words in the left-hand column. Then work from their maths equivalent and try to construct an equation.

Problem Solving—Logic

The other category of Problem Solving questions is logic. These are questions that test the same problem solving skills (selecting relevant information, recognising analogous cases, determining and applying appropriate procedures), but they do not include numerical information.

Logic questions can be further categorised as **statements**, **rules**, or **diagrams** questions. Each will be discussed in detail here.

Logic—Statements

This type of logic question offers two statements. Based on the information in those statements—which can be quite a lot—you will have to deduce one or two things that must be true.

Here is an example:

> Janelle is older than Isidore and Isidore is younger than Benjamin.
> Benjamin is older than Janelle, but younger than Stefan.
>
> Stefan must be:
>
> (A) the youngest;
> (B) younger than Isidore;
> (C) older than Janelle, but younger than Benjamin;
> (D) younger than Isidore and Benjamin;
> (E) the oldest.

In this case, the answer is (E). According to the information given, Stefan is older than the other people mentioned. If you are confused by how to deduce the correct answer based on the statements, refer to the top strategies to improve your skills.

DIFFERENT TYPES OF STATEMENTS ————————————

The statements can usually be described as ranking/directional, describing or situational.

In a *ranking/directional* statement, you may be asked to deduce the rank of people's ages, scores, or other levels, or you may have to deduce a location based on statements indicating direction or distance (east, west, north, south, or closer, farther).

Descriptive statements provide information on the names or characteristics of things and you must deduce what is true based on those statements.

Finally, *situational statements* describe a situation and ask you to verify a result or possible outcome of that situation.

Do not be concerned with memorising these types. The differences among them are usually subtle. Most importantly, the logic used to solve them is the exact same for all three types.

Logic—Rules

As the name implies, this question type offers a set of rules. The answer choices each typically contain a list, an order that is meant to show the outcome of following the given rules. The process of elimination is somewhat simplified with these questions as answer choices that break any of the given rules can immediately be disregarded. Here is an example:

> The order in which 5 teams perform for competition is decided using the number of members on the team and team name. Teams with a number of members that is equal to a multiple of 6 perform first in alphabetical order. Teams with a number of members that is equal to a multiple of 4 perform last in reverse alphabetical order. The only exception to these rules is that the team who won the competition the previous year always perform first. The name and number of team members are listed below.
>
> Sussex Team, 32 members
>
> Midland Team, 8 members
>
> Westfield Team, 30 members
>
> Pritchard Team, 20 members
>
> Cliffside Team, 18 members
>
> If the Cliffside Team won last year, which of the following orders may be correct?
>
> (A) Cliffside, Westfield, Sussex, Pritchard, Midland
>
> (B) Cliffside, Westfield, Midland, Sussex, Pritchard
>
> (C) Cliffside, Sussex, Pritchard, Midland, Westfield
>
> (D) Cliffside, Midland, Pritchard, Sussex, Midland

The correct answer is (A). Only the order of these teams matches all the rules.

Logic—Diagrams

The final type of logic question is based on diagrams. Do not confuse this question type with Data Analysis & Inference questions, which often use diagrams. Instead, Problem Solving diagram questions are very similar to Problem Solving rules questions. Written rules are provided, but diagrams are also included. Again, you will apply the written rules to the graphical information given and use the process of elimination to deduce the correct answer. Here is an example:

A certain clock rings two notes at quarter past the hour, four notes at half past, and six notes at three-quarters past. On the hour, it rings eight notes plus an additional number of notes equal to whatever hour it is.

	:00	:15	:30	:45
1 P.M.	9	2	4	6
4 P.M.	12	2	4	8

Figure 1

	:00	:15	:30	:45
1 P.M.	9	2	4	6
4 P.M.	13	4	2	6

Figure 2

	:00	:15	:30	:45
1 P.M.	9	2	4	6
4 P.M.	12	2	4	6

Figure 3

Which chart shows the number of rings occurring during the 1 P.M. hour and 4 P.M. hour?

(A) Figure 1 only

(B) Figures 1 and 2 only

(C) Figure 3 only

(D) Figures 1 and 3 only

(E) Figure 2 only

The correct answer is choice (C).

THE 6 BASIC PRINCIPLES OF PROBLEM SOLVING

By adopting a systematic approach to Problem Solving, you will have a clear, concise method for thinking your way to a response. You will not waste time by attacking a problem in a tentative or haphazard manner. A systematic approach will ensure that you find the most efficient solution to the problem and that you make as few careless and unnecessary errors as possible.

The 6 basic principles of Problem Solving are:

1. Read through the entire question once.
2. Develop the ability to decipher what is being asked quickly.
3. Outline what information is most relevant.
4. Consider alternative methods.
5. Decide how much effort to put into each question.
6. Guess if you are not sure of the correct answer.

1. Read carefully the entire question once.

This may sound like very simple advice, but it is crucial not to assume anything when problem solving. If you are scanning questions in the Aptitude and Skills section, do not begin sorting out in your head your approach to Problem Solving questions. Take each question as it comes and read the entire question quickly but carefully. If you fail to notice an important detail or relevant information, it renders the following principles useless. Upon first reading, you should also be able to recognise whether your maths or logic skills are being tested.

2. Develop the ability to decipher what is being asked quickly.

With practice, you will quickly recognise exactly what you are being asked. There is a lot of information provided in Problem Solving questions, but the actual question is very specific. Take this Problem Solving maths question, for example:

> Company C sells a line of 25 products with an average retail price of £1,200. If none of these products sells for less than £420, and exactly 10 of the products sell for less than £1,000, what is the greatest possible selling price of the most expensive product?

(A) £2,600
(B) £3,900
(C) £7,800
(D) £11,800
(E) £18,200

If you have followed the first principle, you have read the entire question once, have identified this as a maths question and are now trying to decipher exactly what is being asked. You are not asked simply for a selling price. Nor are you asked to identify the cost of the most expensive item. You are asked to figure out the greatest possible selling price of the most expensive product *given* the information provided. This is where the third principle becomes relevant.

3. Outline what information is most relevant.

As you can see from the previous example, answering exactly what is being asked is impossible without the information found in the question. You will need to use all the relevant details provided to calculate a solution to this problem. As you read the question, key words such as "25 products", "average price of £1,200", "no products less than £420", and "10 products less than £1,000" should have struck you as important.

Make notes about the information you are given and how it is useful for solving the problem. In this case, knowing that the average price of 25 products is £1,200 allows you to calculate the total cost of all 25 items, which is £30,000. The way to maximise the price of the most expensive item is to minimise the prices of the other 24 products. Knowing that 10 of these products sell for less than £1,000, but all sell for at least £420 helps minimise the price of 24 items by selling 10 items at exactly £420. That leaves 14 more that sell for £1,000 or more. In order to keep minimising, you should price these at £1,000. That means that, out of the £30,000 it takes to purchase one of each item, at least 10(£420) + 14(£1,000) = £18,200 is needed in order to purchase the 24 other items. The final, most expensive item can thus cost as much as £30,000 − £18,200 = £11,800. Choice (D) is correct.

4. Consider alternative methods.

If a question seems as if it will take too long to solve, look for shortcuts or other strategies for answering it. Maybe you had no idea where to begin with the previous multi-step question. However, you should remember that with multiple-choice questions, the answer is right in front of you. At the very least, you can test every answer choice against how you think this should be solved (referred to as Backsolving) or you can use the process of elimination. Both of these as well as other alternative methods and shortcuts are found in the Top 10 Strategies for Success with Problem Solving Questions.

5. Decide how much effort to put into each question.

Depending on your progress through the Aptitude and Skills section, you might be better to guess and save time for other questions. For example, if certain types of maths questions are difficult for you, consider guessing on those and allotting more time to other maths or logic questions. You are expected to complete all the questions in a section, so you should move through them quickly to allow time to answer other questions more accurately.

6. Guess if you are not sure of the correct answer.

The way to score a maximum of points on the BMAT is to answer as many questions as you can correctly. However, because there is no penalty for incorrect answers you should never leave a question blank. In the previous example, if you had no idea what the correct answer was, you could guess randomly and still have a 1 in 5 chance of being correct.

THE SAME 6 BASIC PRINCIPLES FOR LOGIC QUESTIONS

The previous section reviewed the basic principles as they applied to a maths question. To be thorough, here is a brief revision of the basic principles as they apply to a logic question.

1. Read carefully the entire question once.

Again, if you fail to notice an important detail or relevant information, the other principles are useless. Read the information quickly and carefully.

2. Develop the ability to decipher quickly what is being asked.

Take this Problem Solving logic question, for example. You might remember it from earlier in the chapter.

> Janelle is older than Isidore and Isidore is younger than Benjamin.
> Benjamin is older than Janelle, but younger than Stefan.
>
> Stefan must be:
>
> (A) the youngest;
> (B) younger than Isidore;
> (C) older than Janelle, but younger than Benjamin;
> (D) younger than Isidore and Benjamin;
> (E) the oldest.

Following the first principle, you should have read the entire question quickly but carefully. You should have deciphered that you are not being asked Stefan's age, but rather, how his age classifies him compared to the others. To do this, you must return to the information in the question to follow the third principle.

3. Outline what information is most relevant.

As you can see from the previous example, answering exactly what is being asked is impossible without the information found in the question. You will need to use all the relevant details provided to calculate a solution to this problem. As you read the question, you should be making notes about each person and their age in relation to the others.

4. Consider alternative methods.

Rather than reading, re-reading, and committing to memory the descriptions of each of the persons mentioned, you can try another method. First, know that the full names are irrelevant. Rather than writing out Janelle, Isidore, Benjamin, and Stefan, you should be using notation such as J, I, B, S. You should also devise a system of highlighting information that makes sense to you. You will learn other alternative methods for answering a question like this in the Top 10 Strategies for Success with Problem Solving Questions.

5. Decide how much effort to put into each question.

Perhaps your ability to follow logic is not as strong as your maths skills. In this case, if you are struggling with deducing the correct answer, you should consider making an educated guess and moving on to another question.

6. Guess if you are not sure of the correct answer.

No matter what, you should always provide an answer for every question. Because logic questions are almost exclusively multiple-choice, you have a 1 in 4 or 1 in 5 chance of guessing the correct answer. Your odds improve even more if you are able to eliminate at least one clearly incorrect answer. Do your best, but if time is running out or you cannot solve the problem, mark an answer and move on.

TOP 10 STRATEGIES FOR SUCCESS WITH PROBLEM SOLVING QUESTIONS

As you prepare for the BMAT, you should review and practise the six basic principles of problem solving so that they become second nature to you. Those principles provide an overall method for attacking Problem Solving questions. Perhaps, though, you are looking for a shortcut or alternative method (principle #4) for answering a specific question. That is where these top strategies come in. They are separated into Problem Solving Maths strategies and Problem Solving Logic strategies.

PROBLEM SOLVING MATHS STRATEGIES

First, we'll take a look at the strategies for Problem Solving Maths. After, we'll look at strategies specific to Logic problems.

Maths Strategy 1—Backsolving

Backsolving is a strategy that allows you to use the answer choices to work backwards through the question. You plug the answer choices into the question to see which one works. The answer choice that agrees with the information in the question stem is correct. You have probably used this strategy unconsciously when you ran into a multiple-choice question that you found difficult. Backsolving can save a great deal of time if you use it wisely. It is an exceptional method for solving questions when you have no idea where to begin on a problem.

Backsolving must be done systematically. Usually answer choices are arranged in ascending or descending order. When that is the case, start Backsolving with choice (B) or choice (D). If that is not the answer, you will usually be able to tell whether the correct answer is larger or smaller, which means you will have narrowed the choices down.

Solve the following problem by Backsolving.

> A crate of apples contains one bruised apple for every 30 apples in the crate. If 3 out of every 4 bruised apples are considered unsaleable, every unsaleable apple is bruised, and there are 12 unsaleable apples in the crate, how many apples are there in the crate?
>
> (A) 270
> (B) 360
> (C) 480
> (D) 600

Start Backsolving with choice (B). Suppose that there are 360 apples in the crate. Then $\frac{360}{30}$ apples, or 12 apples, are bruised. Then $\frac{3}{4}$ of 12 apples, or 9 apples, are unsaleable. This is too few unsaleable apples. So (B) is too small. Eliminate (A) and (B). Now look at (D). Suppose there are 600 apples in the crate. Then $\frac{600}{30}$ apples, or 20 apples, are bruised. Then $\frac{3}{4}$ of 20 apples, or 15 apples, are unsaleable. This is too many unsaleable apples. So (D) is too large. (C) must be correct.

Maths Strategy 2—Pick Numbers

Picking Numbers is a powerful alternative to solving problems by extensive algebraic methods. With this strategy, you pick concrete values for the variables rather than trying to work with unknown variables. Any answer choice that does not work for the concrete values cannot be the correct answer.

How does Picking Numbers work?

- Pick simple numbers to stand in for the variables. The usefulness of the strategy depends in large part on your ability to pick convenient numbers.

- Try all the answer choices, eliminating those that do not agree with the question information. Remember to keep the values you have picked for the variables constant throughout the problem.

- Try different values when more than one answer choice works. Sometimes more than one choice will give the right answer. If that happens, pick some new numbers. The correct choice must work for *all* possible numbers.

- When you encounter a problem that contains variables, Picking Numbers and substituting is often quicker than any mathematical calculation.

Here is the Picking Numbers technique applied to a few problems.

> Carol spends $\frac{1}{4}$ of her savings on a stereo and $\frac{1}{3}$ less than she spent on the stereo for a television. What fraction of her savings did she spend on the stereo and television?

In this case, the common denominator is 12; so let the number 12 (12 pounds) represent Carol's total savings. That means she spends $\frac{1}{4} \times 12$ pounds, or 3 pounds, on her stereo, and $\frac{2}{3} \times 3$ pounds, or 2 pounds, on her television. That comes out to be $3 + 2 = 5$ pounds; that is how much she spent on the stereo and television combined. The question asks what *fraction* of her savings she spent. Because her total savings is 12 pounds, she spent $\frac{5}{12}$ of her savings. Notice how picking a common denominator for the variable (Carol's savings) made it easy to convert each of the fractions ($\frac{1}{4}$ and $\frac{1}{4} \times \frac{2}{3}$ of her savings) to a simple number.

A difficult part of this question is understanding how to figure the price of the television. Remember the second basic principle of problem solving: develop the ability to decipher quickly what is being asked. The television does not cost $\frac{1}{3}$ of her savings, it costs $\frac{1}{3}$ *less* than the stereo; that is, it costs $\frac{2}{3}$ as much as the stereo.

A reasonable estimate would have surely been closer to $\frac{1}{2}$ than to $\frac{1}{4}$. Reasonable estimations are covered later in this section. For now, practice picking numbers for another sample question.

> A car rental company charges for distance travelled as follows: x pounds per kilometre for the first n kilometres and $x + 1$ pounds per kilometre for each kilometre over n kilometres. How much will the charge be, in pounds, for a journey of d kilometres, where $d > n$?
>
> (A) $d(x + 1) - n$
> (B) $xn + d$
> (C) $xn + d(x + 1)$
> (D) $x(n + d) - d$
> (E) $(x + 1)(d - n)$

Reading this question might make it appear difficult, but it becomes much simpler when you substitute numbers for the variables. For instance, suppose you pick $x = 4$, $n = 2$, $d = 5$. The problem now reads: 4 pounds per kilometre for the first 2 kilometres, and 5 pounds a kilometre for each kilometre over 2 kilometres. How much will the charge be for a journey of 5 kilometres?

This problem is easily calculated: the first 2 kilometres cost 2×4 pounds and the remaining 3 kilometres cost 3×5 pounds for a total cost of $8 + 15$, or 23 pounds. Of the answer choices, only (A) has value 23 when $x = 4$, $n = 2$, and $d = 5$.

With the Picking Numbers strategy in mind a seemingly difficult question becomes much easier.

Maths Strategy 3—Avoiding Traps

There are several maths traps to be aware of when taking the BMAT. Here are a few of them, along with methods for avoiding them.

Maths Trap 1: Percent Increase/Decrease

When a quantity is increased or decreased by a percentage more than once, you cannot simply add and subtract the percentages to get the answer. In this kind of percentage problem, the first change is a percentage of the starting amount, but the second change is a percentage of the new amount.

Avoiding the Trap

Do not blindly add and subtract percentages. They can only be added and subtracted when they are of the same amount.

Maths Trap 2: Weighted Averages

You cannot combine averages of different quantities by taking the average of those original averages. In an averages problem, if one value occurs more frequently than others, it is *weighted* more. Remember, the average formula calls for the sum of all the terms divided by the total number of terms.

Avoiding the Trap

Do not just take the average of the averages; work with the sums.

Maths Trap 3: Ratio:Ratio:Ratio

Parts of different ratios do not always refer to the same whole. In the classic ratio trap, two different ratios each share a common part that is represented by two different numbers. However, the two ratios do not refer to the same whole, so they are not in proportion to each other. To solve this type of problem, restate both ratios so that the numbers representing the common part are the same. Then all the parts will be in proportion and can be compared to each other.

Avoiding the Trap

Restate ratios so that the same number refers to the same quantity. Make sure the common quantity in both ratios has the same number in both.

Maths Trap 4: "Least" and "Greatest"

In questions that ask for the *least*, *minimum* or *smallest* something, the choice offering the smallest number is rarely right. In questions that ask for the *greatest*, *maximum* or *largest* something, the choice offering the largest number is very rarely right.

Avoiding the Trap

Consider the constraints and requirements that the nature of the question has placed upon the possible answer. Do not leap to conclusions. In fact, if you ever need to guess on questions asking about the least number, the one place not to go is to the smallest choice and vice versa for questions asking about the largest number.

Maths Trap 5: Percent "of" versus Percent "Less" or "Greater"

Reading too quickly or with insufficient care could lead a test taker to mistake "less than" for "of".

Avoiding the Trap

Be on the lookout for subtleties of wording, especially in questions appearing in the middle or end of a section. Consciously and actively distinguish these three things whenever percent questions arise:

1. *a* percent *of b*;
2. *a* percent *less than b*;
3. *a* percent *greater than b*.

For example:

1. 25 percent *of* 8 means $\frac{1}{4}(8) = 2$;

2. 25 percent *less than* 8 means $8 - \frac{1}{4}(8) = 8 - 2 = 6$;

3. 25 percent *greater than* 8 means $8 + \frac{1}{4}(8) = 8 + 2 = 10$.

Maths Trap 6: Not All Variables Represent Positive Integers

When testing values of variables, do not forget negative numbers and fractions. This is important because negative numbers and fractions between 0 and 1 behave very differently from positive integers.

Avoiding the Trap

When testing the value of variables, consider fractions and negative numbers.

Maths Trap 7: Hidden Instructions

Read the following question:

> At a certain café, Joe ordered 3 rolls and a cup of coffee and was charged £2.25. Stella ordered 2 rolls and a cup of coffee and was charged £1.70. What is the price of 2 rolls?
>
> (A) £0.55
> (B) £1.00
> (C) £1.10
> (D) £1.30
> (E) £1.80

Did you read carefully and avoid the potential trap? You are asked for the price of 2 rolls, not 1 roll. Many Problem Solving questions invite you to misread them. If you are careless when you read the question—for instance, solving for the price of 1 roll in this example—you can be sure that the test maker will include that answer among the four wrong answer choices. Choice (C) is correct.

Avoiding the Trap

Make sure you answer the question that is being asked. Follow the first two principles, reading carefully and deciphering exactly what you are asked. This can prevent you from missing hidden instructions and answering incorrectly.

Maths Strategy 4—The Process of Elimination and Reasonable Estimations

If you simply cannot solve an equation using regular maths or an alternative method, sometimes that is the time to make an educated guess. The key to good guessing on multiple-choice questions is the elimination of wrong answer choices. Some questions will have answer choices that are obviously wrong or do not make sense. If you can eliminate some wrong choices using common sense, you will have improved your chances of guessing the correct answer.

The Process of Elimination

For practice, try to eliminate some answer choices for the following question.

> A container holding 12 millilitres of a solution that is 1 part alcohol to 2 parts water is added to a container holding 8 millilitres of a solution that is 1 part alcohol to 3 parts water. What is the ratio of alcohol to water in the resulting solution?
>
> (A) 2:5
> (B) 3:7
> (C) 3:5
> (D) 4:7
> (E) 7:3

Right away you should eliminate (E). It is the only choice that has more alcohol than water; not only does it stand out from the other answer choices because it is the only one that represents a fraction greater than 1, but it does not make sense because both solutions had less alcohol than water.

You should use common sense to eliminate some other choices. One of the solutions is 1:2 alcohol to water, the other is 1:3. A combination of the two should have a ratio somewhere between 1:2 and 1:3. But (C) and (D) both have a higher proportion of alcohol than the 1:2 solution, so you can eliminate them. Guess (A) or (B); you have a 50 percent chance of being right.

Reasonable Estimation

The process of elimination is not very helpful with short answer questions. For these questions you should rely on reasonable estimations. Obviously, it would be nearly impossible to randomly guess the correct answer. However, using some of the information from the question, even if you are unsure of how to solve it, can help you make a reasonable guess. For example, if a question were to ask you what number is a fractional part of 20,495, a reasonable guess would have to be a number less than 20,495. Although you have narrowed your choices to just a possible solution, you know that a guess lower than that value is more likely to be correct than a guess greater than that value.

PROBLEM SOLVING LOGIC STRATEGIES

Because there are three different types of logic questions (statements, rules, and diagrams), there are different strategies as well.

Statements Strategy 1—Establish an if/then conditional.

The statements found in this type of logic question are often very dense with information. Here is a sample statements question about some fictional animals.

> All lippits are millikins and no millikins are blue. No jobsa is a millikin.

Although there are two sentences, there are really three pieces of information given:

1. All lippits are millikins.
2. No millikins are blue.
3. No jobsa is a millikin.

These facts may be brief, but they contain a lot of information. One way to sort through this information and find out what it really being said is by constructing conditional statements. A conditional statement follows the pattern of

"If BLANK, then BLANK".

By setting up statements in these two clauses, you can understand the logical trigger and logical result. For example:

If you are a lippit, you MUST BE a millikin.

If you are a millikin, you are NOT blue.

If you are a jobsa, you are NOT a millikin.

So, you know that if you are lippit, you must be a millikin. But what happens if you are a millikin? Are you also a lippit? And what if you are blue? What are you?

To answer these questions, or in the case of the BMAT, to test whether an answer choice is true, you must also construct the if/then statements in the other direction.

Statements Strategy 2—Test the if/then statements in both directions.

Remember, the idea is that you must find one or more true statements. So, if you have not answered the question previously posed of whether or not millikins are lippits or what blue animals are or are not, then you have more work to do. In this case, you must test your if/then statements in both directions.

Here is what we mean:

If you are a lippit, you MUST BE a millikin. **AND** If you are NOT a millikin, you are NOT a lippit.

Remember, the statement does not say that all millikins are lippits, but since all lippits are millikins it is a logical conclusion that *some* millikins *might* also be lippits.

If you are a millikin, you are NOT blue. **AND** If you are blue, you are NOT a millikin.

This way you know that if you are blue, you are definitely *not* a millikin.

If you are a jobsa, you are NOT a millikin. **AND** If you are a millikin, you are NOT a jobsa.

This means there is no such thing as an animal that is both jobsa and millikin.

FORMING "IF/THEN" AND ITS OPPOSITE

In each of the preceding examples, we have written the opposite of the "then" statement as the "if" portion. The opposite of the original "if" statement becomes the "then" portion.

"If A, then B". becomes: If NOT B, then NOT A.

Be especially careful with the original wording of if/then statements. Note whether they are already negative, in which case the opposite is a positive statement.

"If A, then NOT B". becomes: If B, then NOT A.

Here are the statements again, followed by a question and answer choices. Use the first two statements strategies to find the correct answers.

> All lippits are millikins and no millikins are blue. No jobsa is a millikin.
>
> Which *two* of the following must be true?
>
> (A) All millikins are lippits.
> (B) No jobsa is a lippit.
> (C) A lippit is a jobsa.
> (D) A lippit is never blue.
> (E) Jobsas are blue.

The answers are (B) and (D). Even with the if/then statements written out, the answers are still not immediately obvious. Choice (B) is correct because it is saying that if you are a jobsa, you are NOT a lippit. If jobsas were lippits, they would also be millikins because all lippits are millikins; the second statement contradicts that, so (B) is true. Choice (D) is slightly more obvious because if lippits were blue then millikins would be blue (since all lippits are millikins). The first statement clearly states that no millikins are blue.

Practice is the best way to improve your logic skills. You can find more statements questions at the end of this chapter.

Statements Strategy 3—Draw your own diagram.

This strategy is most helpful for statements that ask for a rank or location. Here is the same example used earlier in the chapter:

> Gill is older than Isidore and Isidore is younger than Benjamin.
> Benjamin is older than Gill, but younger than Stefan.
>
> Stefan must be:
>
> (A) the youngest;
> (B) younger than Isidore;
> (C) older than Gill, but younger than Benjamin;
> (D) younger than Isidore and Benjamin;
> (E) the oldest.

Because the information you are given involves ranking, in this case ages, choose a system to depict oldest to youngest.

For example, as you read the statements you may translate this into

Statement 1: G > I < B

Statement 2: S > B > G

Immediately, you can use the diagram from Statement 2 to eliminate choices (A) and (D) because your diagram clearly shows that Stefan is not the youngest, nor is he younger than Benjamin.

If you do not want to use the greater/less than symbols, you can put the names in a list that shows their ranking:

S

B

G

I

The main idea is that the diagram you draw should make sense to you. Do not worry about replicating these exact methods, but instead use the ones that help you the most.

Rules Strategy 1—Apply each answer choice systematically to the rules.

This strategy is an application of common sense. The purpose of rules questions is to test each answer choice against the rules given in the question. However, this strategy focuses on having a system. A logical choice is to begin with the first item in the list in choice (A). Proceed with the rest of the items in choice (A) and then repeat the process with choices (B) through (D). Review the sample rules question from earlier in the chapter.

The order in which 5 teams perform for competition is decided on the number of members on the team and team name. Teams with a number of members that is equal to a multiple of 6 perform first in alphabetical order. Teams with a number of members that is equal to a multiple of 4 perform last in reverse alphabetical order. The only exception to these rules is that the team who won the competition the previous year always perform first. The name and number of team members are listed below.

Sussex Team, 32 members

Midland Team, 8 members

Westfield Team, 30 members

Pritchard Team, 20 members

Cliffside Team, 18 members

If the Cliffside Team won last year, which of the following orders may be correct?

(A) Cliffside, Westfield, Sussex, Pritchard, Midland

In this case, the first choice was correct. However, be thorough and always check the other choices systematically to be certain.

(B) Cliffside, Westfield, Midland, Sussex, Pritchard

(C) Cliffside, Sussex, Pritchard, Midland, Westfield

(D) Cliffside, Midland, Pritchard, Sussex, Midland

Diagrams Strategy 1— Apply each answer choice systematically to the rules.

Because diagrams questions are a type of rules questions, you should use the same strategy. Begin with answer choice (A) and test it against the rules and the diagrams provided. Immediately eliminate any choices that do not follow the rules.

Diagrams Strategy 2—Draw your own diagram.

These questions obviously include diagrams. However, that does not mean that you cannot draw your own while reviewing the information provided. For example, pretend that the diagrams provided do not exist. Next, use the information provided to create your own diagram based on the rules. When you are finished, you should find that the figure you drew matches one or more of the diagrams provided. This in turn directs you to the correct answer.

To test this strategy, review the diagrams sample question given earlier in the chapter.

A certain clock rings two notes at quarter past the hour, four notes at half past, and six notes at three-quarters past. On the hour, it rings eight notes plus an additional number of notes equal to whatever hour it is.

	:00	:15	:30	:45
1 P.M.	9	2	4	6
4 P.M.	12	2	4	8

Figure 1

	:00	:15	:30	:45
1 P.M.	9	2	4	6
4 P.M.	13	4	2	6

Figure 2

	:00	:15	:30	:45
1 P.M.	9	2	4	6
4 P.M.	12	2	4	6

Figure 3

Which chart shows the number of rings occurring during the 1 P.M. hour and 4 P.M. hour?

(A) Figure 1 only

(B) Figures 1 and 2 only

(C) Figure 3 only

(D) Figures 1 and 3 only

(E) Figure 2 only

You could test all the values in each of the figures against all the rules given in the question, or you could draw a blank diagram and fill in the information you are given. For example:

	:00	:15	:30	:45
1 P.M.				
4 P.M.	1			

When you have written down the information from the question, your blank diagram should now look like this:

	:00	:15	:30	:45
1 P.M.	9	2	4	6
4 P.M.	12	2	4	6

You can compare this to the diagrams provided and see that only Figure 3 matches and thus, choice (C) is the correct answer. Using this method, you will not have to test all the information in Figures 1 and 2 against the rules.

Now that you have reviewed the basic principles and top strategies of problem solving, test your knowledge by completing these practice questions.

REVIEW QUESTIONS

1. All bacteria are prokaryotes and all prokaryotes are unicellular. No eukaryote is a prokaryote. Which *two* of the following must be true?

    (A) All prokaryotes are bacteria.

    (B) Bacteria are not multi-cellular.

    (C) Prokaryotes are sometimes multi-cellular.

    (D) Eukaryotes are never unicellular.

2. The speed of a train pulling out of a station is given by the equation $s = t^2 + t$, where s is the speed in kilometres per hour, and t is the time in seconds from when the train starts moving. The equation holds for all situations where $0 \leq t \leq 4$. In kilometres per hour, what is the positive difference in the speed of the train 4 seconds after it starts moving compared to the speed 2 seconds after it starts moving?

1	2	3	4
7	5	4	2

3. The diagram shows an example of a 4-digit identification code used by a certain bank for its customers. The digits in the code must be in descending order and no digit can be used more than once in a single code. A digit that is a multiple of 2 can never be used in the second position and a digit that is a multiple of 3 can never be used in the third or fourth position.

1	2	3	4
9	8	7	5
4	3	2	1

Figure 1

1	2	3	4
9	7	5	4
4	3	2	1

Figure 2

1	2	3	4
9	7	4	2
3	2	1	0

Figure 3

1	2	3	4
9	7	5	4
4	3	1	0

Figure 4

Which figure shows the largest and smallest possible codes?

(A) Figure 1
(B) Figure 2
(C) Figure 3
(D) Figure 4

KAPLAN

4. An overnight courier service charges £5.00 for the first 2 grams of a package and £0.75 for each additional gram. If there is a 6% sales tax added to these charges, how much does it cost to send a 6-gram package?

   (A) £4.24

   (B) £8.00

   (C) £8.48

   (D) £9.28

   (E) £10.60

5. Ann and Bob drive separately to a meeting. Ann's average driving speed is greater than Bob's average driving speed by one-third of Bob's average driving speed, and Ann drives twice as many kilometres as Bob. What is the ratio of the number of hours Ann spends driving to the meeting to the number of hours Bob spends driving to the meeting?

   (A) 8:3

   (B) 3:2

   (C) 4:3

   (D) 2:3

6. Each of three charities in Grove Estates has 8 people serving on its board of directors. Exactly 4 people serve on 3 boards each and each pair of charities has 5 people in common on their boards of directors. A total of 13 distinct people serve on one or more boards of directors.

   Which one of the following correctly shows the members of the three boards?

   (A) Board 1: A B C D E F G H   Board 2: A B C D E F J M   Board 3: A B C D F J M

   (B) Board 1: A B C D F H K J   Board 2: A B C D E F H J   Board 3: A B C D J K L M

   (C) Board 1: A B C D K L M N   Board 2: A B C D E M N O   Board 3: A B C D G H I J

   (D) Board 1: A B C D E F H K   Board 2: A B C D E G I L   Board 3: A B C D F G J M

7. In 1966, the operative mortality rate in open heart surgery at a certain hospital was 8.1 per 100 cases. By 1974, the operative mortality rate had declined to 4.8 per 100 cases. If the rate declined by 20% from 1973 to 1974, by approximately what percent did it decline from 1966 to 1973?

   (A) 6%

   (B) 21%

   (C) 26%

   (D) 41%

   (E) 49%

8. At a certain store, each item that normally costs £20.00 or less is on sale for 80% of its normal price, and each item that normally costs more than £20.00 is on sale for 75% of its normal price. If a customer purchases c items, each of which normally costs £15.00, and d items, each of which normally costs £24.00, what is the average (arithmetic mean) amount, in pounds, that he or she pays for each item?

(A) $\dfrac{c+d}{30}$

(B) $\dfrac{12}{c}+\dfrac{18}{d}$

(C) $\dfrac{12c+18d}{2}$

(D) $\dfrac{12c+18d}{c+d}$

(E) $\dfrac{30}{c+d}$

9. On the last exam, Helen earned a lower score than Daniel. Clive earned a higher score than Helen but a lower score than Daniel or Ravi.

Which *two* of the following must be true?

(A) Ravi scored the highest.

(B) Helen had the lowest score.

(C) Clive earned a higher score than Helen or Ravi.

(D) Daniel scored higher than Clive.

(E) Ravi scored the same as Daniel.

10. How many cylindrical oil drums, with a diameter of 1.5 metres and a length of 4 metres, would be needed to hold the contents of a full cylindrical fuel tank, with a diameter of 12 metres and a length of 60 metres?

Answers and Explanations

1. B, D

If you are still familiarising yourself with forming conditional statements, this question is good practice. Using statements strategies 1 and 2, you should have written:

> If you are a bacterium, you are a prokaryote. **AND** If you are NOT a prokaryote, you are NOT a bacterium.
>
> If you are a prokaryote, you are unicellular. **AND** If you are NOT unicellular, you are NOT a prokaryote.
>
> If you are a eukaryote, you are NOT a prokaryote. **AND** If you are prokaryote, you are NOT a eukaryote.

Now, test each answer choice against what you know from the statements.

All bacteria are prokaryotes and all prokaryotes are unicellular. No eukaryote is a prokaryote.

(A) All prokaryotes are bacteria.

This is not true. If you are a bacterium, you are a prokaryote, but the statement does not imply that all prokaryotes are bacteria. They might be, but it is not true.

(B) Bacteria are not multi-cellular.

This is true. If bacteria are prokaryotes and prokaryotes are unicellular, then bacteria are NOT multi-cellular.

(C) Prokaryotes are sometimes multi-cellular.

This is not true. The first sentence states that all prokaryotes are unicellular.

(D) Eukaryotes are never unicellular.

This is true. Prokaryotes are unicellular and eukaryotes are never prokaryotes, therefore eukaryotes are never unicellular.

2. 14

We have an equation that tells us how fast the train is moving at any time: $s = t^2 + t$. For example, when t is 0 (before the train starts moving), the speed is $t^2 + t = 0^2 + 0 = 0$, as we would expect. After one second, the speed would be $t^2 + t = 1^2 + 1 = 2$ kilometres per hour. To answer the question, all we need to do is find the positive difference between the train's speed at 4 seconds and at 2 seconds.

2 seconds: $t = 2$, so $s = t^2 + t = 2^2 + 2 = 4 + 2 = 6$

4 seconds: $t = 4$, so $s = t^2 + t = 4^2 + 4 = 16 + 4 = 20$

The positive difference between the two speeds is $20 - 6 = 14$.

3. D

This is another question where it would be helpful to draw your own diagram. If you do not draw your own diagram, you would have to test the information in each of the four diagrams. Your blank diagram would be:

$$1 \quad 2 \quad 3 \quad 4$$

For the largest number, add digits following the rules. In this case 9, 7, 5, 4. Note that the digits are in descending order, each digit is used only once, the second digit (7) is not a multiple of 2 and the third and fourth digits (5 and 4) are not multiples of 3.

For the lowest number, you must be especially careful. You might be tempted to write 4, 3, 2, 1 because it is in descending order, each digit is used only once, the second digit (3) is not a multiple of 2 and the third and fourth digits (2 and 1) are not multiples of 3. However, the final rule is broken, this is *not* the smallest possible code. The code 4, 3, 1, 0 is smaller and still follows all the same rules.

This question tests your careful reading of the details, as well as your understanding of exactly what is being asked. Even when drawing your own diagram, it might be helpful to test the other options since you may have missed an important detail, in this case that 4, 3, 1, 0, not 4, 3, 2, 1, is the smallest possible code.

4. C

Take it one step at a time. We want to send a 6-gram package. The first 2 grams cost £5.00. Each of the remaining 4 grams costs £0.75. So the total for all 6 grams, exclusive of tax is:

£5.00 + 4(£0.75) = £8.00 To this is added a 6% tax, resulting in a total cost of:

£8.00 + 0.06(£8.00) =

£8.00 + £0.48 = £8.48.

5. B

Picking Numbers is the strategy that works here. Since Ann drives $\frac{1}{3}$ faster than Bob, pick a number for Bob that is a multiple of 3. Why not 3? If you say that Bob drives 3 kilometres per hour, then Ann drives $\frac{1}{3}$ faster, or 4 kilometres per hour.

Now, the other information we have to consider is how far each travels. Ann drives twice as far as Bob. Pick 12 as the number of kilometres she drives (it is a multiple of both 3 and 4, the numbers already chosen—that is usually a good idea). If Ann drives 12 kilometres, then Bob drives 6 kilometres.

So now how much time will each spend driving? Ann will drive 12 kilometres at 4 kilometres per hour:

4 kilometres per hour × x hours = 12 kilometres

$$4x = 12$$
$$x = \frac{12}{4}$$
$$x = 3$$

Bob will drive for 6 kilometres at 3 kilometres per hour:

3 kilometres per hour × x hours = 6 kilometres

$$3x = 6$$
$$x = \frac{6}{3}$$
$$x = 2$$

So the ratio of the amount of time that Ann will drive to amount of time that Bob will drive is 3:2.

6. D

Choice (A) is clearly incorrect because Board 3 has only 7 members and this violates the first rule. In choices (B) and (C) each pair of boards has too many members in common. In choice (B) Board 1 has A, B, C, D, F, and J in common with Board 2. In choice (C) Board 3 has only 4 members in common with Board 2. Only choice (D) shows 13 distinct members with 4 people in common on all three boards (A, B, C, D), as well as a fifth member in common in each pair of boards. For example, Boards 1 and 2 have member E in common, Boards 2 and 3 have member G in common, and Boards 1 and 3 have member F in common.

7. C

To determine the percent decrease in the rate from 1966 to 1973 you need to find the rate for 1973. You know the actual rate for 1974, and since you also know the percent decrease from 1973 to 1974, you can find the 1973 rate. The rate dropped 20% from 1973 to 1974, so the 1974 rate represents $100\% - 20\% = 80\%$ of the 1973 rate. Let the 1973 rate be represented by x, and plug into the percent formula: Percent × Whole = Part, so $.8x = 4.8$, $x = \frac{48}{8} = 6$. So the rate decreased by $8.1 - 6 = 2.1$ from 1966 to 1973. Percent decrease $= \frac{\text{part decrease}}{\text{whole}} \times 100\%$, so $\frac{2.1}{8.1} / \frac{1}{4} \times 100\%$ is approximately $\frac{1}{4} \times 100\%$, or 25%. Choice (C) is closest, and it is the correct answer.

8. D

This is a complicated word problem; translate it one step at a time. Items that are less than or equal to £20.00 are discounted by 80%, items that are over £20.00 are discounted by 75%. The customer purchases c items costing £15.00 and d items costing £24.00, that is, c items discounted by 80% and d items discounted by 75%. The average price then is $\frac{\text{total discounted cost of articles purchased}}{\text{number of articles purchased}}$. Find the average of the discounted prices of all the articles.

80% of £15.00 = £12.00; total amount spent on these c items: £12c

75% of £24.00 = £18.00; the total amount spent on these d items: £18d

$$\text{Average} = \frac{\text{total discounted cost of articles purchased}}{\text{number of articles purchased}}$$

$$= \frac{12c + 18d}{c + d}$$

As you should realise, reading the question carefully is critical. Often, similar terms will be employed and you must keep them straight.

9. B, D

Statements strategy 3, drawing your own diagram, might be helpful with this question. You need to rank each person's score from greatest to least in order to choose which two choices must be true.

First review the two statements: Helen earned a lower score than Daniel. Clive earned a higher score than Helen but a lower score than Daniel or Ravi.

A diagram could show:

$D > C > H$

$R < D$ OR $R > D$ OR $R = D$ (Note, it does not say whether or not Ravi's score is higher than, lower than or equal to Daniel's score, only that Ravi's score is higher than Clive's.)

Now, apply this information to each of the answer choices.

(A) Ravi scored the highest.

This may be true, but it may not be true. This is not one of the correct answers.

(B) Helen had the lowest score.

This is true. Of all the information given, her score is the lowest.

(C) Clive earned a higher score than Helen or Ravi.

This is not true. The second sentence states that Clive earned a higher score than Helen, but a lower score than Ravi.

(D) Daniel scored higher than Clive.

This is true. Clive earned a lower score than Daniel.

(E) Ravi scored the same as Daniel.

Like choice (A), this may be true, but it may not be true, so it is incorrect.

10. 960

To find the number of drums needed to hold the contents of the tank, set the combined volume of all the drums equal to the volume of the tank. The combined volume of the drums is the volume per drum × the total number of drums. The volume of a cylinder is the area of the circular base × the height, and the area of the circular base is equal to π × radius squared. Since the question gives the diameter of each cylinder, you will need to halve each diameter to find the radius, and then you can find the volume. The radius of each drum is $\frac{1.5}{2} = 0.75$ or $\frac{3}{4}$. So, the volume of each drum is $\pi\left(\frac{3}{4}\right)^2(4) = \left(\frac{9}{16}\right)(4)\pi = \frac{9\pi}{4}$. The number of drums is unknown, so use a variable such as x to represent it. So the total volume of the drums is $(x)\frac{9\pi}{4}$. The volume of the tank is $\pi(6^2)(60) = (36)(60)\pi$. So $(x)\frac{9\pi}{4} = (36)(60)\pi$; $x = (36)(60)\pi\left(\frac{4}{9\pi}\right)^4 = (4)(60)(4) = 960$.

Chapter 4: **Understanding Argument**

Imagine you need to convince a patient to undergo a specific course of treatment or persuade administrators to fund research that you believe could make significant advances in your field. How do you present a convincing argument?

Or say an article claims that an experimental drug is highly effective against a particular ailment or that you should use a new system for managing your patient data. Do you accept the article's claims at face value, or do you demand evidence to back up those claims? Do you have the critical thinking skills to evaluate that evidence? And can you spot an illogical argument when you see one?

In these and countless other scenarios, you, as a medical professional, will need to be able to argue effectively and to recognise the effectiveness of other arguments. Hence the Understanding Argument questions on the BMAT.

UNDERSTANDING ARGUMENT QUESTIONS

Each Understanding Argument question has three parts: a brief argument, the question stem, and the answer choices. You can expect approximately 6 of these questions in Section I. They'll look something like this:

Recent surveys show that many people who leave medical school before graduating suffer from depression. Clearly, depression is likely to cause withdrawal from medical school.

Which one of the following, if true, most strengthens the above argument?

(A) Many medical schools provide psychological counselling for their students.

(B) About half of those who leave medical school report feeling depressed after they make the decision to leave.

(C) Depression is very common among management consultants who have a similarly difficult work schedule to those of many young doctors.

(D) Medical students who have sought depression counselling due to family problems leave at a higher rate than the national average.

(E) Career change has been shown to be a strong contributing factor in the onset of depression.

We'll show you the correct answer and explain why the incorrect answers are wrong later in this chapter. First, here is a brief primer on the structure of arguments.

BASIC ARGUMENT STRUCTURE

We tend to think of an argument as a disagreement between two or more people. That's one kind of argument, yes—but not the kind of argument you'll see on the BMAT. In terms of critical thinking, an argument is any text that contains both evidence and a conclusion; it takes a position (conclusion) and offers support (evidence) for that point of view. Your task on the BMAT isn't to agree or disagree with that point of view but to evaluate the effectiveness of that argument.

A conclusion, then, isn't the *ending* or *last part* but rather the main claim or point the author is trying to make. The conclusion can come anywhere in the argument—the beginning (sometimes), middle (on occasion), or end (most often, but definitely not always).

Argument = Evidence + Conclusion

Conclusion: the main point that the author is trying to make

Evidence: the support that the author offers for that conclusion

---

Here's an example:

> Every Wednesday so far this term, Anuj has been late to class. Today is
> Wednesday. Anuj will be late again.

In this simple argument, the first two sentences are the evidence; the last, the conclusion. Based on the two facts (that it's Wednesday and Anuj has been late each previous Wednesday), the author concludes that Anuj will once again be late to class.

As you might guess, your success on Understanding Argument questions absolutely depends upon your ability to correctly identify the conclusion. Usually it will be rather obvious. However, if you have difficulty determining which idea expresses the main point of the argument, ask yourself what the argument adds up to. What does the author want you to think, do or believe? Key words and phrases can also help you identify the conclusion. The following terms generally indicate that a conclusion will follow:

Conclusion Indicators

> thus
>
> therefore
>
> hence
>
> this shows/suggests/implies/proves that
>
> consequently
>
> so
>
> accordingly

These words and phrases, on the other hand, indicate that evidence will follow:

Evidence Indicators

> since
>
> because
>
> for
>
> in view of the fact that

Practice Set 1:

Underline the conclusion in each of the following arguments.

1. One of the best things you can do for your body is add fish oil to your diet. Fish oil lowers blood triglycerides, helps reduce the likelihood of blood clots and helps lower blood pressure. It also reduces inflammation from rheumatoid arthritis and lowers the risk of developing Alzheimer's disease.

2. Many people think of yoga as a passive, leisurely activity that requires little strength or exertion. But yoga can actually provide a rigorous workout of all major (and minor!) muscle groups. It also facilitates better health by reducing stress. Indeed, yoga is a bona fide – and highly beneficial – form of exercise.

3. The debate over year-round school has raised many important issues. Because both parents work in so many families, child care during the summer months can be a real financial and logistical burden. In addition, children often forget much of what they learned over the extended break from school. Year-round school may be a better option than the current system.

4. Sales of organic produce have risen by at least 10% each month over the last six months. Therefore, we should expand all organic product offerings to meet increasing customer demand.

5. Because property taxes are so high in our county, many residents have been moving to neighbouring counties where taxes are significantly lower. We must implement property tax relief measures immediately. If we don't do something to alleviate the tax burden on our residents, our population and property values will continue to decline.

Explanations:

The conclusions are underlined below. Notice how in each example, the other sentences serve to support the conclusion.

1. <u>One of the best things you can do for your body is add fish oil to your diet</u>. Fish oil lowers blood triglycerides, helps reduce the likelihood of blood clots, and helps lower blood pressure. It also reduces inflammation from rheumatoid arthritis and lowers the risk of developing Alzheimer's disease.

2. Many people think of yoga as a passive, leisurely activity that requires little strength or exertion. But yoga can actually provide a rigourous workout of all major (and minor!) muscle groups. It also facilitates better health by reducing stress. <u>Indeed, yoga is a bona fide – and highly beneficial – form of exercise</u>.

3. The debate over year-round school has raised many important issues. Because both parents work in so many families, child care during the summer months can be a real financial and logistical burden. In addition, children often forget much of what they learned over the extended break from school. <u>Year-round school may be a better option than the current system</u>.

4. Sales of organic produce have risen by at least 10% each month over the last six months. <u>Therefore, we should expand all organic product offerings to meet increasing customer demand</u>.

5. Because property taxes are so high in our county, many residents have been moving to neighboring counties where taxes are significantly lower. <u>We must implement property tax relief measures immediately</u>. If we don't do something to alleviate the tax burden on our residents, our population and property values will continue to decline.

Now, in the types of arguments you will encounter on the BMAT – and, indeed, in the majority of arguments you encounter in everyday life – there are often unstated assumptions that connect the evidence to the conclusion. That is, the author provides evidence in the argument, but there's a leap in logic between the evidence and the conclusion. This is called a *non sequitur*. Here's an example:

> Charlotte is very good at science. She will make an excellent doctor.

Clearly there is a gap between the evidence (first sentence) and the conclusion (second sentence) – there's no *stated* connection between the two. But we all know what the author is *thinking*:

> Evidence: Charlotte is very good at science.
>
> Assumption: People who are very good at science make excellent doctors.
>
> Conclusion: She will make an excellent doctor.

Once we identify the underlying assumption, then we can better judge the soundness of the argument. We'll point out the flaws in this argument later in the chapter. Meanwhile, try identifying the unstated assumptions in the following arguments.

Assumption: the idea that connects the conclusion to the stated evidence

Conclusion = Evidence + Assumption(s)

Practice Set 2:

Write the unstated assumption for each argument below.

1. Hector's mother spoke to him in both English and Spanish when he was a baby. That's why he's already able to read at three years old.

2. The average teenager watches four hours of television each day. No wonder obesity is an epidemic among teens.

3. The tank was full when I borrowed Valerie's car, but now it's nearly empty. I'd better fill it up before I return it to her.

Explanations:

Your wording may be different, but your assumptions should convey the ideas expressed below.

1. Children who learn two languages from birth will learn to read at a young age.

2. Many people who watch a lot of television each day are obese.

3. When you borrow something, you should return it in the same condition that it was in when you borrowed it.

TYPES OF UNDERSTANDING ARGUMENT QUESTIONS

Understanding Argument question stems come in five types:

1. Which one of the following is an underlying assumption of the above argument? (Or, more rarely, in plural: *Which of the following are underlying assumptions…*)

Your job is to determine which statement logically connects the evidence to the conclusion by identifying the unstated assumption.

2. Which one of the following is the best statement of the flaw in the above argument?

3. Which one of the following is a reason why this conclusion might be unsafe?

These two kinds of question stems are essentially the same: they both ask you to identify the statement that best expresses the problem with the argument. Why two of a kind? One of the key attitudes universities are looking for in medical students is a tendency to think critically about evidence and conclusions, and in particular about the ramifications a conclusion might have for the community. Thus some questions ask you to think about flaws in general while others help you focus on the consequences of accepting a flawed argument.

4. Which one of the following, if true, most weakens the above argument?

5. Which one of the following, if true, most strengthens the above argument?

For these two questions, the answer choices present new evidence. Assuming the evidence is true, you need to determine which item most undermines or strengthens the conclusion.

Now let's examine each question type in more detail and review specific strategies for each.

Assumption Questions

An assumption, as you know, bridges the gap between an argument's stated evidence and its conclusion. It's a piece of evidence that isn't explicitly stated but that is required for the conclusion to be valid. Whenever you find that a key term appears only in the conclusion, there's one or more unstated assumptions at work.

For example, in the argument about Charlotte, the conclusion uses the term *doctor*, which does not appear in the evidence:

Charlotte is very good at science. She will make an excellent doctor.

Thus we need another statement to connect the two:

People who are very good at science make excellent doctors.

Now, logically and verbally, the parts of the argument are connected.

With an Assumptions question, you will have five assumptions to choose from, and more than one may seem to logically connect evidence and conclusion. The correct answer is always the assumption that is *necessary* to the argument—that is, without that connection, the argument falls apart.

To determine whether a statement is necessary to the argument, you can employ the denial test. Simply negate the statement and see if the argument falls apart. If it does, that's the correct assumption. If, on the other hand, the argument is unaffected, the choice is wrong. Consider the assumption we added to the Charlotte argument. To test whether this is the right assumption (the necessary one), negate it:

No one who is very good at science makes an excellent doctor.

Or

People who are very good at science make lousy doctors.

Based on either version of the negated assumption, can we still conclude that Charlotte would make an excellent doctor? No, we can't. It's possible that she would—but it's just as possible that she wouldn't. By denying the statement, then, the argument falls apart; it's simply no longer valid. And that's our conclusive proof that the statement is a necessary assumption of the argument.

Practice Set 3:

Go back to the assumptions you wrote for Practice 2 and put them through the denial test. If they pass, good for you! If they don't, revise your assumption until it is necessary for the argument.

Strengthen or Weaken Questions

An argument can be strengthened in three ways:

- by adding new evidence
- by proving the validity of existing evidence
- by proving the validity of an unstated assumption

As you can see, you may need to figure out any unstated assumptions before you can deal with how to strengthen an argument.

Let's use Charlotte again as an example.

> Charlotte is very good at science. She will make an excellent doctor.
>
> Which one of the following, if true, most strengthens the above argument?
>
> (A) You cannot become a doctor without successfully completing rigourous science courses.
>
> (B) A survey of successful doctors shows they consistently earned top grades in science at secondary school.
>
> (C) Most of the nation's top doctors report that science was always their favourite subject.
>
> (D) Most science classes are graded on a curve.
>
> (E) Excellent doctors have both extensive scientific knowledge and outstanding people skills.

Perhaps the right answer is obvious to you – but it may not always be. So how do you go about finding the right answer? Here, we know there's an unstated assumption that's essential to the argument. When this is the case, the correct answer is usually the one that validates the unstated assumption (that people who are good at science make excellent doctors). Thus the best answer is (B), which supports that assumption. Choice (A) is true, but it doesn't address the issue of excellence. Choice (C) is irrelevant; the issue isn't whether Charlotte likes science but the fact that she's very good at it. Choice (D) is even further outside the scope of the argument. Choice (E) may be tempting because it pinpoints a flaw in the argument, acknowledging that excellence in a doctor is a combination of factors. But it doesn't answer *this* question, so it is incorrect.

Now let's tackle the other half: how to weaken an argument. You can weaken an argument by:

- demonstrating that stated evidence is invalid
- demonstrating that an unstated assumption is invalid

Again, Charlotte:

> Charlotte is very good at science. She will make an excellent doctor.
>
> Which one of the following, if true, most weakens the above argument?
>
> (A) Many people who are very good at science are not interested in becoming doctors.
>
> (B) Some excellent doctors struggled in their science classes.
>
> (C) Science classes are often challenging for both medical and non-medical students.
>
> (D) Medical students have more difficult science classes than non-medical students.
>
> (E) Scientific knowledge and skill is just one quality of an excellent doctor.

Again, the best answer is the one that addresses the assumption linking the evidence and conclusion. And that choice is (E), which directly weakens the link by pointing out that scientific knowledge alone does not make someone an excellent doctor. Choice (A) may be tempting, but it's outside the scope; the argument doesn't address Charlotte's desire to become a doctor. Choice (B) seems to effectively undermine the argument, but it deals with a different issue: that you can become an excellent doctor even if you struggle in some science classes. That's quite a different matter from whether you will be an excellent doctor simply because you are good at science. Choices (C) and (D) should be more obviously incorrect; they do not address either the issue of being good at science or being an excellent doctor.

As you work through strengthen/weaken questions, remember the following key points:

- Weakening an argument is not the same as *disproving* it, and strengthening it is not the same as *proving* the conclusion to be true. A strengthener simply makes it more likely that the argument is valid while a weakener makes it less likely to be true.

- The wording of these questions always includes *if true*. So always assume the statements in the answer choices to be true, no matter how unlikely they may sound to you. Whether they could be true or not doesn't matter; what matters is what they'd do to the argument if they were.

- Don't be careless. Wrong answer choices in these questions are often worded exactly the opposite of the correct answer. That is, if you're asked to strengthen an argument, it's quite likely that one or more of the wrong answer choices will contain information that actually weakens it.

Practice Set 4:

Recent surveys show that many people who leave medical school before graduating suffer from depression. Clearly, depression is likely to cause withdrawal from medical school.

1. Which one of the following, if true, most strengthens the above argument?

   (A) Many medical schools provide psychological counselling for their students.
   (B) About half of those who leave medical school report feeling depressed after they make the decision to leave.
   (C) Depression is very common among management consultants who have a similarly difficult work schedule to those of many young doctors.
   (D) Medical students who have sought depression counselling due to family problems leave at a higher rate than the national average.
   (E) Career change has been shown to be a strong contributing factor in the onset of depression.

2. Which one of the following, if true, most weakens the above argument?

   (A) A majority of those who withdraw report first feeling depressed after their withdrawal.
   (B) A majority of those who withdraw report feeling uncertain about their ability to practise medicine.
   (C) Law school students who drop out before graduation also report feeling depressed.
   (D) Most students who withdraw from medical school report financial difficulties as their main reason for withdrawal.
   (E) Many medical school students suffer from sleep deprivation.

Answers and Explanations

1. D

It's the best answer because it suggests that when some outside event has brought on depression, leaving becomes more likely in the period subsequent to the depression. This confirms that students who are depressed while in school are more likely to drop out. (A) is irrelevant; the counselling provided may not be for depression, and, in fact, counselling can significantly help depression and would probably make it *less* likely that students would drop out. (B) and (E) support a link between depression and leaving, but in both cases, the depression comes *after* the decision to leave – and that's the *opposite* of what the argument says. (C) is out of the scope of the argument since we're discussing medical students, not young doctors or consultants.

2. A

The argument concludes that depression *causes* withdrawal, which means depression comes first. Choice (A) most weakens the argument because it states that for most students the onset of depression was *after* withdrawal, thereby completely undermining the conclusion. Choices (B) and especially (C) are outside the scope of the argument. Choice (D) may be tempting because it seems logical that many students would withdraw because of difficulties financing the many years of medical school. But that alone is not enough to choose this as the best answer. It may be true, but it doesn't undermine the argument. Remember, we're looking for something to weaken the claim about depression causing withdrawal. Choice (E) interestingly discusses sleep deprivation, which can lead to depression, but that connexion isn't explicitly stated and thus the answer choice does little to impact the argument.

Flaw Questions

This type of question asks you to recognise what's wrong with an argument. There are two basic types.

In the general type, the correct choice will criticise the reasoning of the argument by pointing out a classic fallacy (e.g., "This argument attacks the source of an opinion, not the opinion itself".). In this case, the flaw falls into a general, well-defined category, and the answer choice sticks to the general problem (not using words from the argument).

In the specific type, the correct answer will attack a specific piece of the argument's reasoning. An example of this would be: "The author assumes that all people who are good at science will make excellent doctors". The answer states the specific flaw in terms the argument uses.

In each case, the required skill is the ability to identify the structure of the author's argument – and where the argument goes wrong. So let's review some of the most common weaknesses in arguments.

Five Frequent Flaws

The range of possible flaws in arguments on the BMAT is extensive, but you're most likely to see versions of these five common flaws:

1. Illogical comparisons. These often involve statistical evidence that compares apples and oranges; e.g., a statistic about all of a school's students in one statement may be compared to a statistic about first-year students in another. Or it could involve the author "projecting" the qualities of one group onto another. Here's an example:

In recent years, attacks by Dobermans on small children have risen dramatically. Last year saw 35 such attacks in the continental United States alone, an increase of almost 21% over the previous year's total. Clearly, it is unsafe to keep dogs as pets if one has small children in the house.

Which one of the following is the best statement of the flaw in the above argument?

(A) It offers a justification for euthanising dangerous pets.

(B) It ignores the possibility that the injured children instigated the attacks by hurting the dogs.

(C) It does not provide statistics of attacks by other kinds of dogs.

(D) It does not acknowledge the percentage of Dobermans that are properly trained and no harm to humans.

(E) It assumes that the behaviour toward small children exhibited by Dobermans is representative of dogs in general.

Clearly the problem with this argument is expressed in choice (E): it projects the characteristics of a limited population (Dobermans) onto a general population (dogs in general) – and that's poor logic. Apples and oranges.

2. Jumping to conclusions. As you've seen, many arguments are based on unstated assumptions. Sometimes those assumptions just don't make sense, so there remains a gap between the evidence and conclusion. Here's an example:

A whopping 85% of our students say they are concerned about adequate nutrition. Clearly we need to change our lunch menu.

In this argument, the author quite obviously jumps to the conclusion that the students are unhappy with school lunches and the lunches should be changed to address student concerns. The argument falls apart when you articulate the unstated assumption:

Students who are concerned about adequate nutrition are also unhappy with the lunch menu.

Put it through the denial test, and you'll see that the argument doesn't make sense – the assumption fails to logically connect the evidence and conclusion.

Another kind of jumping-to-conclusions argument is one that draws a conclusion based on insufficient evidence. For example:

I ate at the new restaurant in town yesterday, and my dinner was awful. Don't ever eat there. The food is terrible.

If you go back to the restaurant two or three more times and each time the food is awful, then you have enough evidence to reasonably conclude the food is terrible. But just one trip, tasting just one meal, doesn't give you a wide enough base to draw this conclusion. Maybe the regular cook was out that night; maybe he or she was there but was feeling sick. There could be many reasons for one bad experience.

3. Irrelevance. In this case, one or more ideas are irrelevant – they fall outside the scope of the argument or issue. Let's take the Doberman example:

> In recent years, attacks by Dobermans on small children have risen dramatically. Last year saw 35 such attacks in the continental United States alone, an increase of almost 21% over the previous year's total. Clearly, the breeding of Dobermans should be more strictly regulated.

Are Dobermans being bred to be more violent? It's highly unlikely. The issues of breeding and regulations for breeders are irrelevant; they have nothing to do with attacks on children.

4. Failure to consider alternatives. These arguments overlook alternative reasons or explanations. Here's an example:

> Jenny went to visit Mike. Mike was sick with a cold. The next day, Jenny came down with a cold. She must have caught the cold from Mike.

Maybe she did – and maybe she didn't. Maybe *she* had the cold first and passed it to Mike before she showed any symptoms. Maybe they both got it from someone else – or from two different people. There are several equally viable alternatives.

5. Stereotypes or generalisations. Finally, we come back to the argument about Charlotte. Here it is again:

> Charlotte is very good at science. She will make an excellent doctor.

Notice how this argument makes a big – and erroneous – generalisation about people who are good at science. Indeed, beware any time you see an argument that makes a blanket statement about a group. Words like *all, every, none, always,* and *never* are all-inclusive and don't allow for exceptions. But there are always exceptions, and an absolute greatly weakens an argument.

Practice Set 5:

Read each argument below carefully. Determine which flaws, if any, are in the argument. Arguments may have more than one flaw.

Flaws:

(A) Illogical comparisons.

(B) Jumping to conclusions.

(C) Irrelevance.

(D) Failure to consider alternatives.

(E) Stereotypes or generalisations.

1. Every Wednesday, Anuj is late to class because he works. This week, he wasn't late. He must have lost his job.

2. Every week Anuj is late to class, and he never seems to be prepared. It must be because he's on the football team.

3. Anuj has never missed a class. Now he's missed class for two weeks in a row. He must have dropped out.

4. One hundred men aged 20-65 tried ProTen, a probiotic dietary supplement. Three-quarters reported feeling more energetic after taking ProTen once a day for two weeks. ProTen is clearly a proven energy booster for men and women.

Answers and Explanations

1. B and D

This argument jumps to the conclusion that Anuj lost his job. He's only arrived on time once; anything could account for that anomaly. Thus it also fails to consider alternative explanations.

2. C and E

Though a rigourous sports team schedule may make it difficult for an athlete to keep up with schoolwork, it's unlikely that it would make a student perpetually unprepared for class. That makes the football connexion irrelevant. The author also seems to be suggesting that football players don't care about academics, and that's an ignorant stereotype.

3. B and D again

This argument has a little more evidence upon which to base the conclusion (Anuj has clearly missed more than one class). Still, that's not enough to assume that he's dropped out. Once again, the author fails to consider alternative explanations. Maybe Anuj is on holiday, or a business trip, or severely ill. There are many other possibilities.

4. A and D

These 100 men are not representative of all men *and* women, so the argument is guilty of irrelevant comparison. It also fails to consider other causes for the men's increase in energy.

TOP 5 STRATEGIES FOR UNDERSTANDING ARGUMENT QUESTIONS

1. Read the question stem first.

Always read the question stem before you read the argument. The stem tells you what to look for in the argument (an assumption, a flaw, a way to weaken or strengthen the argument). Previewing the stem allows you to set the tone of your attack on each stimulus, saving time.

2. Read actively.

As you read the arguments on the BMAT, *read actively*. Identify and underline the conclusion. If the conclusion seems complex, restate it in your own words. This will not only help you get the author's point in the first place, but it'll also help you hold on to it until you've found the correct answer.

Reading actively also means reading *critically*. As you read, question the argument. Does the author's position seem valid? Why or why not?

Don't allow yourself to fall into the bad habits of the passive reader – reading solely for the purpose of getting through the stimulus. Those who read this way invariably find themselves having to read the stimuli twice or even three times. Then they wonder why they run out of time on the section. Read the stimuli right the first time – with a critical eye.

3. Answer the question being asked.

It's disheartening when you fully understand the argument and then lose the point by supplying an answer to a question that wasn't asked. For example, when you're asked for an assumption, it does you no good to jump on the answer choice that paraphrases the conclusion. Likewise, if you're asked for the flaw in the argument, don't be fooled into selecting a choice that looks like a piece of the author's evidence.

When asked why they chose a particular wrong answer, students sometimes respond by saying such things as, "Well, it's true, isn't it?" and "Look, it says so right there", pointing to the stimulus. Well, that's simply not good enough. The question stem doesn't ask, "Which one of the following looks familiar to you?" or "Which one of the following is true?" It asks for something very specific, and it's your job to find the answer that meets that request.

As you work, be on the lookout for "reversers" – words such as *not* and *except* which can be easy to miss but entirely change what you're looking for among the choices.

Don't forget to predict the answer!

---

4. Stay within the scope of the argument.

One of the most important strategies for Understanding Argument questions is the ability to focus in on the scope of the argument. The majority of wrong choices in this section are distractors. They are tempting because they seem logical and/or may be true, but they are outside the scope of the argument.

Some common examples of scope problems are choices that are too narrow, too broad, or literally have nothing to do with the author's points. For example, take another look at the Doberman argument (the answers have been slightly modified this time):

> In recent years, attacks by Dobermans on small children have risen dramatically. Last year saw 35 such attacks in the continental United States alone, an increase of almost 21% over the previous year's total. Clearly, it is unsafe to keep dogs as pets if one has small children in the house.
>
> Which one of the following is an underlying assumption of the above argument?
>
> (A) No reasonable justification for these attacks by Dobermans on small children has been discovered.
>
> (B) Other household pets, such as cats, don't display the same violent tendencies that dogs do.
>
> (C) The number of attacks by Dobermans on small children will continue to rise in the coming years.
>
> (D) Dobermans are more dangerous than any other pet.
>
> (E) The behaviour toward small children exhibited by Dobermans is representative of dogs in general.

Hopefully you immediately identified choices B and D as outside the scope of the argument. The argument is about Dobermans and their attacks on children; it is not about other pets.

Similarly, when considering the assumptions behind an argument, make sure you limit yourself to the *argument's* assumptions, not *your* assumptions. You may have your own opinions about the subject or outside knowledge, but they are, for the purposes of the BMAT, irrelevant. However valid or correct your knowledge or opinions may be, they can lead you to choose an incorrect answer.

Recognising scope problems is a great way to eliminate wrong answers quickly.

5. Eliminate wrong choices first if you have to guess.

Any wrong choice you can eliminate improves your chance of choosing the correct answer. One or more of the wrong answer choices on any question will fall into patterns that, with practice, you'll quickly recognise. On Understanding Argument questions, common wrong answer types include:

Outside scope. Just as arguments can be flawed by having evidence that's outside the scope of the argument, one or more answer choices are likely to be irrelevant. (This can be true for any question type, not just flaw questions.)

Extreme. Choices using words like *always, never, none, all* and *every* are usually wrong. There's almost always an exception, and these answers rule out those exceptions, thereby weakening the argument.

Distortion. Some choices use language or ideas from the stimulus, but distort them conspicuously.

Half right, half wrong. Some choices join a correct statement with an incorrect one; don't be hasty and choose your answer without reading the entire choice.

Reversals. These choices are exactly the opposite of the correct one. These are especially common in questions that ask for exceptions or in the strengthen/weaken question type.

Irrelevant comparisons. Answer choices may also employ this common flaw: comparing apples to oranges.

REVIEW QUESTIONS

For this review, we ask two questions about each argument to help you get deeper into the structure of each argument. On the BMAT, however, and in the practice tests in this book, you should expect to see only one question per argument.

Questions 1-2 refer to the following argument.

> A study of twenty overweight men revealed that each man experienced significant weight loss after adding SlimDown, an artificial food supplement, to his daily diet. For three months, each man consumed one SlimDown portion every morning after exercising, and then followed his normal diet for the rest of the day. Clearly, anyone who consumes one portion of SlimDown every day for at least three months will lose weight and will look and feel his best.

1. Which one of the following is an underlying assumption of the above argument?

   (A) The men in the study will gain back the weight they lost if they discontinue the SlimDown programme.

   (B) No other dietary supplement will have the same effect on overweight men.

   (C) The daily exercise regimen was not responsible for the effects noted in the study.

   (D) Women will not experience similar weight reductions if they adhere to the SlimDown programme for three months.

   (E) Overweight men will achieve only partial weight loss if they do not remain on the SlimDown programme for a full three months.

2. Which one of the following, if true, most strengthens the above argument?

   (A) The men in the study were only slightly overweight before they began the SlimDown programme.

   (B) The men in the study exercised regularly before beginning the SlimDown programme.

   (C) The men in the study had a strong positive attitude toward the SlimDown programme.

   (D) The regular diet of the men in the programme was balanced and healthy.

   (E) None of the men in the programme had ever used a weight loss supplement before.

Questions 3-4 refer to the following argument.

Dr. Kells is a better physician than Dr. Li. This is obvious because in a recent survey their mutual patients rated Dr. Kells as the better physician.

3. Which one of the following is an underlying assumption of the above argument?

   (A) Patient rating is a valid indicator of the quality of a physician.

   (B) Patients will rate a doctor as "better" if they feel more comfortable with that doctor.

   (C) The better doctor will be the one with greater experience.

   (D) The better doctor is the one from whose care patients benefit more.

   (E) There are no doctors better than Dr. Kells.

4. Which one of the following is the best statement of the flaw in the above argument?

   (A) It assumes Dr. Li and Dr. Kells practise the same kind of medicine.

   (B) Surveys are untrustworthy because questions can be biased to encourage certain answers.

   (C) Patient satisfaction is just one measure of a physician's quality.

   (D) We do not know on what characteristics the patients rated the doctors.

   (E) We do not know how many patients were surveyed.

KAPLAN

Questions 5-6 refer to the following argument.

The rate of violent crime in a particular U.S. state is up 30% from last year. The fault lies entirely in the court system: recently our judges' sentences have been so lenient that criminals can now do almost anything without fear of a long prison term.

5. Which of the following are underlying assumptions of the above argument?

    I. People take potential prison terms into account before they commit a crime.
    II. Judges' decisions can have a serious impact on crime rates.
    III. The judicial system is inefficient and corrupt.

(A) I only

(B) II only

(C) III only

(D) I and II

(E) II and III

6. Which one of the following, if true, most weakens the above argument?

(A) 85% of the other states in the nation have lower crime rates than this state.

(B) White-collar crime in this state has also increased by over 25% in the last year.

(C) 35% of the police in this state have been laid off in the last year due to budget cuts.

(D) Polls show that 65% of the population in this state oppose capital punishment.

(E) The state has appointed 25 new judges in the last year to compensate for deaths and retirements.

Questions 7 and 8 refer to the following argument.

World War II had a profound effect on the growth of nascent businesses. The Acme Packaging Company netted only £10,000 in the year before the war. By 1948, it was earning almost 10 times that figure.

7. Which one of the following is an underlying assumption of the above argument?

(A) Acme's growth rate is representative of other nascent businesses during the same time period.

(B) An annual profit of £10,000 was not especially high at the time.

(C) Wars inevitably stimulate a nation's economy.

(D) Rapid growth for nascent businesses is especially desirable.

(E) Acme was in business for less than two years before the war began.

8. Which one of the following is the best statement of the flaw in the above argument?

(A) It does not say how long the company was in business.

(B) Inflation could account for such a steep growth in revenue.

(C) Many other factors could have accounted for Acme's wartime success.

(D) The company profited from the suffering of others during wartime.

(E) Revenues are the prime indicator of a company's growth.

ANSWERS AND EXPLANATIONS

1. C

The conclusion states that people who consume SlimDown will lose weight – it does not mention exercise or diet. Thus the author must assume that exercise was not a factor in the weight loss of the participants. (Clearly this is a rather faulty assumption.) Choices (A) and (B) are outside the scope; there's no mention of other supplements or the potential to regain weight after stopping the programme. Choice (D) is incorrect as it states the opposite of what the argument assumes. The author states that "anyone" who goes on the SlimDown programme will lose weight, so that means men *and* women. Choice (E) may be tempting because it sounds logical, but it does not fill the gap between evidence and conclusion.

2. B

Logic should tell you that exercise was likely to be at least partially responsible for the significant weight loss of the men participating in the SlimDown programme, even though the argument gives SlimDown all the credit. Thus the best way to strengthen the argument is to get rid of that flaw. Choice (B) effectively eliminates exercise from the equation; if the men were already on a regular exercise programme, something else – SlimDown – would have been responsible for their weight loss. Choice (D) addresses diet, which of course is also an important factor in weight gain or loss, but the argument specifically states that the men followed their normal diet while on the SlimDown programme. Thus it doesn't matter whether that diet was healthy or not; it's not a factor in the argument. Choice (A) is illogical, since the study states that the men experienced "significant" weight loss – not likely if they were only slightly overweight. While a positive attitude would likely have some impact on weight loss, choice (C) is irrelevant in terms of the argument, as is choice (E).

3. A

This short argument concludes that Dr. Kells is a better physician than Dr. Li. The evidence, which is very brief, is that their patients rate Kells as a better doctor. As always in an Assumption question, we're looking for the missing piece that ties the evidence (that patients rate Kells the better doctor) to the conclusion (that Kells *is* the better doctor). If the ratings of patients provide a solid basis for determining who is the better doctor, then the argument is solid. That's a perfect match for (A). (B) does nothing to tie ratings to actual quality. Instead, it introduces a new factor, the patients' comfort level with a doctor, which is outside scope. Likewise, (C) and (D) introduce new factors ("greater experience" and "from whose care patients benefit more") without filling the gap between ratings and actual quality. (E) needn't be true for the argument to be valid; the conclusion claims only that Kells is better than Li, not better than everyone.

4. C

However important patient satisfaction may be, it is still just one measure of the quality of a physician. But the conclusion rests on the assumption that patient ratings alone is a valid means for measuring the better doctor. Whether the doctors practise the same or different kinds of medicine is irrelevant; the issue is how their quality is measured, so choice (A) is incorrect. Choice (B) may be true – surveys can be biased – but again, the argument revolves around the matter of patient ratings. Choices (D) and (E) also deal with the matter of the survey, and were this a more developed argument, it might deal with these issues. However, as the argument stands, it only rests on one key assumption which is not addressed in these two answers.

5. D

From one piece of evidence (the 30% increase in violent crime), the author concludes that judges are at fault because their lenient sentences make criminals feel they can get away with anything. There's a significant gap in this argument, and two assumptions fill the void: that people take potential prison terms into account before they commit a crime and that judges' decisions can have a serious impact on crime rates. Reverse the assumptions to see they are both necessary: if judges' decisions *didn't* have a serious impact, then the author couldn't claim that the increase in crime was the judges' fault. Likewise, if people *didn't* take prison terms into account, then the author couldn't claim that "criminals can now do almost anything without fear of a long prison term". The author may feel that the judicial system is inefficient and corrupt (choice III), but that is not within the scope of this argument.

6. C

If we can show that something besides the court system may explain the increase in crime (if we can show a different cause for the same effect), we would weaken the argument. The author, after all, assumes that there is no other cause. Choice (A) is a classic faulty comparison. The argument does not compare one country to another. The argument's scope is the crime rate increase in this country only. In (B), the fact that white collar crime is also on the rise is more of a strengthener than a weakener—maybe it is the leniency in the courtroom that is responsible for the overall crime surge. (C) presents an alternative explanation for the increase in crime. Maybe it is not the judges at all but the fact that there are fewer police officers on the street. As for (D), what if 65% of the people in the country opposed capital punishment? What if 100% did? The fact is irrelevant and outside the scope of the argument. (E) tells us that numerous judges have been replaced in the last year. It is possible that the new judges are more lenient, but this would only strengthen the author's conclusion.

7. A

The author uses the single case of Acme to conclude that the war profoundly affected "nascent businesses". This assumes that Acme's growth rate is typical, or representative of such businesses (choice A); otherwise, why hold it up as an example? As for (B), the author needn't assume that £10,000 isn't much of a profit. Maybe he thinks it started out high and got even higher. (C), which brings up other wars, is beyond the scope – the argument only concerns World War II. (D) is tricky, but it's not assumed. Notice that the author claims only that World War II had a profound, not salutary, effect on nascent businesses, so we don't know just how he feels about rapid growth rates. As for (E), being in business less than two years would make Acme a nascent business, but the argument doesn't rest on a specific assumption of the length of time before the war that the company existed. The argument is valid so long as Acme is representative of other young businesses, whether they were in business two years or just two months.

8. C

Obviously being at war would have a wide-ranging impact on a country's economy. But there could be other reasons for Acme's tremendous growth. There's no evidence in the argument that Acme's packaged goods were used in any way in the war effort. We do not need to know exactly how long Acme was in business (A), unless it were to demonstrate that Acme was not a nascent business at the beginning of the war; but that is not the purpose of the statement. Choice (B) makes an illogical statement (inflation would mean that the rise was *less* impressive); it is a flaw, but not of the argument. Choice (D) attempts to lure you by engaging your emotions, but it is outside the scope of the argument (besides, we don't know anything about what Acme produced or how the business was run). (E) actually helps validate the argument; if revenues are a prime indicator of growth, then Acme did indeed do well. This does not state a flaw in the argument.

Chapter 5: **Data Analysis and Inference— Statistical and Graphical**

This chapter reviews the essentials for mastering the Data Analysis & Inference questions pertaining to statistics and graphs on the Biomedical Admissions Test. Question format and structure, as well as basic principles and strategies are found here. Test what you have learned by completing the practice questions found at the end of the chapter.

QUESTION FORMAT AND STRUCTURE

Data Analysis & Inference questions require you to analyse and interpret information, to make deductions and inferences, and to reach valid conclusions based on the information provided. These twelve questions are based on three types of information: verbal, statistical and graphical. The following chapter details how to handle verbal information, namely reading passages. This chapter will focus on statistical and graphical information such as charts, graphs, tables and other data. To understand Data Analysis & Inference questions it is not necessary to differentiate between the different types of graphical information. Throughout this chapter, the generic term "graphs" applies to any statistical or graphical information that may be found in these questions.

Data Analysis & Inference Forms	Number of Questions	Time Allowed
Verbal*	3–5	—
Statistical	3–5	—
Graphical	3–5	—
	TOTAL: 12 (approximate)	TOTAL: 15 minutes

*NOTE: This table covers the entire Data Analysis section; however, this chapter reviews only the statistical and graphical forms as they apply to this section. Verbal/Reading Comprehension forms will be covered in the following chapter.

Data Analysis & Inference questions are not found in a distinct section of the BMAT. While completing the 35 questions in the Aptitude Section of the BMAT, these questions are interspersed with Problem Solving questions and Understanding Argument questions. There are no specific instructions for Data Analysis & Inference questions.

Multiple-Choice and Short Answer Questions

Like most questions on the BMAT, Data Analysis & Inference questions are found in two formats: multiple-choice or short answer. In multiple-choice format, the question is followed by possible answer choices. Questions may have as many as six answer choices (A–F), but they are more likely to have five (A–E), or four answer choices (A–D). For this format, you must select which is the correct answer among the possibilities listed. In some cases, there will be more than one correct answer. These questions instruct you to "choose all that apply".

Although not as common, the short answer format is also used for Data Analysis & Inference questions. In this format, no answer choices are provided. You are responsible for deducing and writing the correct answer to the question. As a rule, you should always review your answers since you will not be able to compare your answer with a provided answer choice. You should never leave a short answer question blank. Remember, there is no penalty for incorrect responses and the answer can be found somewhere among the information provided.

Four Question Structures

When you encounter a Data Analysis & Inference question, it is likely to be based on four question structures. These are referred to here as: graphs within questions, graphs as answer choices, graphs with single questions, and graphs with multiple questions. These structures are not mutually exclusive. For example, you may have a graph followed by several questions, one of which has graphs as answer choices.

Graphs within Questions

In this question structure, the graph is found within the question. You will have to review the information provided and answer the question that follows.

Graphs as Answer Choices

Here, the graph is not found only within the question. The question itself will be text and each of the answer choices will contain a graph relating to this information.

Graphs Followed by Single Questions

In some cases, a graph is followed by a single question. The information in the graph is used once to answer this question.

Graphs with Multiple Questions

Occasionally, one graph is followed by as many as four questions. To answer these questions it is especially important to familiarise yourself with the graph so that you are able to answer all the questions that pertain to it. When many questions follow a single graph, each question is still worth only one point.

ELEMENTS OF A GRAPH

When you have to review the contents of a graph, it is important to familiarise yourself with its elements. Each is detailed here.

Introductory Information

On the BMAT, many questions begin with a sentence or paragraph that explains or supplements the graph. Here is an example of introductory text: The following pie chart shows the percentage of income spent on various expenses and taxes.

Title

This tells you the topic of the graph or chart: what the information means. The title is usually clear and concise; you should always read it first. On the BMAT, the title may be replaced by the introductory information.

Units

The units of the graph will often be given with the title of the graph, or by the relevant scale on a graph, or column on a chart. Make sure you understand the units before you answer the questions. In particular, look out for things like "(in millions of pounds)" underneath the title; this kind of thing is very common on the BMAT, and very easy to miss.

Scales

The scale will usually appear along the side and bottom of a bar or line graph, and tells you how many units each mark along the side signifies. Check to see where the scale starts—it need not start at zero. You may be given more than one line or set of bars on one graph; if so, they may have different scales. Check the right-hand side of the graph to make sure—that is where a second scale would be.

Keys

If a graph contains information for several different groups or factors, there is often a key to differentiate between them. For example, a bar graph may have bars that are shaded in black and in grey. The key should let you know, for example, that bars shaded in black refer to one thing, while bars shaded in grey refer to another. Keys are often found on the side of or below a graph. It may be a small detail, but it can affect your answers greatly.

SCIENCE-RELATED GRAPHS AND STATISTICS ————————————

If a graph in a Data Analysis & Inference question presents scientific information, rest assured that you are *not* tested specifically on your knowledge of biology, chemistry, or physics. Section 2 of the BMAT, Scientific Knowledge and Applications, is where you find these types of questions. In the Aptitude and Skills section of the BMAT, the data or graphs may cover science topics, but you are not tested on this subject.

TYPES OF GRAPHS—A BRIEF OVERVIEW

Chapter 23, Mathematics reviews in detail several maths topics, including data interpretation. Here is a brief discussion of this topic.

Tables

Tables share many of the characteristics of graphs, except for the visual advantages—you can estimate values from a graph, but not from a table. Tables can be enormous and complicated, but the basic structure is always the same: columns and rows. Here is an example of a very simple one (much simpler than those that appear on the BMAT):

JOHN'S INCOME: 2000–2004

YEAR	INCOME
2000	£30,000
2001	£32,000
2002	£28,000
2003	£25,000
2004	£38,000

Bar Graphs

These can be used to show visually the information that would otherwise appear in a table. On a bar graph, the *height* of each column shows its value. Here is the information from the previous table presented as a bar graph:

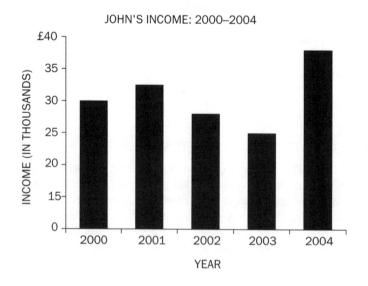

JOHN'S INCOME: 2000–2004

When you look at a bar graph you can see the relative values by looking at the height of each bar. By glancing at the previous graph, for example, it is easy to see that John's income in 2004 was almost double his income in 2003. Note that it is easy to see these values because the scale starts at zero; the scale could just as easily start somewhere *other* than zero.

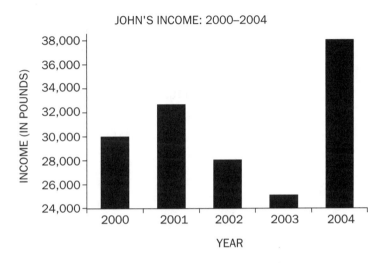

JOHN'S INCOME: 2000–2004

This graph presents the same information, but now it is not possible to estimate as before. At a glance it is still clear that his 2004 income exceeded 2003, but it is not possible to quickly estimate the ratio. In order to find some numerical value from a bar graph, find the correct bar (such as 2004 income), and move horizontally across from the top of the bar to the value on the scale on the left. For example, John's 2004 income was approximately £38,000. Notice that this is different from a table, which lists John's *exact* income.

Line Graphs

Line graphs follow the same principle as bar graphs, except the values are presented as points, rather than bars.

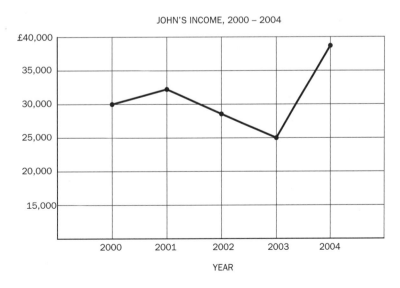

JOHN'S INCOME, 2000 – 2004

As with bar graphs, the value of a particular year is the vertical distance from the bottom of the graph to the line. In addition, you can see the relative value of the described amounts by looking at their heights—with the caveat that the base must be zero in order to estimate ratios.

Pie Charts

A pie chart shows how things are distributed; the fraction of a circle occupied by each piece of the "pie" indicates what fraction of the whole it represents. Usually, the pie chart will identify what percent of the whole each piece represents.

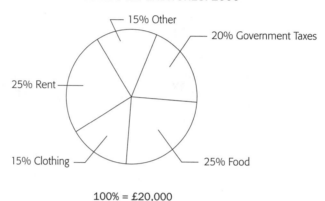

JOHN'S EXPENDITURES: 2000

100% = £20,000

The total size of the whole pie is usually given under the graph, either as "TOTAL = £3,547" or "100% = £5.9 billion" or whatever.

Pie charts often travel in pairs. If so, be sure that you do not attempt to compare slices from one chart with slices from another. For instance, suppose you encounter another pie chart for John's expenditures, one covering 2004.

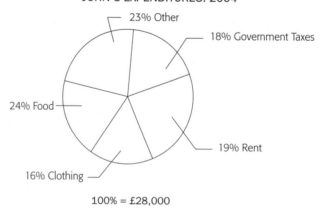

JOHN'S EXPENDITURES: 2004

100% = £28,000

Part III: How to Approach the Aptitude and Skills Section
Data Analysis and Inference—Statistical and Graphical | **85**

A careless glance might suggest that he paid less in government taxes in 2004 than in 2000. This is not the case. His 2000 taxes were a greater percentage of his income than were his 2004 taxes, but his 2004 income was much greater than his 2000 income. In fact, he paid about £1,000 *more* in taxes in 2004 than in 2000. Since the totals for the two charts are different, the pieces of the pie are not directly comparable.

Multiple Graphs

On the BMAT some questions may present more than one graph. Be certain to review each graph individually and all graphs as a group to ensure that you are deducing the correct information.

Here are two charts or graphs that are related in some way.

STUCK LIFTS IN COUNTRY *X*

Year	Stuck
2000	432
2001	459
2002	621
2003	645

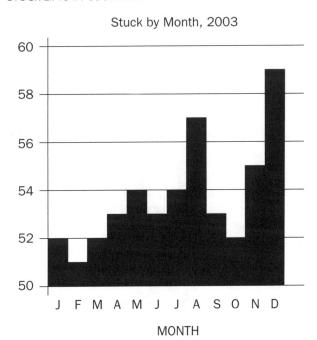

Here, the table covers stuck lifts, while the accompanying bar graph presents the information by month for 2003.

What can be more confusing is when you are given two graphs (either two line graphs or two bar graphs) occupying the same space. Sometimes both graphs will refer to the same vertical scale; other times, one graph will refer to a scale on the left, the other graph to a scale on the right.

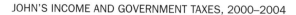

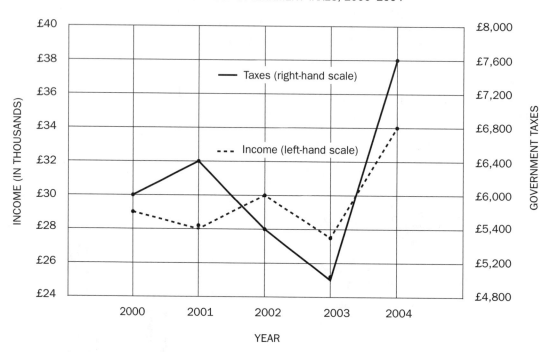

Here is the same graph of John's income, but with new information added. Presented here is not only John's income for a given year, but also the amount of government taxes for that year. The income refers to the left-hand scale; the taxes to the right-hand scale. At this point, obviously, the number of potential questions has risen dramatically.

Double graphs are not really any more difficult than single graphs as long as you do not confuse the scales. Learn to double-check that you are using the correct scale when working with double graphs. If you find yourself getting confused, slow down and give yourself a chance to sort things out.

INFERENCE

Data Analysis & Inference questions obviously test your inference skills. First, you should understand the difference between data analysis and inference. The former means that you must analyse the information to find the answer to a question. Inference is more subtle. You will have to analyse the information but you will have to make an inference, or educated guess, as to an outcome or conclusion. If you have to make an inference, you will have to understand what the data is implying, not just exactly what it is presenting.

Here is a sample inference question based on the graphs found earlier in this chapter:

Which of the following statements can be inferred from the charts?

1. John paid more in government taxes in 2004 than in 2000.
2. John paid a higher percentage of his income in total taxes in 2000 than in 2004.
3. John's medical expenditures were greater in 2004 than in 2000.

(A) 1 only
(B) 2 only
(C) 1 and 2 only
(D) 1 and 3 only
(E) 1, 2, and 3

You have to understand the scope of the graph, and the difference between what MUST be true and what MIGHT be true. In the previous question, the first statement can be inferred from the information, as seen before: the percentage paid in government taxes decreased, but the actual amount of government taxes paid increased. Statement 2 cannot be inferred for a simple reason: it refers to *total* taxes, while the pie charts only concern *government* taxes. A subtle distinction, you might think, but you have to learn to look for these in inference questions. If the questions all say "government taxes" and then one suddenly says "total taxes", there must be a reason; the question is written to test how carefully you are reading. Finally, statement 3 is not inferable either; medical expenditures must fall into the "other" category, and although the total "other" category increased between the two years, there is no reason to assume that *every* expenditure within that category also increased. Perhaps he had *no* medical expenditures in 2000. Only the first statement can legitimately be inferred, and the answer is **(A)**.

Because inference questions are often in the 1, 2, 3 format, you can always use the answer choices to your benefit. For instance, in the previous question, if you realise that statement 2 is not inferable, you do not even have to look at statement 1: every answer choice except for **(B)** includes it. You know that statement 1 *must* be true. So you can save time, and concentrate on statement 3. This will often happen on such questions; as you decide the truth of the statements, eliminate answer choices.

MATHS

As opposed to questions that test your inference skills, questions that test your data analysis skills often test your maths skills as well. Some of the most commonly tested maths topics found in Data Analysis & Inference questions are:

- ratios and rates
- probability (simple and compound)
- percentages
- averages

Of course, other maths topics that relate to data interpretation can be tested. For a thorough review of mathematics, review Section VII.

Here is an example of this question type:

The graph here shows the types of medical treatments used by patients complaining of flu-like symptoms. This data was collected over a year-long period to the nearest 4%. The graph shows the percentage of each type of treatment used. Data is recorded separately for men and women. The total annual flu-like symptom occurrence rates are 8,000 per 10,000 women and 4,000 per 10,000 men. There are an equal number of men and women in this given population.

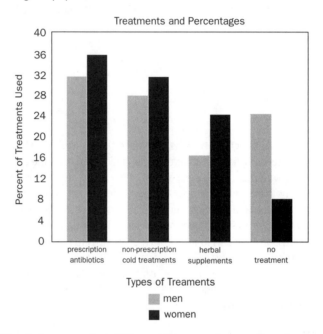

What is the numerical difference between the number of men who use no treatment and the number of women who use prescription antibiotics?

(A) 990

(B) 1,120

(C) 1,440

(D) 1,920

(E) 2,560

The correct answer is **(D)**.

GRAPHICAL INTERPRETATION AND UNDERSTANDING

This question type encompasses both data analysis skills and inference skills. Questions that test your graphical interpretation and understanding usually include graphs as answer choices. If the answer choices are not graphs, the questions are usually asking you to identify some other non-mathematical information from the graph. Here is a sample question with graphs as answer choices:

Which of the following shows the percentage of treatments for men with flu-like symptoms?

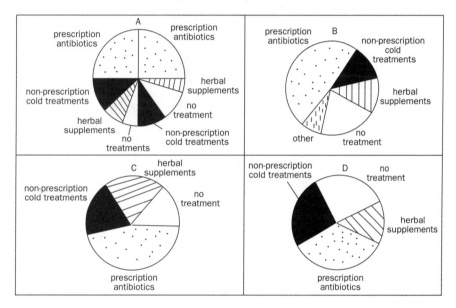

The correct answer is **(D)**.

Here is a sample question that asks you to identify non-mathematical information from the graph:

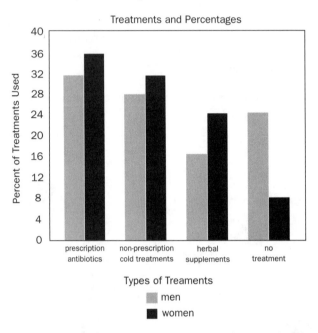

By percentage, which treatments are used less by men than by women? (Choose all that apply)

(A) prescription antibiotics

(B) herbal supplements

(C) no treatment

(D) non-prescription cold treatments

The correct answers are **(A)**, **(B)** and **(D)**. Do not think that this is a maths question because the term "percentage" is used. The question is really just asking you to compare the heights of the different bars.

THE 5 BASIC PRINCIPLES OF DATA ANALYSIS & INFERENCE

A systematic approach is the best way to solve Data Analysis & Inference questions. Do not waste time by answering a question in a scattered way. You should also never attempt to answer a question without first reviewing the graph. A systematic method will ensure that you understand exactly what each graph is displaying and that you answer all the questions quickly and efficiently.

The 5 basic principles of Problem Solving are:

1. Read carefully through the entire question once.

2. Review every element of every graph, especially if they are found in the question.

3. Know exactly what is being asked.

4. Research the correct answer.

5. Guess if you are not sure, but always use the process of elimination.

1. Read carefully through the entire question once.

This principle may sound familiar because it was also the first principle of problem solving. Clearly, there is nothing more important than reading through the entire question carefully to have the right foundation for answering Data Analysis & Inference questions. Work quickly, but efficiently. Even though the data is typically displayed using graphs, there is often some text that describes the graph or provides additional information that will be needed to answer the questions. Make certain you have reviewed all of the content provided in the question before you start to answer it.

2. Review every element of every graph, especially if they are found in the question.

When facing a graph for the first time, you must review every element. This includes but is not restricted to the:

- introductory information
- title
- units
- scales
- keys

To answer correctly, you must have all the information provided. Missing a crucial detail such as the scale of a graph could result in a series of incorrect answers.

If the graphs are found in the answer choices, it is not as critical to review all the elements of all the graphs. After all, unless specified, there is only one correct answer and once you have found it and checked it against the information provided, you can mark your answer and move on.

3. Know exactly what is being asked.

This is another principle that was stressed in the previous chapter: you must know exactly what you must answer. Read the question carefully so you are not calculating the ratio of men to women, when the question requires the ratio of women to men. Look again at this example:

> Which treatments are used less by men than by women? (Choose all that apply)
>
> (A) prescription antibiotics
> (B) herbal supplements
> (C) no treatment
> (D) non-prescription cold treatments

If you did not read carefully, you may have interpreted the question as which treatments men use more. If that were the question, the answer would be **(C)**, when the answers are actually **(A)**, **(B)**, and **(D)**—the treatments *women* use more. Careless reading and not understanding what you are answering will prevent you from earning a top score. Be especially careful of questions that ask you to compare two pieces of information. Finding the percentage of something rather than the percentage less something will never yield the correct answer.

4. Research the correct answer.

BMAT Data Analysis & Inference questions are written so that you cannot answer the question without first reviewing the text and graphs provided. When you know exactly what is being asked, it is time to start your research to deduce the correct answer.

For example, you are not expected to know the numerical difference between the number of men who use no treatment and the number of women who use prescription antibiotics on your own. You are expected to deduce this information from the graph, so always go back to it and research the correct answer.

Look again at the sample question from earlier in the chapter:

The graph here shows the types of medical treatments used by patients complaining of flu-like symptoms. This data was collected over a year-long period to the nearest 4%. The graph shows the percentage of each type of treatment used. Data is recorded separately for men and women. The total annual flu-like symptom occurrence rates are 8,000 per 10,000 women and 4,000 per 10,000 men. There are an equal number of men and women in this given population.

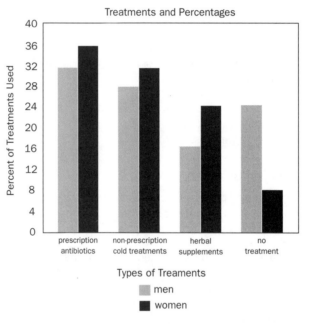

What is the numerical difference between the number of men who use no treatment and the number of women who use prescription antibiotics?

(A) 990

(B) 1,120

(C) 1,440

(D) 1,920

(E) 2,560

To answer this question you need to refer to the introductory text, which shows that the total annual flu-like symptom occurrence rates were 8,000 per 10,000 women and 4,000 per 10,000 men. You also need to review the graph to find out that 24% of men used no treatment and that 36% of women used prescription antibiotics to treat flu-like symptoms.

Even if a question is not maths-based and asks you to make an inference, you can still test whether your conclusion is logical based on the information provided. Avoid careless errors by always using the graphs to research the correct answer.

5. Guess if you are not sure, but always use the process of elimination.

The way to score a maximum of points on the BMAT is to answer correctly as many questions as you can. However, because there is no penalty for incorrect answers you should never leave a question blank. Even if you have no idea what the correct answer is, always make a guess.

To make your best guess on multiple-choice questions, try to eliminate incorrect answer choices. Some questions will have answer choices that are obviously incorrect or do not make sense. If you can eliminate some incorrect choices using common sense, you will have improved your chances of guessing the correct answer.

The process of elimination is as helpful with short answer questions. For these questions you should rely on reasonable guesses. For example, if a graph displays a range of 10 years and you are asked to write the year in which the percent increase was the greatest, you will actually have a 1 in 10 chance of guessing the correct year. Review the graph again and make a reasonable guess of the correct answer.

TOP 3 STRATEGIES FOR SUCCESS WITH DATA ANALYSIS & INFERENCE QUESTIONS

The principles will help you throughout the Aptitude and Skills section of the BMAT, but you may find that you need certain methods and tips for answering Data Analysis & Inference questions. Here are the top 3 strategies for success with these questions.

Strategy 1—Use alternative methods: Backsolving or estimation

If you are trying to answer a maths-based Data Analysis & Inference question, you can often use one of these shortcuts to find the answer quickly.

Backsolving

If you already read Chapter 3 then you know that Backsolving is a great strategy for solving maths questions. Here is a brief review.

Remember that Backsolving is a strategy that allows you to use the answer choices to work backward through the question. You plug the answer choices into the question to see which one works. The answer choice that agrees with the information in the question stem is correct. Backsolving is a true time-saving method.

Hopefully you also remember that Backsolving must be done systematically. Usually answer choices are arranged in ascending or descending order. When that is the case, start Backsolving with choice **(B)** or choice **(D)**. If that is not the answer, you will usually be able to tell whether the correct answer is larger or smaller, which means you will have narrowed the choices down.

Estimation

You can often estimate on BMAT graph problems. But before you estimate, check your units: are they in hundreds? thousands? Always make sure the scales start at zero.

In general, try to find precise values only as a last resort: remember, the BMAT tests to see whether you understand the basic concepts behind graphs.

Since you know how the Backsolving strategy works from the Problem Solving chapter, practise estimation on this question found earlier in the chapter.

The graph here shows the types of medical treatments used by patients complaining of flu-like symptoms. This data was collected over a year-long period to the nearest 4%. The graph shows the percentage of each type of treatment used. Data is recorded separately for men and women. The total annual flu-like symptom occurrence rates are 8,000 per 10,000 women and 4,000 per 10,000 men. There are an equal number of men and women in this given population.

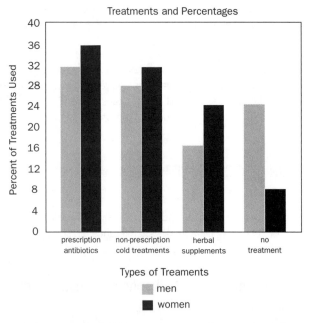

What is the numerical difference between the number of men who use no treatment and the number of women who use prescription antibiotics?

(A) 990

(B) 1,120

(C) 1,440

(D) 1,920

(E) 3,560

To make the maths easier, round the percentage of men who use no treatment (24%) to 25%; (.25)(4,000) = 1,000. Next, round the percentage of women who use prescription antibiotics (36%) to an even 40%; (.4)(8,000) = 3,200. Find the difference between the two: 3,200 − 1,000 = 2,200. Even this very rough estimation has allowed you to eliminate choices **(A)** and **(E)** for being far too low and high, respectively. The closest answer to your estimate is **(D)**, but you should calculate the exact difference which is (.24)(4,000) – (.36)(8,000) = 1,920. Choice **(D)** is correct.

AVOIDING TRAPS—A QUICK REVIEW

Remember these traps from the Problem Solving chapter. They may appear on some Data Analysis & Inference questions.

Maths Trap 1: Percent Increase/Decrease: When a quantity is increased or decreased by a percentage more than once, you cannot simply add and subtract the percentages to get the answer.

Maths Trap 2: Weighted Averages: Do not combine averages of different quantities by taking the average of those original averages. In an averages problem, if one value occurs more frequently than others, it is *weighted* more.

Maths Trap 3: Ratio:Ratio:Ratio: In the classic ratio trap, two different ratios each share a common part that is represented by two different numbers. However, the two ratios do not refer to the same whole, so they are not in proportion to each other. To solve this type of problem, restate both ratios so that the numbers representing the common part are the same.

Maths Trap 4: "Least" and "Greatest": In questions that ask for the *least*, *minimum* or *smallest* something, the choice offering the smallest number is rarely right. In questions that ask for the *greatest*, *maximum* or *largest* something, the choice offering the largest number is very rarely right.

Maths Trap 5: Percent "of" versus Percent "Less" or "Greater": Consciously and actively distinguish these three things whenever percent questions arise:

  1. a percent of *b*;

  2. a percent less than *b*;

  3. a percent greater than *b*.

Maths Trap 6: Not All Variables Represent Positive Integers: When testing values of variables, do not forget negative numbers and fractions. This is important because negative numbers and fractions between 0 and 1 behave very differently from positive integers.

Maths Trap 7: Hidden Instructions: Always read carefully to avoid a potential trap. Make sure you know exactly what you are being asked.

Strategy 2—Never answer a question from memory

No matter how long you have studied a question or graph, you should never answer a question without first referring to the graph. When answering a block of questions based on a single graph, you may feel as though you know the answer to the final question without having to look yet again at the graph. Resist this temptation and always do your research (principle #4). Exam writers are savvy and know exactly the kinds of mistakes that test takers are likely to make. Do not be one of those test takers.

Strategy 3—Always check your answer against the information provided

It may seem a waste of time to check your answer to every question, but your accuracy leads to more points and a higher BMAT score. Not only should you refer to the graph when you are answering the question, but once you have chosen your answer, take a few moments to ensure that you have answered correctly. There is no benefit in assuming your choice is correct when you can compare it to the information provided and hopefully know it is correct. Again, exam writers are clever people, who know how to write answer choices that are similar so as to distract you from the correct one.

Finally, if you are answering an inference question, make sure that the statements you chose MUST BE true and not just MIGHT BE true.

Now that you have reviewed the basic principles and top strategies of data analysis and inferences, test your knowledge by completing these practice questions.

REVIEW QUESTIONS

FORESTED LAND BY REGION IN THE
CONTINENTAL UNITED STATES

Region	Land Area (1,000 acres)	Area Forested (1,000 acres)	Percent Forested
New England	40,119	32,460	81
Mid Atlantic	87,813	50,686	58
Lake States	207,952	53,011	25
Central	241,425	42,871	18
South	474,906	185,514	39
Pacific Coast	570,253	214,274	38
Rocky Mountain	546,959	136,378	25
Total U.S.	2,169,427	715,194	33

1. Which of the regions listed has the least amount of forested land?

   _____

2. The following scatter plot shows the heights and weights of various students in a health class.

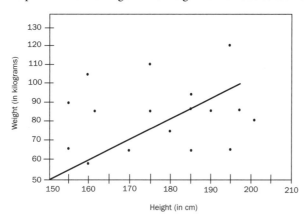

What is the average between the tallest and shortest person on the scatter plot?

(A) 90 cm

(B) 165 cm

(C) 177.5 cm

(D) 184.5 cm

Questions 3–6 refer to the following information.

AFRICAN LANGUAGES OF KENYA BY LINGUISTIC FAMILY

NUMBER OF MOTHER-TONGUE SPEAKERS[1]

I. Major Bantoid Languages		II. Major Nilotic Languages		III. Major Kushitic Languages	
1. Kikuyu	4,602,000	A. Western Nilotic		1. Somali	225,000
2. Luhya	3,045,000	1. Luo	2,810,000		
3. Kamba	2,479,000	B. Eastern Nilotic			
4. Gusii	1,356,000	1. Kalenjin	2,374,000		
5. Meru	1,207,000	2. Masai	346,000		
6. Nyika	1,053,000	3. Turkana	297,000		
7. Embu	260,000	4. Sambur	106,000		————
TOTAL	14,002,000	TOTAL	5,933,000	TOTAL	225,000

Mother-Tongue Speakers of Unlisted African Languages: 1,309,000

Population of Kenya: 22,020,000

[1]All Kenyans are assumed to have exactly one mother tongue.

[2]Includes speakers of non-African languages as mother tongue.

3. Other than mother-tongue speakers of an unlisted language, how many Kenyans have an Eastern Nilotic language as their mother tongue?

   (A) 106,000
   (B) 2,374,000
   (C) 2,810,000
   (D) 3,123,000

4. Approximately what percent of the Kenyan population has as their mother tongue one of the seven listed Bantoid languages?

   (A) 47%
   (B) 52%
   (C) 64%
   (D) 67%
   (E) 70%

5. What is the approximate ratio of mother-tongue Masai speakers to mother-tongue Turkana and mother-tongue Sambur speakers combined in Kenya?

   (A) 3 : 1
   (B) 7 : 6
   (C) 1 : 1
   (D) 3 : 4
   (E) 7 : 8

6. Which of the following statements must be true based on the information in the table?

   1. In Kenya, a greater number of people speak languages other than those listed in the table than the number of people who speak Eastern Nilotic languages.
   2. You cannot determine how many Kenyans speak non-African languages.
   3. A percentage of Kenyans who speak Nyika also speak Somali.

   (A) 1 only
   (B) 2 only
   (C) 2 and 3 only
   (D) All of the above
   (E) None of the above

7. These graphs show the rates of different types of cells (H, I, J, K) in an experiment testing the effect of temperature on growth.

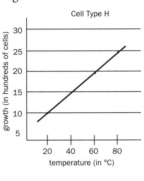

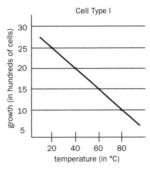

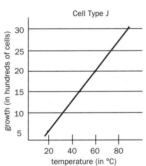

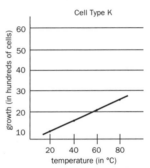

Which two cell types have the same rate of growth depending on temperature?

(A) H and I

(B) H and K

(C) I and J

(D) J and K

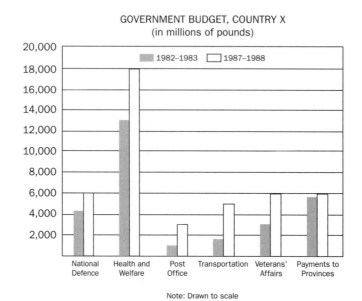

GOVERNMENT BUDGET, COUNTRY X
(in millions of pounds)

Note: Drawn to scale

8. How many of the given categories did NOT see an increase of at least 25 percent in 1987–88 over 1982–83?

(A) 0

(B) 1

(C) 2

(D) 3

ANSWERS AND EXPLANATIONS

1. New England

Scan the "Area Forested" column for the smallest value. New England has the smallest entry: 32,460 thousand acres; therefore, it is the answer.

2. C

Since you are looking for height (tallest and shortest) you should only look at points that are farthest right or left on the graph. The tallest person is 200 cm and the shortest person is 155 cm—even though this value is not explicitly labelled, you should know that the point between 150 and 160 is 155. Find the average by adding these amounts and dividing by 2; $155 + 200 = 355$; $\frac{355}{2} = 177.5$ cm. The maths skills required to solve this are actually quite basic, but you have to know how to read the scatter plot to determine the values you should use.

3. D

At the bottom of the Nilotic (Nilo-Saharan) column there are 5,933,000 speakers of Nilotic languages total. Of these 2,810,000 speak Luo, a Western Nilotic language, while the rest are the Eastern Nilotic speakers in question. Subtract the Luo speakers from the total to find the number of Eastern Nilotic speakers, but do it roughly to save time. (The answer choices are not that close together.) The difference is a little more than 3 million; 3,123,000 must be the answer.

4. C

The percent will be the total number of speakers for the seven listed Bantoid languages divided by the total population of Kenya. At the bottom of the first column, the total number of Bantoid speakers is about 14 million, while the total population of the country is about 22 million. So the percent sought after is around $\frac{14}{22}$. This fraction must be a little LESS than $\frac{2}{3}$ or $66\frac{2}{3}$%, since $\frac{14}{21} = \frac{2}{3}$. The best choice is 64%.

5. E

The answer choices are not very close together here, so it is best to use estimation. You are looking for the ratio of Masai speakers to Turkana and Sambur combined. These are all Eastern Nilotic languages, so you should focus on the Nilotic column. This says that there are 346,000 mother-tongue Masai speakers in Kenya, or about 350,000. The number of Turkana and Sambur mother-tongue speakers is 297,000 + 106,000 or about 400,000. The ratio you are looking for is about $\frac{350,000}{400,000} = \frac{35}{40} = \frac{7}{8}$ or 7 : 8.

6. B

You are asked to make inferences about what **must be** true based on the information in the graph. Test each statement:

1. In Kenya, a greater number of people speak languages other than those listed in the table than the number of people who speak Eastern Nilotic languages.

This is not true. You must read the information below the table to answer this. It reads: "Mother-Tongue Speakers of Unlisted African Languages: 1,309,000". You should compare this number to the number of people who speak Eastern Nilotic languages: 3,120,000. More people speak Eastern Nilotic languages than the number of people who speak unlisted African languages.

2. You cannot determine how many Kenyans speak non-African languages.

This is true. By using the given population of Kenya and subtracting the total number of speakers of major Bantoid languages, major Nilotic languages, major Kushitic languages, and other unlisted African languages, you can determine the number of Kenyans who speak a non-African language *as a mother tongue*. However, the statement does not specify. Therefore, it is true that you cannot determine how many Kenyans speak non-African languages in general.

3. A percentage of Kenyans who speak Nyika also speak Somali.

This may be true, but does not have to be true. The table presents information about mother-tongue languages only. It does not mention whether or not members of the population speak more than one language. This statement is not always true.

The answer is choice **(E)**, none of the above.

7. B

The important thing to note in the question is that you are not looking for graphs that look the same, you are looking for two graphs that show the same *rate*. In this example you should pay careful attention to the rates that each graph shows. You should immediately eliminate any answer choice that has "I" in it. Cell type I has a negative rate of growth, while the others have positive rates of growth. This limits your possible choices to **(B)** and **(D)**. Look closely at the graphs for types H and K. They both show a positive correlation, but the slope (rate) appears to be less in K. However, you should examine the graph closely. Notice that the scale of growth in centimetres in H is in increments of 5 and the scale in K is in increments of 10. If you noticed this, then you would have seen that although the graphs look different, they are actually showing the same information: at 20 degrees there are 1,000 cells, at 40 degrees there are 1,500 cells, and so on.

8. B

You are, in effect, looking for which categories show an increase of less than 25%. Estimate to make your work easier. National defence grew from a little more than 4 billion to about 6 billion. Well, if it had increased exactly 25%, then that would mean an increase of about 1 billion. Since it increased significantly more than that, you know it must have increased more than 25%. Health and Welfare grew from about 13 billion to 18 billion, an increase of about 5 billion. Since 5 billion is more than 25% of 13 billion, Health and Welfare is not what you want, either. You can dismiss the next three categories, Post Office, Transportation, and Veterans' Affairs, very quickly; just by looking at the graph, you should see that each department saw an increase of more than 25%. That leaves you with Payments to Provinces, and that too, you can evaluate very quickly, because there the increase was so slight it was obviously less than a 25% increase. That last category was the only one that did *not* see an increase of 25% in spending; therefore, the answer is 1, choice **(B)**.

Chapter 6: **Data Analysis & Inference–Verbal**

About a quarter of your Data Analysis & Inference questions will be based on a reading passage rather than charts or graphs. The text, approximately 750 words, is likely to be about a scientific topic and have plenty of scientific terms and statistics.

If this sounds like bad news to you, we have plenty of good news to counter it. For one thing, the reading comprehension strategies you'll need to answer the questions about the passage are basic. For another, there will be only one reading passage on the exam followed by just three to five questions. It's a small portion of the test, and you'll get through it quickly.

Of course, you want to do your best. This chapter shows you what the reading comprehension questions will be like and the strategies you can use to answer them correctly.

QUESTION TYPES

Despite the variety in question stems, BMAT reading comprehension questions will generally be one of three basic types:

1. **Main idea**. These often ask you to identify the statement that best summarises the main idea of a paragraph or larger part of the text. Question stems might look like the following:

    > Which of the following statements best summarises the author's objection to mandatory counselling?

    > Which of the following best expresses the implications of the study's findings?

2. **Specific facts or details**. You can expect the majority of reading comprehension questions to ask you about specific facts or details from the text. The question stems can take many forms. Here are some possibilities:

    > Which of the following extraction techniques was most successful?

    > Which of the following is NOT a health benefit of fish oil?

Keep in mind that this type of question may also ask you to calculate the solution to a specific problem based on figures presented in the text.

3. **Inference**. The third type of question will ask you to draw some kind of conclusion based on evidence from the text. It may ask you for a prediction or a projection. For example:

    > Based on the results of the study, if the study had included women over the age of 65, how might the results have differed?

    > The author of the article would most likely support which of the following courses of action?

FINDING THE "ACCURATE" ANSWER

Your exam may include the following question stem:

> Which of the following statements may we safely conclude to be accurate?

At a glance, this sounds like an inference question because it asks you to draw a conclusion. And there's a good chance it will be an inference question. But be aware that this stem can also be used for main idea and specific detail questions as well, and answer choices can include a wide range of possibilities.

Your best bet? Immediately eliminate the answer choices you know are incorrect. Then look for answers that accurately paraphrase statements from the passage. If there isn't an accurate paraphrase of an idea or detail from the text, then find the answer that makes a logical inference based on the passage. (Remember, distractors will often distort ideas from the text – so make sure you read answer choices carefully.)

Finding the Main Idea

The first thing to remember about the main idea of a passage is this: the main idea is not the same as the *subject* of the passage. The subject tells us what the passage is *about*; the main idea tells us what the author is trying to say *about* that subject. For example, the following paragraph is *about* spasms in paralysed muscles. The main idea goes farther; what idea *about* those spasms does the paragraph convey?

Paralysed muscles may still move regularly as a result of muscle spasms. Muscle spasms can occur whenever the skin below the level of paralysis is stimulated. The stimulated nerve cells send a reflex message to the brain, which then interprets the signal. If the stimulus is determined not to be dangerous, the brain responds with an inhibitory signal that cancels the reflex, but scar tissue on the spinal cord prevents that inhibitory signal from reaching the stimulated muscles. The muscles therefore continue to contract, resulting in a spasm.

The paragraph tells us exactly what *causes* spasms in paralysed muscles.

Subject: spasms in paralysed muscles

Main idea: spasms in paralysed muscles are caused by blocked inhibitory signals

The second thing to remember about the main idea is that it encompasses the whole passage. That is, it serves as a kind of "umbrella" under which all of the other ideas in the passage fit. Notice how every sentence in the muscle spasm paragraph falls under the umbrella of the main idea; it directly supports that idea, offering specific facts and details to explain the physiology of muscle spasms.

Incorrect answer choices in main idea questions will often be too narrow, focusing on a specific fact or detail, or overly broad, casting too wide a net over the text.

Too narrow: scar tissue blocks inhibitory signals from the brain (focuses only on the blockage)

Too broad: spinal cord injuries prevent effective communication between nerve cells and the brain (includes all kinds of spinal cord communication issues)

Answer choices that are too specific to be a main idea are often supporting ideas from the passage. Supporting ideas can often be distinguished from main ideas by these introductory words or phrases:

for example	in particular
for instance	specifically
furthermore	such as
in addition	

For example, notice how the supporting ideas are introduced in the following paragraph:

> Muscle spasms offer several benefits to those with spinal cord injuries. An increase in spasms, **for example**, often indicates a problem that people with paralysis would otherwise not be able to sense, **such as** the onset of a urinary tract infection. **In addition**, spasms help maintain circulation as well as muscle size and bone strength.

Each one of these supporting ideas can be eliminated in your search for the main idea, because they are too specific to serve as an umbrella for the whole paragraph.

Topic sentences.

Sometimes the main idea is clearly expressed in a topic sentence. The first sentence in the paragraph above – *Muscle spasms offer several benefits to those with spinal cord injuries* – is a topic sentence, stating the main idea that is supported by the rest of the paragraph.

Like the conclusion in an argument, the topic sentence can be anywhere – at the beginning, in the middle, or at the end. Often, writers will begin with a topic sentence and then follow it with several sentences providing support for that idea. Or writers may lead with their supporting ideas and build up to the main idea. On occasion, a topic sentence can even be found in the middle of the paragraph.

<u>Muscle spasms offer several benefits to those with spinal cord injuries</u>. An increase in spasms, for example, often indicates a problem that people with paralysis would otherwise not be able to sense, such as the onset of a urinary tract infection. In addition, spasms help maintain circulation as well as muscle size and bone strength.

An increase in muscle spasms often indicates a problem that people with paralysis would otherwise not be able to sense, such as the onset of a urinary tract infection. In addition, spasms help maintain circulation as well as muscle size and bone strength. <u>Thus muscle spasms offer several benefits to those with spinal cord injuries</u>.

An increase in muscle spasms often indicates a problem that people with paralysis would otherwise not be able to sense, such as the onset of a urinary tract infection. That's one of <u>several important benefits of muscle spasms for those with spinal cord injuries</u>. Spasms also help maintain circulation as well as muscle size and bone strength.

Implied main idea.

Of course, writers don't always state the main idea so clearly. Often it is suggested or *implied*, and you have to work out the overriding idea of the passage.

That means you have to be a detective, looking for clues in word choice, tone, structure, and the facts and ideas presented. Based on all that you see, what idea might serve as an umbrella for the passage? Make sure the umbrella is the right size (not too specific or overly broad).

Practice

Read the following paragraph and then answer the question that follows.

> People who suffer from depression have lower levels of the neurotransmitter serotonin than people who are not depressed. Because vitamin B_6 is essential in the synthesis of serotonin and other neurotransmitters, researchers have been trying to determine whether B_6 supplements can alleviate the symptoms

of depression. Studies to date, however, have not proven supplementation to be effective.

Which sentence best expresses the main idea of this paragraph?

(A) People with depression should not take vitamin B_6 supplements.

(B) Vitamin B_6 supplements do not appear to alleviate symptoms of depression.

(C) Vitamin B_6 is essential for serotonin, which is deficient in people who suffer from depression.

(D) People with depression have problems with neurotransmitters.

Answer: B

This is the only sentence that can serve as an umbrella for the paragraph; it's what everything adds up to. Choice A makes an inappropriate inference; the study has determined that supplements are not effective in alleviating the symptoms of depression, but that doesn't mean that people with depression should not take vitamin B_6 supplements as they might be useful in alleviating other symptoms. The statements in choice C are correct, but they cannot serve as an umbrella for the other sentences; instead, they simply paraphrase specific facts stated in the first two sentences. The final choice, on the other hand, is overly broad; the low levels of serotonin and vitamin B_6 are just one kind of neurotransmitter problem. Choice D allows for a much wider discussion than is covered in the paragraph.

Identifying Specific Facts and Details

At least two of your reading comprehension questions are likely to ask you about specific facts or details in the text. Why the emphasis on specific facts and details? Well, one sign of a good reader is the ability to know where to look within a text for specific information and to be able to find that information quickly and accurately. You aren't expected to memorise every detail in the passage. But you are expected to know how to scan for key words and ideas and to distinguish between main ideas and their support.

Because these questions will often deal with statistics cited in the passage, you'll need to be extra careful about reading the question stem and answer choices, which will often distort or negate information from the text. Be sure you know exactly what you're looking for. For example, if you had the question:

Which of the following is NOT a benefit of muscle spasms?

You'd need to make sure you identify the item that is *not* mentioned in the passage. Be careful to stay within the framework of the text. If you have outside knowledge – for example, if you know that muscle spasms can help prevent osteoporosis – that doesn't make the answer correct if it isn't written in or implied by the passage.

Drawing Inferences

An inference is a conclusion based upon evidence. The key to drawing correct inferences from a text is to be sure your inferences are based *on evidence in the passage*. Make sure you can back up your inference with specific facts and details evidence from the text. For inference questions, there are almost always answer choices that you may know to be true based on your own experience or outside knowledge or that are logical conclusions *not* founded on information in the text. These will never be the correct answer.

For example, read the two paragraphs about muscle spasms and then answer the question that follows:

Paralysed muscles may still move regularly as a result of muscle spasms. Muscle spasms can occur whenever the skin below the level of paralysis is stimulated. The stimulated nerve cells send a reflex message to the brain, which then interprets the signal. If the stimulus is determined not to be dangerous, the brain responds with an inhibitory signal that cancels the reflex, but the scar tissue on the spinal cord prevents that inhibitory signal from reaching the stimulated muscles. The muscles therefore continue to contract, resulting in a spasm.

Muscle spasms offer several benefits to those with spinal cord injuries. An increase in spasms, for example, often indicates a problem that people with paralysis would otherwise not be able to sense, such as the onset of a urinary tract infection. In addition, spasms help maintain circulation as well as muscle size and bone strength.

Which of the following statements can we safely conclude to be accurate?

(A) Over time, spasm signals can help reduce the amount of scar tissue on the spinal cord.

(B) Occasional muscle spasms are normal even in people without spinal cord injuries.

(C) Medication to stop spasms should only be taken if spasms are severe.

(D) People with paralysis should see a doctor whenever they have increased spasms.

Choice **(A)** may be tempting because it is hopeful, but nothing in the passage indicates that spasms have any effect on the size of the scar tissue blocking communication paths in the spinal cord. Choice **(B)** may be tempting because we know it to be true; we've all had an occasional eye twitch or leg spasm. But there's nothing in the passage to bring us to this conclusion, because the passage is solely about spasms in those with paralysis. In fact, if anything, the passage would lead us to the opposite inference, since people without spinal cord injuries lack the scar tissue that blocks the inhibitory signal. Choice **(D)** is also tempting, but it is a distortion. The passage tells us that spasms often indicate a problem, but an increase in spasms doesn't necessarily mean there is a problem; it could simply mean that the paralysed area is being overstimulated. Thus it is not a fully logical conclusion. Only choice **(C)** presents a logical inference based on the passage. The second paragraph tells us the numerous benefits of muscle spasms. Therefore, it is safe to assume that spasms should only be minimised if they are severe.

TOP 5 READING COMPREHENSION STRATEGIES

Whatever the question type, use these five strategies to earn your best score on this part of the exam.

Strategy 1—Map the Text

The single most beneficial strategy is to map the passage as you read.

When you create a text map, you create a guide that you can use to find the specific information you'll need to answer the questions that follow. Mapping the text also improves comprehension because it forces you to pay greater attention to the text as you read and synthesise the main idea of each paragraph as you move through the passage.

To create your text map, *briefly* note the main idea or topic of each paragraph, either in the margins or on a separate piece of paper. Do *not* include details; your map should consist only of key words and ideas. You don't have time to go into detail, and there's no need – the map will serve as your guide for finding any details you'll need later (why write details for all seven paragraphs when the questions will only ask about details in paragraphs two and five?). Don't bother writing complete sentences, either; a few words will do to give you the gist of the paragraph. Here's an example:

> Muscle spasms offer several benefits to those with spinal cord injuries. An increase in spasms, for example, often indicates a problem that people with paralysis would otherwise not be able to sense, such as the onset of a urinary tract infection. In addition, spasms help maintain circulation as well as muscle size and bone strength.

Now you try. Here's a test-length passage. Read it actively and map it as you go. We've done the first paragraph for you as an example.

Juvenile Rheumatoid Arthritis

One in three Americans is affected by arthritis, and most cases are chronic. There are more than 100 different types of arthritis and related conditions. The causes of most types are unknown, and while some treatments are effective in alleviating symptoms, lack of understanding of the origins of the disease has thus far prevented the development of more effective diagnosis, treatments, and preventative measures.

benefits of spasms

According to the Arthritis Foundation, approximately 285,000 children in the United States have arthritis. The most common form of arthritis in children is juvenile rheumatoid arthritis (JRA). The Cincinnati Children's Medical Centre is currently sponsoring a multi-year study involving over 250 children in six hospitals to try to determine the causes of JRA. The study will use multiple blood samples and patient surveys to determine whether there is a genetic factor that causes JRA to express in some children and not others or whether JRA is caused by extra-genetic factors such as diet, viral infections or environment.

many kinds, causes unknown

Understanding any form of arthritis requires an understanding of joint structure. Joints are lined with a tissue called synovium, which secretes a lubricant that helps the joint move smoothly and easily (synovial fluid). The spongy cartilage at the end of bones works as a shock absorber to prevent bones from rubbing together. Joints are supported by surrounding muscles and tendons. Different types of arthritis can affect different parts of the joint and can change the shape or alignment of the joint.

Osteoarthritis (OA), also called degenerative arthritis, is the most common type of arthritis and involves the breakdown of cartilage and bone. The most commonly affected areas include fingers and the weight-bearing joints (knees, feet, hips, back). Onset is typically after age 45.

With rheumatoid arthritis (RA), on the other hand, an abnormality in the body's immune system causes inflammation of the joint, beginning in the synovium and sometimes damaging cartilage and bone. Joints are often affected equally on both sides of the body. Most commonly affected areas are hands, wrists, feet, knees, ankles, shoulders, neck, jaw and elbows. RA affects women more than men.

There are three types of juvenile rheumatoid arthritis: polyarticular JRA, pauciarticular JRA, and systemic onset JRA. Polyarticular JRA affects five or more joints and affects girls more frequently than boys. If onset of the disease occurs in teenagers, the symptoms may more closely resemble adult rheumatoid arthritis. The small joints of fingers and hands are most often affected, although the weight-bearing joints can also be affected, and joints are often symptomatic on both sides of the body. Symptoms include a low-grade fever; a positive blood test for rheumatoid factor (RF); rheumatoid nodules, most commonly on the elbow; and anaemia. Damage to the affected joints is possible.

Pauciarticular JRA affects four or fewer joints and favours the large joints, especially the knees, ankles, and elbows. Unlike polyarticular JRA, pauciarticular JRA will often affect a particular joint only on one side of the body. Children with pauciarticular JRA have the highest risk of developing *uveitis*, chronic inflammation of the eye. Young girls with pauciarticular JRA and antinuclear antibodies (ANA) in the blood are particularly at risk. There are often no symptoms of uveitis until severe damage to the eye has already occurred, so children with pauciarticular JRA should be seen by an ophthalmologist at regular intervals, even when the arthritis is in remission. In most cases, pauciarticular JRA is not chronic; most children with the disease will stop experiencing symptoms by their teenage years. Because the disease is limited to fewer joints, it's also the most manageable form of JRA while patients are symptomatic.

The least common and most debilitating form of JRA is systemic onset JRA. This disease affects the entire body and may affect internal organs as well as joints. Symptoms of this form include high spiking fevers (103°F) that may last for weeks or even months, a rash of pale red spots on the chest and thighs (and occasionally other parts of the body) and joint inflammation. The rash and joint inflammation may accompany the fever but may be intermittent and/or appear weeks later. Less common symptoms of systemic onset JRA include inflammation of the outer lining of the heart or lungs, inflammation of the heart or lungs themselves, anaemia, and enlarged lymph nodes, liver or spleen. While the systemic symptoms of the disease usually resolve, the arthritis itself will usually be chronic.

Diagnosis of JRA is a multi-step process of elimination as many other diseases must first be ruled out. To make a diagnosis, a complete health history to determine the length and character of the existing symptoms is required along with a physical examination of any joint inflammation, rashes, nodules or eye problems that may suggest JRA. Laboratory tests for suspected cases of JRA include erythrocyte sedimentation (sed) rate, antinuclear antibody test (ANA), rheumatoid factor test (RF), HLA-B27 typing, complete blood count (CBC) and urinalysis. In addition, paediatricians should order X-rays of the affected joints to check for evidence of joint damage.

Here's how we mapped the passage. Your map may be worded differently, but your notes for each paragraph should capture the same key concepts with similar brevity.

P1: many kinds, causes unknown

P2: JRA most common in kids; study 4 genetic cause

P3: joint structure

P4: osteoarthritis

P5: rheumatoid arthritis

P6: polyarticular jra – many joints

P7: pauciarticular jra – few joints, uveitis, not chronic

P8: systemic jra – internal organs

P9: multi-step diagnosis

Notice how brief the mapping notes are and how they capture the main topics covered in each paragraph. The only ones that have some detail are paragraphs 6, 7 and 8 so that you don't have to re-read those paragraphs to remember the key differences between the three types of JRA. That's all you need to go back to the passage and find the specific information and details you need for each question.

Strategy 2—Keep Moving

Time is of the essence, so you must read efficiently – and that means you must read for main ideas, not details. Once you've gleaned the main idea of a paragraph and noted it on your map, move on. Don't get bogged down trying to remember specific details. This may sound contradictory since most of your questions will be about specific facts and details, but it's not. After all, you'll only be asked about two or three specific things – so it's a waste of time and energy to try to remember them all. If you create a map as you go, you'll be able to quickly find the information you need once you know exactly *what* information you need.

Strategy 3—Read Question Stems Carefully

Time is of the essence, but if you read question stems too quickly, you're liable to make costly errors. Use key words from the question stems to find out exactly what sort of answer you need. Are you looking for a specific fact or detail? Do you need to summarise the main idea? Are you being asked to draw a conclusion?

For example, if a question asks:

Which of the following is NOT used in the diagnosis of JRA?

The key word diagnosis should send you immediately to the last paragraph, where you can find the specific details about diagnosing JRA. The key word *not* also tells you to look for the answer choice that is not stated in the paragraph.

Distractors may seduce you by using exact words or phrases from the text. But if you read the answer choices carefully, you'll often find that they distort the original idea or do not directly answer the question being asked.

Strategy 4—Predict the Answer

Whenever the question allows, predict the answer to the question before you look at the answer choices. This way you're not as likely to get misled by distractors. Use your map to locate the part of the text that should contain your answer. Once you've made your prediction, read the answer choices and choose the one that best matches your prediction.

Some question stems won't allow you to predict an answer without reading the choices. For example, for the common stem *Which of the following statements can we safely conclude to be accurate?*, there's no getting around it: you simply must read each answer choice and determine whether it is accurate or not, based on the information in the passage.

Strategy 5—Read Answer Choices Carefully

Finally, read each answer choice carefully. Remember that distractors are designed to trick you. Some will seem correct because they use exact words or phrases from the text, but on a closer look, you may see that the idea has been distorted or negated. For example, the underlined words in the following answer choice come straight from the passage about benefits of spasms:

> Over time, spasm signals can help reduce the amount of <u>scar tissue on the spinal cord.</u>

The use of the exact words from the text gives the answer choice false authority; it seems right because of the repetition, but the first part of the sentence renders it false. If you skim over the answer choices, however, those familiar words may be enough to lead you to the wrong answer choice.

Don't forget the power of elimination. Narrow down the pool of possible answer choices by eliminating the ones you're sure are incorrect.

REVIEW QUESTIONS

Ready to practise? Here are two passages and eight questions like those you'll see on the BMAT. The first is the passage you've already read about JRA. Read it again and create another map – see how quickly you can do it this time. Then answer the questions that follow. Do the same for the next passage, then check your answers against ours at the end of the chapter.

Juvenile Rheumatoid Arthritis

One in three Americans is affected by arthritis, and most cases are chronic. There are more than 100 different types of arthritis and related conditions. The causes of most types are unknown, and while some treatments are effective in alleviating symptoms, lack of understanding of the origins of the disease has thus far prevented the development of more effective diagnosis, treatments and preventative measures.

According to the Arthritis Foundation, approximately 285,000 children in the United States have arthritis. The most common form of arthritis in children is juvenile rheumatoid arthritis (JRA). The Cincinnati Children's Medical Center is currently sponsoring a multi-year study involving over 250 children in six hospitals to try to determine the causes of JRA. The study will use multiple blood samples and patient surveys to determine whether there is a genetic factor that causes JRA to express in some children and not others or whether JRA is caused by extra-genetic factors such as diet, viral infections or environment.

Understanding any form of arthritis requires an understanding of joint structure. Joints are lined with a tissue called synovium, which secretes a lubricant that helps the joint move smoothly and easily (synovial fluid). The spongy cartilage at the end of bones work as a shock absorber to prevent bones from rubbing together. Joints are supported by surrounding muscles and tendons. Different types of arthritis can affect different parts of the joint and can change the shape or alignment of the joint.

Osteoarthritis (OA), also called degenerative arthritis, is the most common type of arthritis and involves the breakdown of cartilage and bone. The most commonly affected areas include fingers and the weight-bearing joints (knees, feet, hips, back). Onset is typically after age 45.

With rheumatoid arthritis (RA), on the other hand, an abnormality in the body's immune system causes inflammation of the joint, beginning in the synovium and sometimes damaging cartilage and bone. Joints are often affected equally on both sides of the body. Most commonly affected areas are hands, wrists, feet, knees, ankles, shoulders, neck, jaw and elbows. RA affects women more than men.

There are three types of juvenile rheumatoid arthritis: polyarticular JRA, pauciarticular JRA, and systemic onset JRA. Polyarticular JRA affects five or more joints and affects girls more frequently than boys. If onset of the disease occurs in teenagers, the symptoms may more closely resemble adult rheumatoid arthritis. The small joints of fingers and hands are most often affected, although the weight-bearing joints can also be affected, and joints are often symptomatic on both sides of the body. Symptoms include a low-grade fever; a positive blood test for rheumatoid factor (RF); rheumatoid nodules, most commonly on the elbow; and anaemia. Damage to the affected joints is possible.

Pauciarticular JRA affects four or fewer joints and favours the large joints, especially the knees, ankles, and elbows. Unlike polyarticular JRA, pauciarticular JRA will often affect a particular joint only on one side of the body. Children with pauciarticular JRA have the highest risk of developing uveitis, chronic inflammation of the eye. Young girls with pauciarticular JRA and antinuclear antibodies (ANA) in the blood are particularly at risk. There are often no symptoms of uveitis until severe damage to the eye has already occurred, so children with pauciarticular JRA should be seen by an ophthalmologist at regular intervals, even when the arthritis is in remission. In most cases, pauciarticular JRA is not chronic; most children with the disease will stop experiencing symptoms by their teenage years. Because the disease is limited to fewer joints, it's also the most manageable form of JRA while patients are symptomatic.

The least common and most debilitating form of JRA is systemic onset JRA. This disease affects the entire body and may affect internal organs as well as joints. Symptoms of this form include high spiking fevers (103°F) that may last for weeks or even months, a rash of pale red spots on the chest and thighs (and occasionally other parts of the body) and joint inflammation. The rash and joint inflammation may accompany the fever but may be intermittent and/or appear weeks later. Less common symptoms of systemic onset JRA include inflammation of the outer lining of the heart or lungs, inflammation of the heart or lungs themselves, anaemia, and enlarged lymph nodes, liver or spleen. While the systemic symptoms of the disease usually resolve, the arthritis itself will usually be chronic.

Diagnosis of JRA is a multi-step process of elimination as many other diseases must first be ruled out. To make a diagnosis, a complete health history to determine the length and character of the existing symptoms is required along with a physical examination of any joint inflammation, rashes, nodules or eye problems that may suggest JRA. Laboratory tests for suspected cases of JRA include erythrocyte sedimentation (sed) rate, antinuclear antibody test (ANA), rheumatoid factor test (RF), HLA-B27 typing, complete blood count (CBC) and urinalysis. In addition, paediatricians should order X-rays of the affected joints to check for evidence of joint damage.

1. Which of the following statements may we safely conclude to be accurate?

   (A) All forms of JRA are likely to have the same cause.

   (B) Researchers believe certain genetic factors may predispose children to JRA.

   (C) Once the causes of JRA are identified, researchers will develop a blood test to diagnose the disease.

   (D) Arthritis in children is far more common than most people realise.

2. Which of the following best summarises the main difference between osteoarthritis (OA) and rheumatoid arthritis (RA)?

   (A) OA affects the joints while RA affects the immune system.

   (B) OA affects the elderly while RA affects children and teens.

   (C) OA involves the deterioration of joints while RA involves inflammation of joints.

   (D) OA is easier to diagnose than RA.

3. Most children with pauciarticular JRA can be expected to:

   (A) suffer from uveitis

   (B) fully recover from the disease

   (C) experience symptoms periodically throughout their lifetime

   (D) have antinuclear antibodies in the blood

4. All of the following are true of uveitis EXCEPT:

   (A) It is most likely to afflict children with pauciarticular JRA.

   (B) It may damage the eye without any visible symptoms.

   (C) It can be active in patients even when other arthritis symptoms are in remission.

   (D) It is more likely to afflict boys than girls.

5. Based on the article, it is reasonable to conclude that:

   (A) children in early stages of JRA may be misdiagnosed with other ailments

   (B) doctors need to be more educated about treatment options for patients with JRA

   (C) early eye problems may predispose children to pauciarticular JRA

   (D) blood tests for suspected cases of JRA are sometimes cost-prohibitive

Does Acupuncture Work? Scientific Evidence Is Mounting

While Eastern medicine has long touted the benefits of acupuncture, Western medicine has long been sceptical of its efficacy in treating the wide range of ailments acupuncture has traditionally been used to address. But recent research is showing those sceptics hard scientific evidence that acupuncture works. More importantly, research is beginning to reveal exactly how this ancient practice helps heal the body.

One of the oldest medicinal traditions, acupuncture has been practiced in China for over 2,500 years. In acupuncture, very fine needles – as thin as a human hair – are inserted into the skin at precise locations and secured with gentle twisting or pumping movements. During a typical 20-40 minute treatment, the patient usually relaxes on a table, often under a heat lamp, with soft music playing in the background.

The location of the needles depends upon the ailment(s) being treated. One patient may have needles from forehead to feet while in another the needles may be concentrated in the hands and torso. There are 401 acupoints on the body which run along the *Qi* meridians. The Chinese believe that Qi is the body's energy force, and when its flow is disrupted, pain or illness results. Acupuncture is believed to restore balance to the flow of the Qi by reopening blocked pathways and redirecting disturbed energy.

The hundreds of thousands of Americans who have undergone acupuncture treatments know that it works, but until recently, there has been no hard scientific evidence of acupuncture's efficacy. But a 1999 study conducted by scientists at the University of Medicine and Dentistry of New Jersey (UMDNJ) used brain imaging to prove that acupuncture *does* work to relieve pain. The researchers compared brain images of 12 people experiencing pain with images taken after receiving an acupuncture treatment. Following the treatment, researchers found, the images showed 60-70% less experience of pain in the brain.[1] Similarly, a 2004 study by the National Institutes of Health, published in the *Annals of Internal Medicine*, concluded that acupuncture reduced pain by 40% and generated a 40% improvement in knee function for arthritis patients.[2] By 14 weeks into the study, the patients receiving real acupuncture reported a sharp drop in pain in comparison with patients receiving sham acupuncture (where patients cannot determine whether or not the acupuncture needles are actually inserted).

In another study, researchers at the Vermont College of Medicine examined the acupuncture technique of manipulating the needles once they have been inserted into the skin. Published in the *Journal of Applied Physiology* in 2002, the study found that twisting the needle causes a kind of "ripple effect" along the Qi pathway. The volunteers in the study were needled on eight acupuncture points on one side of the body and on the other side in areas not along the Qi meridians. When the computerised needles were twisted in the same direction, they were 167% harder to pull out than if not twisted; needles twisted back and forth were 52% harder to pull out.[3] Researchers also found that it was significantly harder to remove the needles placed in acupoints than those that were not placed along the meridian. The explanation? The researchers believe the tiny needles actually wind up tiny strands of the connective tissue found in the space between muscles and in nerve bundles, where typical acupoints lie.[3]

While this study may not prove anything, it does begin to help researchers understand what happens physiologically during an acupuncture treatment. And that can help Eastern and Western doctors alike become more effective practitioners.

Sources:

[1] "Brain imaging suggests acupuncture works, study says". *CNN.com*. 1 December, 1999. http://archives.cnn.com/1999/HEALTH/12/01/brain.acupuncture.

[2] "Acupuncture 'works for arthritis.'" *BBC News*, UK edition. 21 December, 2004. http://news.bbc.co.uk/1/hi/health/4111047.stm.

[3] Denoon, Daniel. "Why Acupuncture Works", *WebMD.com*. 11 January, 2002. http://www.webmd.com/content/article/17/1668_51359.

6. Acupuncture needles are placed along Qi meridians because:

   (A) that's where muscles are most tense

   (B) it is where muscle and nerve bundles meet

   (C) it makes the needles harder to pull out

   (D) they are believed to be the main pathways of the body's energy

7. The author's main goal in this article is to:

   (A) convince readers to try acupuncture

   (B) explain what is known about the biomechanics of acupuncture

   (C) point out key differences in Eastern and Western medical practices

   (D) urge more scientific studies of acupuncture

8. Which of the following statements can we safely conclude to be accurate?

   (A) acupuncture works primarily because patients *believe* it works, not because of any physiological changes the needles create in the body

   (B) the efficacy of acupuncture is scientifically unprovable

   (C) acupuncture works on a fundamental biomechanical level in the body

   (D) Eastern medicine is more effective than Western medicine

Answers and Explanations

1. B

Though the three types of JRA are forms of rheumatoid arthritis affecting children, the symptoms and severity of the three types vary greatly. Researchers are hoping to find a genetic trigger for the disease, but that doesn't mean it would be the same for all types of JRA. Because the passage emphasises the lack of understanding of the causes of arthritis, and because there is no specific indication that researchers suspect the same cause for all types of JRA, choice A is not a logical inference. Choice **(B)**, however, is an accurate statement. The passage states that researchers are trying to "determine whether there is a genetic factor that causes JRA to express in some children and not others"; choice **(B)** essentially paraphrases this statement. Choice **(C)** may be tempting because the opening paragraph states that not knowing the causes of arthritis has "prevented the development of more effective diagnosis, treatments and preventative measures" and the last paragraph lists a series of blood tests used to confirm a JRA diagnosis. But that doesn't mean that once the cause (or causes) of JRA are found, a blood test will be developed to diagnose the disease. Researchers may find other, more effective techniques for diagnosis. Choice D may be true – in fact, you may have had no idea that children even get arthritis. But that doesn't make it a logical inference *based on the passage*. Nowhere does the text discuss the general public's knowledge of arthritis in children.

2. C

If you created a good map, you should be able to go directly to paragraphs 4 and 5 to find the answer to this specific fact/detail question. OA "involves the breakdown of cartilage and bone" while RA "causes inflammation of the joint". Thus **(C)** is the correct answer. Choice **(A)** seems reasonable because it points out that RA affects the immune system, but it also suggests that only OA affects the joints – an effective distractor. Both OA and RA, however, affect the joints, just in different ways, so **(A)** is incorrect. JRA affects children and teens; OA and RA both affect adults, so **(B)** is incorrect. (Note how this distractor attempts to distort the issue of age.) And while we know that JRA can be difficult to diagnose, there is no indication in the passage of whether OA is more difficult to diagnose than RA.

3. B

While children with pauciarticular JRA are more likely to suffer from uveitis than children with other forms of JRA, that doesn't mean that most children with pauciarticular JRA will *get* uveitis; they simply have "the highest risk" of developing the disease. Thus choice **(A)** is incorrect. Paragraph 7 tells us that "in most cases, pauciarticular JRA is not chronic". That means B is correct; most children with pauciarticular JRA will fully recover. It also means that **(C)** is incorrect, for if it is not chronic, they will not experience symptoms throughout their lifetime. Choice **(D)** may be tempting, because the paragraph mentions patients having antinuclear antibodies in the blood. But take a closer look: the passage tells us that young girls with ANA are at greatest risk for developing uveitis. That means that not all children with pauciarticular JRA have ANA in their blood.

4. D

Once again, the question and your map should send you to paragraph 7, the only paragraph that discusses uveitis. The paragraph states that young girls with ANA in the blood "are particularly at risk", which indicates that girls are more likely to develop uveitis than boys. Thus **(D)** is the correct answer. Choices **(A)**, **(B)** and **(C)** state true facts about uveitis mentioned in the paragraph.

5. A

The last paragraph describes the lengthy process of diagnosing JRA. It is therefore reasonable to assume that JRA may be misdiagnosed at first (A), since "many other diseases must first be ruled out". The passage does not discuss treatment of JRA, so no assumption about doctors' knowledge of treatments (B) is reasonable. Choice **(C)** is an interesting distractor because it reverses the truth; children with pauciarticular JRA are predisposed to eye problems, not the other way around. Finally, blood tests *may* be costly, but there is no evidence of this in the passage, and without that knowledge we certainly can't conclude that they are cost-prohibitive, so **(D)** is incorrect.

6. D

The distractors here may be particularly tricky, so careful reading is even more important. The third paragraph tells us that acupoints "run along the Qi meridians", that Qi "is the body's energy force", and that acupuncture "restore[s] balance to the flow of the Qi by reopening blocked pathways and redirecting disturbed energy". Thus **(D)** is correct. There's no discussion of the level of tension of muscles in the body, so choice **(A)** is incorrect. The study discussed in paragraph 5 states that acupoints typically lie "in the space between muscles and in nerve bundles", but that doesn't explain why needles are placed along the meridians, so choice **(B)** is incorrect. The same paragraph tells us that needles were harder to pull out when they were placed along the meridian, but there's no indication in the article that making needles harder to pull out is desirable and would thus be a reason to place them on the meridians; it only states the fact that they *were* harder to pull out, so **(C)** is also incorrect.

7. B

While readers may be convinced to try acupuncture after reading this article (A), that's clearly not the main goal of the text. If it were, the author would spend most of the time highlighting the benefits of the practice. Instead, the focus is on what has been learned about the biomechanics of acupuncture: what is scientifically known about how it works in the body. Thus **(B)** is correct. While acupuncture is an ancient Chinese practice, there is no comparison of Eastern and Western medical practices, so **(C)** is incorrect. Finally, the author does not anywhere encourage the further study of acupuncture, so **(D)** is likewise incorrect.

8. C

Choices **(A)** and **(B)** directly contradict the passage, which cites two scientific studies that show evidence of the physiological changes that occur during acupuncture treatments. True, the studies are limited, and there may be a psychological factor at work in some patients, but neither of these negate the fact that the studies have been conducted and have had significant and tangible results. Choice **(D)** is a dangerous conclusion since the passage only discusses one practice of Eastern medicine and does not make any direct comparisons to any form of Western medicine. Only **(C)** is a logical assumption that is supported by the findings in the two studies discussed in the passage.

PART IV

Essential Biology Review

Chapter 7: **Cell Activity**

This chapter covers the major topics relating to cell activity, including how molecules move into and out of the cell membrane, cell division and the cell cycle. Practice questions at the end of the chapter will test your knowledge of these topics.

CELL THEORY

The role of the cell in modern biology is so inherent in the way we view life that is easy to overlook its importance. Cells were unknown until the development of the microscope in the seventeenth century allowed scientists to see cells for the first time. Matthias Schleiden and Theodor Schwann proposed that all life was composed of cells in 1838, while Rudolph Virchow proposed in 1855 that cells arise only from other cells. The **cell theory** based on these ideas unifies all biology at the cellular level and may be summarized as follows:

- All living things are composed of cells.
- All chemical reactions of life occur in cells or in association with cells.
- Cells arise only from pre-existing cells.
- Cells carry genetic information in the form of DNA. This genetic material is passed from parent cell to daughter cell.

PLASMA MEMBRANE

The **plasma membrane** is an important component of cellular structure. The plasma membrane (also called the **cell membrane**) encloses the cell and exhibits **selective permeability**; it regulates the passage of materials into and out of the cell. To carry out the biochemical activities of life, life must retain some molecules inside the cell and keep other material out of the cell. This is what the selective permeability of the membrane provides.

How does the membrane create selective permeability, restricting the flow of material into and out of the cell? The lipid membrane itself is one factor responsible for the control of material into and out of the cell, in addition to proteins in the membrane. With the membrane itself, the hydrophobic interior of the membrane prevents charged or very polar molecules from diffusing across the membrane, although noncharged small molecules such as water, oxygen and carbon dioxide diffuse freely through the membrane. The proteins within the membrane also allow material to pass in and out of the cell. Cell membrane proteins contain both ion channels that act as selective pores for ions and receptors that bind signalling molecules outside of the cell and send signals into the cell. They also carry out the functions of cell adhesion and nutrient transport.

MEMBRANE TRANSPORT ACROSS THE PLASMA

It is crucial for a cell to control what enters and exits it. In order to preserve this control, cells have developed the mechanisms described here.

Permeability-Diffusion Through the Membrane

Traffic through the membrane is extensive, but the membrane is selectively permeable; substances do not cross its barrier indiscriminately. A cell is able to retain many small molecules and exclude others. The sum total of movement across the membrane is determined by **passive diffusion** of material directly through the membrane and selective transport processes through the membrane that require proteins.

Diffusion/Passive Transport

Diffusion is the net movement of dissolved particles down their concentration gradients, from a region of higher concentration to a region of lower concentration. **Passive diffusion** does not require proteins since it occurs directly through the membrane. Since molecules are moving down a concentration gradient, no external energy is required.

Facilitated Diffusion

The net movement of dissolved particles down their concentration gradient—with the help of carrier proteins in the membrane—is known as **facilitated diffusion**. This process does not require energy. Ion channels are one example of membrane proteins involved in facilitated diffusion, in which the channel creates a passage for ions to flow through the membrane down their concentration gradient. These ions will not flow through the membrane on their own. Some ion channels are always open for ions to flow through them, while other ion channels open only in response to some stimulus, such as a change in the voltage across the membrane or the presence of a molecule like a neurotransmitter that opens the channel.

Active Transport

Active transport is the net movement of dissolved particles against their concentration gradient with the help of transport proteins. This process requires energy, and is necessary to maintain membrane potentials in specialized cells such as neurons. The most common forms of energy to drive active transport are ATP or a concentration gradient of another molecule. Active transport is used for the uptake of nutrients against a gradient.

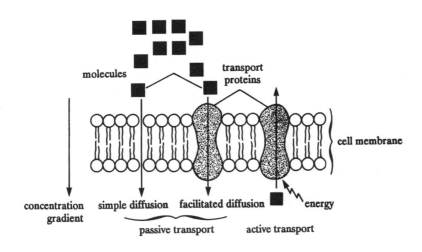

MOVEMENT ACROSS MEMBRANES

Osmosis

Osmosis is the simple diffusion of water from a region of lower solute concentration to a region of higher solute concentration. Water flows to equalize the solute concentrations. If a membrane is impermeable to a particular solute, then water will flow across the membrane until the differences in the solute concentration have been equilibrated. Differences in the concentration of substances to which the membrane is impermeable affect the direction of osmosis.

Water diffuses freely across the plasma membrane. When the cytoplasm of the cell has a lower solute concentration than the extracellular medium, the medium is said to be **hypertonic** to the cell; water will flow out, causing the cell to shrink. On the other hand, when the cytoplasm of a cell has a higher solute concentration than the extracellular medium, the medium is **hypotonic** to the cell, and water will flow in, causing the cell to swell. If too much water flows in, the cell may lyse. Red blood cells, for example, lyse when put into distilled water. Finally, when solute concentrations are equal inside and outside, the cell and the medium are said to be **isotonic**. There is no net flow of water in either direction.

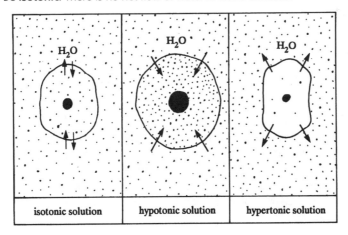

OSMOSIS

CELL DIVISION

Cell division is the process by which a cell doubles its organelles and cytoplasm, replicates its DNA, and then divides in two. For unicellular organisms, cell division is a means of reproduction, while for multicellular organisms it is a method of growth, development and replacement of worn-out cells.

THE CELL CYCLE

The four stages of the cell cycle are designated as **G1**, **S**, **G2**, and **M**. The first three stages of the cell cycle are **interphase** stages, that is, they occur between cell divisions. The fourth stage, **mitosis**, includes the actual cell division.

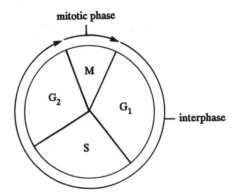

Interphase

This is by far the longest part of the cell cycle. A cell normally spends at least 90 percent of the cycle in interphase.

G_1 stage (Presynthetic Gap)

This stage is one of intense biochemical activity and growth. The cell doubles in size and new organelles such as mitochondria, ribosomes, endoplasmic reticulum and centrioles are produced. A typical cell proceeds through the G_1 stage, passing a **restriction point**, after which it is committed to continue through the rest of the cell cycle and divide. However, some cells, including specialized skeletal muscle cells and nerve cells, never pass this point, instead entering a nondividing phase sometimes referred to as **G_0**.

S stage (Synthesis)

In the synthetic stage each chromosome is replicated so that during division, a complete copy of the genome can be distributed to both daughter cells. After replication, the chromosomes consist of two identical **sister chromatids** held together at a central region called the **centromere**. The ends of the chromosome are called the **telomeres**. Note that after DNA replication, the cell still contains the diploid number (2N) of chromosomes, but since each chromosome now consists of two chromatids, cells entering G_2 actually contain twice as much DNA as cells in G_1.

G₂ — rendered as: G_2 *stage (Postsynthetic Gap)*

G_2 *stage (Postsynthetic Gap)*

The cell continues to grow in size, while assembly of new organelles and other cell structures continues.

M Stage (Mitotic Stage)

This stage consists of mitosis and **cytokinesis**. Mitosis is the division and distribution of the cell's DNA to its two daughter cells such that each cell receives a complete copy of the original genome. Cytokinesis refers to the division of cytoplasm that follows.

MITOSIS AND ASEXUAL REPRODUCTION

Asexual reproduction is any method of producing new organisms in which fusion of nuclei from two individuals (fertilization) does not take place. The fusion of nuclei from two parent individuals to create a new individual is **sexual reproduction**. In **asexual reproduction**, only one parent organism is involved. The new organisms produced through asexual reproduction form daughter cells through mitotic cell division and are genetically identical, clones of their parents. Asexual reproduction serves primarily as a mechanism for perpetuating primitive organisms and plants, especially in times of low population density. Asexual reproduction can allow more rapid population growth than sexual reproduction, but does not create the great genetic diversity that sexual reproduction does.

Four Stages of Mitosis

Mitosis is the division and distribution of the cell's DNA to its two daughter cells. The daughter cells are an exact replica of the original parent cell. Although mitosis is a continuous process, four stages are discernible: **prophase, metaphase, anaphase,** and **telophase**.

Prophase

The chromosomes condense, the centriole pairs separate and move toward opposite poles of the cell, and the spindle apparatus forms between them. The nuclear membrane dissolves, allowing spindle fibres to enter the nucleus, while the nucleoli become less distinct or disappear. Kinetochores, with attached kinetochore fibres, appear at the chromosome centromere.

Metaphase

The centriole pairs are now at opposite poles of the cell. The kinetochore fibres interact with the fibres of the spindle apparatus to align the chromosomes at the **metaphase plate** (equatorial plate), which is equidistant to the two poles of the spindle fibres.

Anaphase

The centromeres now split, so that each chromatid has its own distinct centromere, thus allowing the sister chromatids to separate. The telomeres are the last part of the chromatids to separate. The sister chromatids are pulled toward the opposite poles of the cell by the shortening of the kinetochore fibres.

Telophase

The spindle apparatus disappears. A nuclear membrane forms around each set of chromosomes and the nucleoli reappear. The chromosomes uncoil, resuming their interphase form. Each of the two new nuclei has received a complete copy of the genome identical to the original genome and to each other. Cytokinesis occurs.

See the following figure for a summary of mitosis.

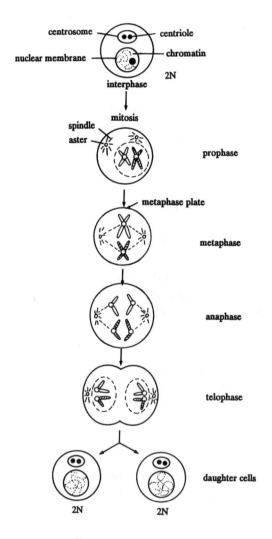

SEXUAL REPRODUCTION

Most multicellular animals and plants reproduce sexually, as do as many protists and fungi. **Sexual reproduction** involves the union of a **haploid cell** from two different parents to produce diploid offspring. These haploid cells are the **gametes**, sex cells produced through mitosis in males and females. Gametes have a single copy of the genome (one of each chromosome), and diploid cells have two copies of the genome (two of each chromosome). In humans, all of the cells of the body are diploid, with the exception of the gametes. When the male gamete (the sperm) and the female gamete (the egg) join, a **zygote** is formed that develops into a new organism genetically distinct from both its parents. The zygote is the diploid single cell offspring formed from the union of gametes.

MORE ABOUT THE HUMAN REPRODUCTIVE SYSTEM ————————

Although some topics of sexual reproduction are reviewed here, Chapter 8, Human Biology and Anatomy includes additional information on the human reproductive system.

Sexual reproduction ensures genetic diversity and variability in offspring. Since sexual reproduction is more costly in energy than asexual reproduction, the reason for its overwhelming prevalence must be that genetic diversity is worth the effort. Sexual reproduction does not create new alleles, though. Only mutation can do that. Sexual reproduction increases diversity in a population by creating new combinations of alleles in offspring and therefore new combinations of traits. Genetic diversity is not an advantage to an individual, but allows a population of organisms to adapt and to survive in the face of a dynamic and unpredictable environment.

The diversity created by sexual reproduction occurs in part during meiotic gamete production and in part through the random matching of gametes to make unique individuals. The range of mechanisms involved in sexual reproduction in animals, including humans, are detailed here.

Gamete Formation

Specialized organs called gonads produce gametes through meiotic cell division. Male gonads, **testes**, produce male gametes, **spermatozoa**, while female gonads, **ovaries**, produce **ova**. A cell that is committed to the production of gametes, although it is not itself a gamete, is called a **germ cell**. The rest of the cells of the body are called **somatic cells**. Only the genome of germ cells contributes to gametes and offspring. A mutation in a somatic cell, for example, may be harmful to that cell or the organism if it leads to cancer, but a mutation in a somatic cell will not affect offspring since the mutation will not be found in germ cell genomes. Germ cells are themselves diploid and divide to create more germ cells by mitosis, but create the haploid gametes through meiosis.

MEIOSIS

In asexual reproduction, a single diploid cell (or cells) is used to create new identical copies of an organism. In sexual reproduction, two parents contribute to the genome of the offspring and the end result is genetically unique offspring. To do this requires that each parent contributes a cell with one copy of the genome. **Meiosis** is the process whereby these sex cells are produced.

As in mitosis, the gametocyte's chromosomes are replicated during the S phase of the cell cycle. The first round of division (**meiosis I**) produces two intermediate daughter cells. The second round of division (**meiosis II**) involves the separation of the sister chromatids, resulting in four genetically distinct haploid gametes. In this way, a diploid cell produces haploid daughter cells. Since meiosis reduces the number of chromosomes in each cell from *2n* and *1n*, it is sometimes called **reductive division**.

Each meiotic division has the same four stages as mitosis, although it goes through each of them twice (except for DNA replication). The stages of meiosis are detailed in the following paragraphs.

Interphase

Gametocyte chromosomes are replicated during the S phase of the cell cycle, while the centrioles replicate at some point during interphase.

Prophase

During this stage, chromatin condenses into chromosomes, the spindle apparatus forms, and the nucleoli and nuclear membrane disappear. Homologous chromosomes (matching chromosomes that code for the same traits, one inherited from each parent) come together and intertwine in a process called **synapsis**. Since at this stage each chromosome consists of two sister chromatids, each synaptic pair of homologous chromosomes contains four chromatids, and is therefore often called a **tetrad**.

Sometimes chromatids of homologous chromosomes break at corresponding points and exchange equivalent pieces of DNA; this process is called **crossing over** or **recombination**. Note that crossing over occurs between homologous chromosomes and not between sister chromatids of the same chromosomes. The chromatids involved are left with an altered but structurally complete set of genes.

The chromosomes remain joined at points called **chiasmata** where the crossing over occurred. Such genetic recombination can "unlink" linked genes, thereby increasing the variety of genetic combinations that can be produced via gametogenesis. Recombination among chromosomes results in increased genetic diversity within a species. Note that sister chromatids are no longer identical after recombination has occurred.

Metaphase I

Homologous pairs (tetrads) align at the equatorial plane of the dividing cells, and each pair attaches to a separate spindle fibre by its kinetochore.

Anaphase I

Homologous pairs separate and are pulled to opposite poles of the cell. This process is called **disjunction**, and it accounts for a fundamental Mendelian law (see Chapter 9, Genetics and Evolution). During disjunction, each chromosome of paternal origin separates (or disjoins) from its homologue of maternal origin, and either chromosome can end up in either daughter cell. Thus, the distribution of homologous chromosomes to the two intermediate daughter cells is random with respect to parental origin. Each daughter cell will have a unique pool of alleles provided by a random mixture of maternal and paternal origin. These genes may code for alternative forms of a given trait.

Telophase I and Cytokinesis

A nuclear membrane forms around each new nucleus. At this point, each chromosome still consists of sister chromatids joined at the centromere. Next, the cell divides through cytokinesis into two daughter cells, each of which receives a nucleus containing the haploid number of chromosomes. Between cell divisions there may be a short rest period, or interkinesis, during which the chromosomes partially uncoil.

Prophase II

The centrioles migrate to opposite poles and the spindle apparatus forms.

Metaphase II

The chromosomes line up along the equatorial plane once again. The centromeres divide, separating the chromosomes into pairs of sister chromatids.

Anaphase II

The sister chromatids are pulled to opposite poles by the spindle fibres.

Telophase II

Finally, a nuclear membrane forms around each new haploid nucleus. Cytokinesis follows and two daughter cells are formed. Thus, by the time meiosis is completed, four haploid daughter cells are produced per gametocyte. In females, only one of these becomes a functional gamete.

The following diagram summarizes the various stages of meiosis I and meiosis II. Notice that the random distribution of homologous chromosomes in meiosis, coupled with crossing over in prophase I, enables an individual to produce gametes with many different genetic combinations. Every gamete gets one copy of each chromosome, but the copy of each chromosome found in a gamete is random. For example, each gamete has a chromosome #9, but this chromosome can be either of the two copies of this chromosome. With 22 autosomal chromosomes, this factor alone allows for 222 possible gametes, not including the additional genetic diversity created by recombination. This is why sexual reproduction produces genetic variability in offspring, as opposed to asexual reproduction, which produces identical offspring. The possibility of so many different genetic combinations is believed to increase the capability of a species to evolve and adapt to a changing environment.

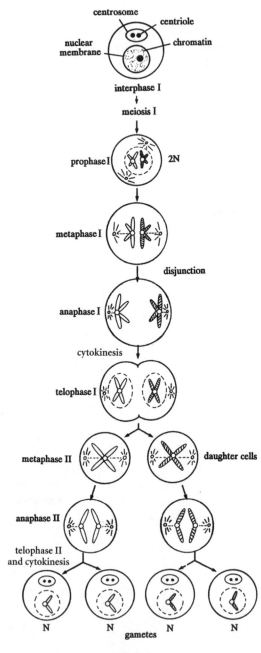

MEIOSIS

MITOSIS V. MEIOSIS

Mitosis:

- Produces diploid cells from diploid cells
- Occurs in all dividing cells
- Does not involve the pairing up of homologous chromosomes
- Does not involve crossing over (recombination)

Meiosis:

- Produces haploid cells from diploid cells
- Occurs only in sex cells (gametocytes)
- Involves the pairing up of homologous chromosomes at the metaphase plate, forming tetrads
- Involves crossing over

REVIEW QUESTIONS

1. A process that cannot take place in a haploid cell is

   (A) mitosis
   (B) meiosis
   (C) ATP production
   (D) DNA replication

2. Which statement about the plasma membrane is false?

   (A) It serves as a selectively permeable barrier to the external environment.
   (B) It serves as a mediator between the internal and external environments.
   (C) In eukaryotes, it contains the cytochrome chain of oxidative phosphorylation.
   (D) It contains phospholipids as a structural component.
   (E) It contains proteins that in some cases span the membrane.

3. Meiosis differs from mitosis in that

   I. two cell divisions take place
   II. DNA replicates during Interphase
   III. haploid cells are produced from diploid cells

   (A) I only
   (B) II only
   (C) III only
   (D) I and III
   (E) I, II, and III

Answers and Explanations

1. B

A cell that is *n* (haploid) cannot undergo meiosis to become 1/2*n*. Choices (A) and (D) are incorrect, however, because haploid organisms undergo mitosis to grow. An example of such an organism is a braconid wasp. These animals in the haploid form are males (*n*); females (2*n*) are only formed when a female mates.

2. C

The plasma membrane separates the cellular contents from the environment. It is responsible for the permeability of the membrane—in other words, for what is allowed in and out of the cell. The fluid mosaic model of the plasma membrane states that this membrane is a bilayer of phospholipids interspersed with proteins acting as receptors, pores, and channels. The pores and channels cross the entire membrane. The cytochrome chain referred to in the correct answer is actually located in the cristae (the inner membrane) of the mitochondria.

3. D

Meiosis has two divisions that create four haploid cells from one diploid cell, while mitosis results in two diploid cells from one diploid cell. Both mitosis and meiosis replicate DNA during interphase.

Chapter 8: **Human Biology and Anatomy**

Chapter 8 covers the topics of human biology and anatomy. As multicellular organisms have evolved into larger and more complex forms over time, their cells have become more removed from the external environment and more specialized toward one specific function. These specialized cells form **tissues**, cells with a common function and often a similar form. Cells from different tissues come together to form **organs**, large anatomical structures made from several tissues working together toward a common goal. Organs in turn are part of organ systems, including systems for digestion, respiration, circulation, immune reactions, excretion, reproduction, the nervous system and the endocrine system. Practice questions at the end of the chapter test your understanding and knowledge of these important systems.

MUSCULOSKELETAL SYSTEM

The musculoskeletal system forms the basic internal framework of the vertebrate body. Muscles and bones work in close coordination to produce voluntary movement. In addition, bone and muscle perform a number of other independent functions.

Skeletal System

The skeleton functions primarily in the physical support of an organism. In contrast to the external skeleton (**exoskeleton**) of arthropods, vertebrates have an internal skeleton, or **endoskeleton**. The mammalian skeleton is divided into the **axial** and **appendicular** skeletons. The axial skeleton is the basic framework of the body, consisting of the skull, the vertebral column, and the rib cage. The appendicular skeleton consists of the limb bones and the pelvic and pectoral girdles. In addition to providing the lever upon which skeletal muscles act during locomotion, the skeleton surrounds and protects delicate organs such as the brain and the spinal cord. Furthermore, skeletal bone marrow houses much of the body's blood-forming elements. The two major components of the skeleton are **cartilage** and **bone**.

Cartilage

Cartilage is a type of connective tissue that is softer and more flexible than bone. It is composed of a firm but elastic matrix called **chondrin**, which is secreted by specialized cells called **chondrocytes**. Cartilage is the principal component of embryonic skeletons in higher animals. During mammalian development, however, much of it hardens and calcifies into bone. Cartilage is retained in adults in places where firmness and flexibility are needed. For example, in humans, the external ear, the nose, the walls of the larynx and trachea, and the skeletal joints contain cartilage. Most cartilage is avascular (i.e., contains no blood or lymph vessels) and is devoid of nerves; it receives nourishment from capillaries located in nearby connective tissue and bone via diffusion through the surrounding fluid.

Bone

Bone is a specialized type of mineralized connective tissue that has the ability to withstand physical stress. Ideally designed for body support, bone tissue is hard and strong, while at the same time, somewhat elastic and lightweight.

There are two basic types of bone: **compact bone** and **spongy bone**. Compact bone is dense bone that does not appear to have any cavities when observed with the naked eye. Spongy bone, also called **cancellous bone**, is much less dense, and consists of an interconnecting lattice of bony spicules (trabeculae); the cavities in between the spicules are filled with **yellow** and/or **red bone marrow**. Yellow marrow is inactive and infiltrated by adipose tissue; red marrow is involved in blood cell formation.

The bones of the appendages are called the **long bones**.

Muscular System

Muscle tissue consists of bundles of specialized contractile fibres held together by connective tissue. There are three morphologically and functionally distinct types of muscle in mammals: **skeletal muscle**, **smooth muscle**, and **cardiac muscle**.

Skeletal Muscle

Skeletal muscle is responsible for voluntary movements and is innervated by the **somatic nervous system**. A muscle is a bundle of parallel fibres. Each fibre is a multinucleated cell created by the fusion of several mononucleate embryonic cells. The nuclei are usually found at the periphery of the cell. Embedded in the fibres are filaments called **myofibrils**, which are further divided into contractile units called **sarcomeres**.

Skeletal muscle has striations of light and dark bands, and is therefore also referred to as **striated** muscle. Skeletal muscle fibres can be characterized as either red or white. **Red fibres** (slow-twitch fibres) have a high **myoglobin** content (a protein resembling haemoglobin) and many mitochondria. They derive their energy primarily from aerobic respiration and are capable of sustained and vigorous activity. **White fibres** (fast-twitch fibres) are anaerobic and therefore contain less myoglobin and fewer mitochondria than red fibres. White fibres have a greater rate of contraction than red fibres; however, white fibres fatigue more easily.

Smooth Muscle

Smooth muscle is responsible for involuntary actions and is innervated by the **autonomic nervous system**. Smooth muscle is found in the digestive tract, bladder, uterus, and blood vessel walls, among other places. Smooth muscle cells possess one centrally located nucleus. While smooth muscle cells also contain actin and myosin filaments, these filaments lack the organization of skeletal sarcomeres; consequently, smooth muscles lack the striations of skeletal muscle.

Cardiac Muscle

The muscle tissue of the heart is composed of cardiac muscle fibres. These fibres possess characteristics of both skeletal and smooth muscle fibres. As in skeletal muscle, actin and myosin filaments are arranged in sarcomeres, giving cardiac muscle a striated appearance. However, cardiac muscle cells generally have only one or two centrally located nuclei. Cardiac muscle is innervated by the autonomic nervous system, which serves only to modulate its inherent beat, since cardiac muscle, like smooth muscle, is myogenic.

REPRODUCTIVE SYSTEM

Chapter 7 covered some aspects of sexual reproduction, but this section focuses on the organs of the human reproductive system.

Human Male Reproductive System

The male gonads, called the **testes**, contain two functional components: the **seminiferous tubules** and the **interstitial cells (cells of Leydig)**. Sperm are produced in the highly coiled seminiferous tubules, where they are nourished by **Sertoli cells**. The interstitial cells, located between the seminiferous tubules, secrete **testosterone** and other **androgens** (male sex hormones). The testes are located in an external pouch called the **scrotum**, which maintains testes temperature 2 to 4°C lower than body temperature, a condition essential for sperm survival. Sperm pass from the seminiferous tubules into the coiled tubules of the **epididymis**. Here they acquire motility, mature, and are stored until **ejaculation**. During ejaculation they travel through the **vas deferens** to the ejaculatory duct and then to the **urethra**. The urethra passes through the **penis** and opens to the outside at its tip. In males, the urethra is a common passageway for both the reproductive and excretory systems.

Sperm is mixed with **seminal fluid** as it moves along the reproductive tract; seminal fluid is produced by three glands: the **seminal vesicles**, the **prostate gland**, and the **bulbourethral glands**. The paired seminal vesicles secrete a fructose-rich fluid that serves as an energy source for the highly active sperm. The prostate gland releases an alkaline milky fluid that protects the sperm from the acidic environment of the female reproductive tract. Finally, the bulbourethral glands secrete a small amount of viscous fluid prior to ejaculation; the function of this secretion is not known. Seminal fluid aids in sperm transport by lubricating the passageways through which the sperm will travel. Sperm plus seminal fluid is known as **semen**.

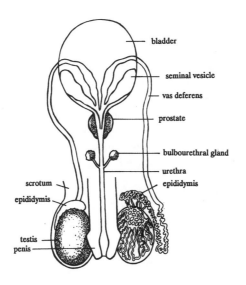

Human Female Reproductive System

The female gonads, called the **ovaries**, produce eggs (**ova**), and secrete the hormones oestrogen and progesterone. The ovaries are found in the abdominal cavity, below the digestive system. The ovaries consist of thousands of **follicles**; a follicle is a multilayered sac of cells that contains, nourishes, and protects an immature ovum. It is actually the follicle cells that produce oestrogen. Once a month, an immature ovum is released from the ovary into the abdominal cavity and drawn into the nearby **fallopian tube**. The inner surface of the fallopian tube is lined with cilia that create currents that move the ovum into and along the tube. Each fallopian tube opens into the upper end of a muscular chamber called the **uterus**, which is the site of fetal development. The lower, narrow end of the uterus is called the **cervix**. The cervix connects with the **vaginal canal**, which is the site of sperm deposition during intercourse and is also the passageway through which a baby is expelled during childbirth. The external female genitalia is referred to as the **vulva**. Note that in the mammalian (placental) female, the reproductive and excretory systems are distinct from one another; i.e., the urethra and the vagina are not connected.

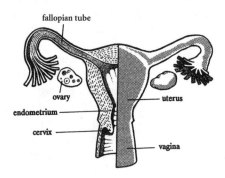

The Menstrual Cycle

The **menstrual cycle** is a repeating sequence of events in the tissues and hormones of the female body. We will describe the process in humans. The key hormones in the menstrual cycle are GnRH from the hypothalamus, FSH and LH from the pituitary, and **oestrogen** and **progesterone** from the ovary, each regulating the secretion of the other hormones as part of the menstrual cycle. GnRH stimulates FSH and LH secretion, which in turn stimulate the production of oestrogen and progesterone. Oestrogen and progesterone inhibit the production of FSH and LH as well as GnRH usually, with a key exception that is required for ovulation. Oestrogen and progesterone also regulate the tissues in the uterus involved in the menstrual cycle.

There are four stages in the menstrual cycle:

- The follicular stage
- Ovulation
- The corpus luteum (luteal) stage
- Menstruation

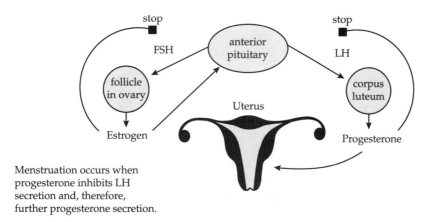

MENSTRUAL CYCLE

In the **follicular stage** of menstruation, FSH (follicle stimulating hormone) from the anterior pituitary gland stimulates a follicle to mature and produce oestrogen. Oestrogen promotes thickening of the uterine lining to support an embryo if fertilization occurs. This stage lasts approximately nine to ten days.

When the follicle is mature, a surge in LH secretion from the pituitary causes **ovulation**, the release of the ovum from an ovary. The LH surge is a key factor in ovulation and ovulation will not occur without it. Constant high levels of oestrogen block the LH surge and block ovulation. This is the mechanism by which the birth control pill acts.

After ovulation, the remains of the follicle in the ovary create the **corpus luteum**. Lutenizing hormone from the pituitary stimulates the corpus luteum to produce progesterone and oestrogen, which stimulates vascularization (growth of blood vessels) and lining formation of the uterus in preparation for implantation of the fertilized egg. This stage lasts 12 to 15 days. Then, if no fertilization or implantation has occurred, the increased oestrogen and progesterone block LH production. Without LH, the corpus luteum atrophies and progesterone levels fall. Without progesterone, the thickened, spongy uterine wall that had been prepared for implantation breaks down. The degenerating tissue, blood, and unfertilized egg are passed out as **menstrual flow**. This stage lasts approximately four days, bringing the total to 28 days for the entire cycle.

If fertilization occurs, the developing placenta produces HCG (**human chorionic gonadotrophic hormone**), which maintains the corpus luteum. The corpus luteum then continues to make progesterone and oestrogen. Progesterone prevents menstruation and ensures that the uterine wall is thickened so that embryonic development can occur and pregnancy can continue. With time, the placenta develops and takes over the production of oestrogen and progesterone for the duration of pregnancy.

Internal Development of an Embryo during Pregnancy

Fertilization and embryo development occur within the mother. This internal development utilizes a placenta to sustain the embryo. The **placenta** includes tissues of both the embryo and the mother. It is the site at which exchange of food, oxygen, waste and water can take place.

In placental animals, there is no direct contact between the bloodstreams of the mother and the embryo. Transport is accomplished by diffusion and active transport between juxtaposed blood vessels of the mother and embryo in the placenta. The eggs of placental animals are very small, since the embryo is only briefly maintained until a placental connection is completed. Humans, for example, have no yolk, but they do have a yolk sac.

The **umbilical cord** that attaches the embryo to the placenta is composed completely of tissues of embryonic, not maternal, origin. This cord contains the umbilical artery and vein. As in birds and reptiles, the amnion of placental mammals provides a watery environment to protect the embryo from shock.

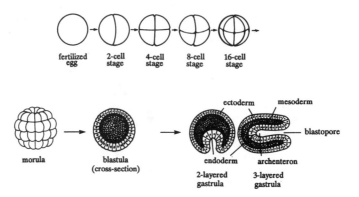

Postembryonic Development

The development of the embryo to the adult is termed **maturation**. Maturation involves cell division, differentiation, increase in size and development of a distinctive adult shape. Maturation can be interrupted, such as in the metamorphosis of arthropods, or uninterrupted, as in mammals. Differentiation of cells is complete when all organs reach adult form. Further cell division is needed only for repair and replacement of tissues. In humans, growth occurs rapidly in children, followed by sexual maturation during puberty.

DIGESTIVE SYSTEM

Digestion consists of the degradation of large molecules into smaller molecules that can be absorbed into the bloodstream and used directly by cells. **Intracellular digestion** occurs within the cell, usually in membrane-bound vesicles. **Extracellular digestion** refers to a digestive process that occurs outside of the cell, within a lumen or tract. Mammals have a one-way digestive tract known as the **alimentary canal**. Mammalian digestive tracts tend to be complex, and are organized into regions specialized for the digestion and absorption of specific nutrients.

The human digestive tract begins with the **oral cavity**, and continues with the **pharynx**, the **esophagus**, the **stomach**, the **small intestine**, and the **large intestine**. Accessory organs, such as the **salivary glands**, the **pancreas**, the **liver**, and the **gall bladder**, also play essential roles in the digestive process.

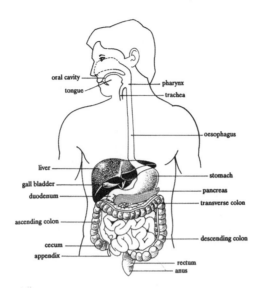

HUMAN DIGESTIVE TRACT

The Oral Cavity

The oral cavity (the mouth) is where mechanical and chemical digestion of food begins. **Mechanical digestion** is the breakdown of large food particles into smaller particles through the biting and chewing action of teeth (mastication). While mechanical digestion does not lead to changes in the molecular composition of food, the total surface area of the food is increased, allowing for faster and more efficient enzymatic action. **Chemical digestion** refers to the enzymatic breakdown of macromolecules into smaller molecules, and begins in the mouth when the salivary glands secrete saliva. Saliva lubricates food to facilitate swallowing, and provides a solvent for food particles. Saliva is secreted in response to a nervous reflex triggered by the presence of food in the oral cavity. Saliva contains the enzyme **salivary amylase (ptyalin)**, which hydrolyses starch into simple sugars. However, since food does not remain in the mouth for long, only a small portion of starch is hydrolysed there. The muscular **tongue**, containing the taste buds, manipulates the food during chewing, rolls it into a ball called a **bolus** and pushes the bolus into the pharynx.

The Pharynx

The pharynx is the cavity that leads food from the mouth into the esophagus. The pharynx also functions in respiration as the passageway through which air enters the trachea. During swallowing, the opening of the trachea is covered by a flap called the **epiglottis**, thereby preventing food particles from going down the wrong passageway.

The Oesophagus

The oesophagus is the muscular tube leading from the pharynx to the stomach. Food is moved down the oesophagus by rhythmic waves of involuntary muscular contractions called **peristalsis**. When a wave of peristalsis spreads down the oesophagus, a specialized ring of muscle in the lower oesophagus opens, allowing food to enter the stomach. Following the peristaltic wave, this muscle, called the **lower oesophageal sphincter** or **cardiac sphincter**, returns to its normal closed state, thus preventing the regurgitation of stomach contents into the oesophagus.

The Stomach

The stomach, a large, muscular organ located in the upper abdomen, stores and partially digests food. The walls of the stomach are lined by the thick gastric mucosa, which contains the **gastric glands** and **pyloric glands**. The gastric glands are stimulated by nervous impulses from the brain, which responds to the sight, taste and/or smell of food. The gastric glands are composed of three types of secretory cells: **mucous cells**, **chief cells** and **parietal cells**.

Mucous cells secrete mucus, which protects the stomach lining from the harshly acidic juices (pH = 2) present in the stomach. **Gastric juice** is composed of the secretions of the chief cells and the parietal cells. Chief cells secrete **pepsinogen**, the zymogen of the protein-hydrolysing enzyme **pepsin**. Parietal cells secrete **hydrochloric acid (HCl)**. HCl kills bacteria, dissolves the intercellular "glue" holding food tissues together, and facilitates the conversion of pepsinogen to pepsin. Pepsin hydrolyses specific peptide bonds to yield polypeptide fragments. The pyloric glands secrete the hormone **gastrin** in response to the presence of certain substances in food. Gastrin stimulates the gastric glands to secrete more HCl, and also stimulates muscular contractions of the stomach, which churn food. This churning produces an acidic, semifluid mixture of partially digested food known as **chyme**.

At the junction of the stomach and the small intestine is the muscular **pyloric sphincter**, which regulates the passage of chyme from the stomach into the small intestine via alternating contractions and relaxations. Although nutrient absorption occurs in the small intestine, alcohol and certain drugs (e.g., aspirin) can be directly absorbed into the systemic circulation through capillaries in the stomach wall.

The Small Intestine

Chemical digestion is completed in the small intestine. The small intestine is divided into three sections: the **duodenum**, the **jejunum**, and the **ileum**. In order to maximize the surface area available for digestion and absorption, the intestine is extremely long (greater than six metres in length) and highly coiled. In addition, numerous fingerlike projections called **villi** extend out of the intestinal submucosa, and tiny cytoplasmic projections called **microvilli** project from the surface of the individual cells lining the villi. The total surface area of the small intestine is approximately 300 m^2.

The Large Intestine

The large intestine is approximately 1.5 m long, and consists of three parts: the **caecum**, the **colon**, and the **rectum**. The caecum is a blind outpocketing at the junction of the small and large intestines. At the tip of the caecum is a small, fingerlike projection called the **appendix**. The appendix is a **vestigial structure** containing lymphoid tissue that is often surgically removed if it becomes infected. The colon functions in the absorption of salts and the absorption of any water not already absorbed by the small intestine. If digested matter moves through the colon too quickly, too little water is absorbed, causing diarrhaea and dehydration. Alternatively, if movement through the bowels is too slow, too much water is absorbed, causing constipation. The rectum stores **faeces**, which consist of bacteria (particularly **E. coli**), water, undigested food, and unabsorbed digestive secretions (e.g., enzymes and bile). The **anus** is the opening through which wastes are eliminated and is separated from the rectum by two sphincters that regulate elimination.

RESPIRATORY SYSTEM

Respiration is a broad term referring to the exchange of gases between an organism and its external environment, the transport of these gases within the organism and the diffusion of gases into and out of cells. (Cellular respiration refers to the role that these gases play in generating energy at the cellular level.) Aerobic organisms exchange CO_2 generated during cellular respiration for O_2 obtained from the external environment. Higher vertebrates have developed respiratory systems whereby gas exchange occurs at a single **respiratory surface**, the **lungs**.

Respiratory Anatomy

In the human respiratory system, air enters the lungs after travelling through a series of respiratory airways, as outlined in the following figure. Air enters the respiratory tract through the **external nares** (nostrils), and then travels through the nasal cavities, where it is filtered by mucous and nasal hairs. It then passes through the pharynx and into a second chamber called the **larynx**. Ingested food also passes through the pharynx en route to the oesophagus. To ensure that food does not accidentally enter the larynx and induce choking, a piece of tissue called the epiglottis covers the glottis (the opening to the larynx) during swallowing, thereby channelling food into the oesophagus. Air passes from the larynx into the cartilaginous **trachea**, which divides into two bronchi, one entering the right lung, the other entering the left. Both the trachea and bronchi are lined by ciliated epithelial cells, which filter and trap particles inhaled along with the air. The bronchi repeatedly branch into smaller bronchi, the terminal branches of which are called **bronchioles**. Each bronchiole is surrounded by clusters of small air sacs called **alveoli**. Gas exchange between the lungs and the circulatory system occurs across the very thin walls of the alveoli. Each alveolus is coated with a thin layer of liquid containing **surfactant**, and is surrounded by an extensive network of capillaries. Surfactant lowers the surface tension of the alveoli and facilitates gas exchange across the membranes. Three hundred million alveoli provide approximately 100 m^2 of moist respiratory surface for gas exchange.

Following gas exchange, air rushes back through the respiratory pathway and is exhaled.

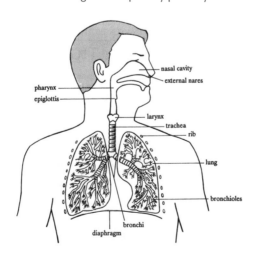

RESPIRATORY SYSTEM

Ventilation

Ventilation of the lungs (breathing) is the process by which air is inhaled and exhaled. The purpose of ventilation is to take in oxygen from the atmosphere and eliminate carbon dioxide from the body. The ventilating mechanism is dependent upon pressure changes in the **thoracic cavity**, the body cavity that contains the heart and lungs. The thoracic cavity is separated from the abdominal cavity by a muscle known as the **diaphragm**, and is bounded on the sides by the chest wall.

CARDIOVASCULAR SYSTEM

Higher organisms rely on a complex **cardiovascular system** to transport respiratory gases, nutrients and wastes to and from cells. A secondary circulatory system, the **lymphatic system**, collects excess body fluids and returns them to the cardiovascular circulation.

Cardiovascular Anatomy

The human cardiovascular system is composed of a muscular four-chambered **heart**, a network of **blood vessels**, and the **blood** itself. The right side of the heart pumps deoxygenated blood into the lungs via the pulmonary arteries. Oxygenated blood returns from the lungs to the left side of the heart via the pulmonary veins. It is then pumped into the **aorta**, which branches into a series of arteries. The arteries branch into **arterioles**, and then into microscopic capillaries. Exchange of gases, nutrients and cellular waste products occurs via diffusion across capillary walls. The capillaries then converge into venules, and eventually into veins, leading deoxygenated blood back toward the right side of the heart. Blood returning from the lower body and extremities enters the heart via the **inferior vena cava**, while deoxygenated blood from the upper head and neck region flows through the **jugular vein** and into the **superior vena cava**, which also leads into the heart. Oxygenated blood is supplied to heart muscle by the **coronary arteries**. The first branches off the aorta; **the coronary veins** and **coronary sinus** return deoxygenated blood to the right side of the heart.

In systemic circulation there are three special circulatory routes, referred to as **portal systems**, in which blood travels through *two* capillary beds prior to returning to the heart. There is a portal system in the liver (hepatic portal circulation), in the kidneys and in the brain (hypophyseal portal circulation).

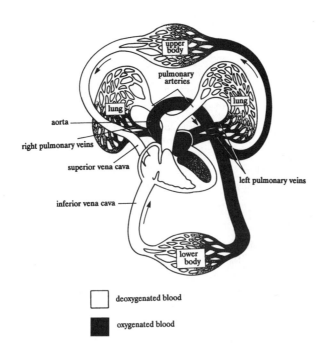

deoxygenated blood

oxygenated blood

The Heart

The heart is the driving force of the circulatory system. The right and left halves can be viewed as two separate pumps: the right side of the heart pumps deoxygenated blood into pulmonary circulation (toward the lungs), while the left side pumps oxygenated blood into systemic circulation (throughout the body). The two upper chambers are called **atria** and the two lower chambers are called ventricles. The atria are thin-walled, while the **ventricles** are extremely muscular. The left ventricle is more muscular than the right ventricle because it is responsible for generating the force that propels systemic circulation and because it pumps against a higher resistance.

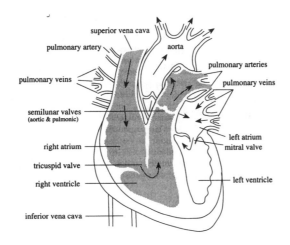

Blood Vessels

The three types of blood vessels are arteries, veins and capillaries. **Arteries** are thickly-walled, muscular, elastic vessels that transport oxygenated blood away from the heart—except for the pulmonary arteries, which transport deoxygenated blood from the heart to the lungs. **Veins** are relatively thinly-walled, inelastic vessels that conduct deoxygenated blood towards the heart—except for the pulmonary veins, which carry oxygenated blood from the lungs to the heart. Much of the blood flow in veins depends on their compression by skeletal muscles during movement, rather than on the pumping of the heart. Venous circulation is often at odds with gravity; thus larger veins, especially those in the legs, have valves that prevent backflow. **Capillaries** have very thin walls composed of a single layer of endothelial cells across which respiratory gases, nutrients, enzymes, hormones and wastes can readily diffuse. Capillaries have the smallest diameter of all three types of vessels; red blood cells must often travel through them single file.

Composition of Blood

On the average, the human body contains 4–6 litres of blood. Blood has both liquid (55%) and cellular components (45%; formed elements). **Plasma** is the liquid portion of the blood. It is an aqueous mixture of nutrients, salts, respiratory gases, wastes, hormones, and blood proteins (e.g., immunoglobulins, albumin and fibrinogen). The cellular components of the blood are **erythrocytes**, **leukocytes** and **platelets**.

Erythrocytes (Red Blood Cells)

Erythrocytes are the oxygen-carrying components of blood. An erythrocyte contains approximately 250 million molecules of **haemoglobin**, each of which can bind up to four molecules of oxygen. Erythrocytes have a distinct biconcave, disklike shape, which gives them both increased surface area for gas exchange and greater flexibility for movement through those tiny capillaries. Erythrocytes are formed from stem cells in the bone marrow, where they lose their nuclei, mitochondria, and membranous organelles. Since erythrocytes lack mitochondria, they are anaerobic and obtain their ATP via glycolysis alone. Once mature, erythrocytes circulate in the blood for about 120 days, after which they are phagocytised by special cells in the spleen and liver. There are about five million erythrocytes per mm^3 of blood.

Leukocytes (White Blood Cells)

Leukocytes arise from stem cells in the marrow of long bones. Leukocytes are larger than erythrocytes and have protective functions. The number of leukocytes in the blood varies widely; there are normally 5,000–10,000 leukocytes per mm^3 of blood, but this number substantially increases when the body is battling an infection. There are three types of leukocytes: **granular leukocytes**, **lymphocytes** and **monocytes**. Granular leukocytes (**neutrophils**, **basophils** and **eosinophils**) play key roles in inflammation, allergic reactions, pus formation and the destruction of invading bacteria and parasites. Lymphocytes play an important role in the **immune response**; they are produced in the lymph nodes, tonsils, spleen, appendix, thymus and bone marrow, and are involved in the production of **antibodies**. The two types of lymphocytes are **B lymphocytes** and **T lymphocytes**. Monocytes phagocytise foreign matter and organisms such as bacteria. Some monocytes migrate from the blood to tissue, where they mature into stationary cells called **macrophages**. Macrophages have greater phagocytic capability than monocytes.

Platelets

Platelets are cell fragments approximately 2–3 μm in diameter and are also formed in the bone marrow. Platelets lack nuclei and function in clot formation. There are about 250,000–500,000 platelets per mm^3 of blood.

Blood Antigens

Erythrocytes have characteristic cell-surface proteins (**antigens**). Antigens are macromolecules that are foreign to the host organism and trigger an immune response.

Transport of Gases

Erythrocytes transport O_2 throughout the circulatory system. Actually, it is the haemoglobin molecules in erythrocytes that bind to O_2. A haemoglobin molecule is composed of four polypeptide chains, each containing a prosthetic haeme group. Each haeme group is capable of binding to one molecule of oxygen. Thus, each haemoglobin molecule is capable of binding to four molecules of O_2. The binding of O_2 at the first haeme group induces a conformational change that facilitates the binding of O_2 at the other three haeme groups. Similarly, the unloading of O_2 at one haeme group facilitates the unloading of O_2 at the other three haeme groups.

Transport of Nutrients and Wastes

Amino acids and simple sugars are absorbed into the bloodstream at the intestinal capillaries and transported to the liver via the hepatic portal vein. After processing, they are transported throughout the body. Fats enter the lymphatic system through lymph capillaries in the small intestine and drain into the bloodstream at the large veins of the neck, thereby bypassing the liver. Throughout the body, metabolic waste products (e.g., water, urea and carbon dioxide) diffuse into capillaries from surrounding cells; these wastes are then delivered to the appropriate excretory organs.

The exchange of materials is greatly influenced by the balance between the **hydrostatic pressure** and the **osmotic pressure** of the blood and tissue fluids. The hydrostatic pressure at the arteriole end of the capillaries is greater than the hydrostatic pressure of the surrounding tissue fluids (interstitial fluid). This causes fluid to move out of the capillaries at the arteriole end. However, because blood has a higher solute concentration than the tissue fluid, osmotic pressure causes fluid to move back into the capillaries at the venule end.

Clotting

When platelets come into contact with the exposed collagen of a damaged vessel, they release a chemical that causes neighboring platelets to adhere to one another, forming a platelet plug. Subsequently, both the platelets and the damaged tissue release the clotting factor **thromboplastin**. Thromboplastin, with the aid of its cofactors calcium and vitamin K, converts the inactive plasma protein **prothrombin** to its active form, **thrombin**. Thrombin then converts **fibrinogen** (another plasma protein) into **fibrin**. Threads of fibrin coat the damaged area and trap blood cells to form a **clot**. Clots prevent extensive blood loss while the damaged vessel heals itself. People suffering from the genetic disease **haemophilia** lack one of the agents involved in clot formation and bleed excessively, even from minor cuts and bruises.

The Lymphatic System

The lymphatic system is a secondary circulatory system distinct from cardiovascular circulation. Its vessels transport excess interstitial fluid, called **lymph**, to the cardiovascular system, thereby keeping fluid levels in the body constant. **Lymph capillaries** (lacteals) collect fats by absorbing chylomicrons in the small intestine and transporting them to cardiovascular circulation. Lymph capillaries are closed at one end and lead into other lymph vessels that have valves to prevent the backflow of lymph. These lymph vessels then converge in the region of the upper chest and neck, where they drain into the large veins of the cardiovascular system. Lymph flow is regulated by contraction of neighboring skeletal muscles and rhythmic contractions of the lymphatic vessels themselves. **Lymph nodes** are swellings along lymph vessels containing phagocytic cells (leukocytes) that filter the lymph, removing and destroying foreign particles.

HOMEOSTASIS

Homeostasis is the process by which a stable internal environment within an organism is maintained. Some important homeostatic mechanisms include the maintenance of a water and solute balance (**osmoregulation**), the removal of metabolic waste products (**excretion**), the regulation of blood glucose levels and the maintenance of a constant internal body temperature (**thermoregulation**). In mammals, the primary homeostatic organs are the **kidneys**, the **liver**, the **large intestine** and the **skin**.

The Kidneys

The kidneys regulate the concentration of salt and water in the blood through the formation and excretion of urine. The kidneys are bean-shaped and are located behind the stomach and liver.

Osmoregulation

Filtration, **secretion** and **reabsorption** are the three processes that regulate salt and water balance in the blood.

Filtration

Blood pressure forces 20% of the blood plasma entering the glomerulus into the surrounding Bowman's capsule. The fluid and small solutes entering the nephron are called the **filtrate**. The filtrate is isotonic with blood plasma. Molecules too large to filter through the glomerulus, such as blood cells and albumin, remain in the circulatory system.

Secretion

The nephron secretes substances such as acids, bases and ions from the interstitial fluid into the filtrate by both passive and active transport. Secretion maintains blood pH, potassium concentration in the blood and nitrogenous waste concentration in the filtrate.

Reabsorption

Essential substances (glucose, salts and amino acids) and water are reabsorbed from the filtrate and returned to the blood. This results in the formation of concentrated urine, which is hypertonic to the blood.

Hormonal Regulation

Hormonal regulation plays a key role in urine formation. Two hormones that regulate water reabsorption are **aldosterone** and **ADH**.

Aldosterone

Aldosterone, which is produced by the adrenal cortex, stimulates both the reabsorption of Na^+ from the collecting duct, and the secretion of K^+. Na^+ reabsorption increases water reabsorption, leading to a rise in blood volume, and hence a rise in blood pressure. In a person suffering from **Addison's disease**, aldosterone is produced insufficiently or not at all. This causes overexcretion of urine with a high Na^+ concentration, which causes a considerable drop in blood pressure. Aldosterone secretion is regulated by the **renin-angiotensin system**.

ADH (antidiuretic hormone)

ADH, also known as **vasopressin**, is formed in the hypothalamus and stored in the posterior pituitary (see Endocrine System). As an "antidiuretic", it causes increased water reabsorption. It acts directly on the collecting duct, increasing its permeability to water. The amount of ADH produced is dependent on plasma osmolarity. A high solute concentration in the blood causes increased ADH secretion, while a low solute concentration in the blood reduces ADH secretion. Alcohol and caffeine inhibit ADH secretion, causing excess excretion of dilute urine and dehydration.

Excretion

By the time filtrate exits the nephron, most of the water has been reabsorbed. The remaining fluid, composed of urea, uric acid and other wastes, leaves the collecting tubule and exits the kidney via the **ureter**, a duct leading to the bladder. Urine is stored there until it is excreted from the body through the **urethra**. In a healthy individual, the nephron reabsorbs all of the glucose entering it, producing glucose-free urine. The urine of a diabetic, however, is not glucose-free. The high blood glucose concentration in a diabetic overwhelms the nephron's active transport system, leading to the excretion of glucose in the urine.

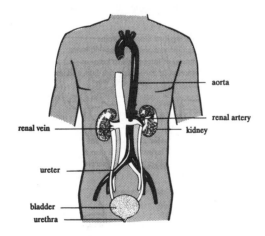

The Liver

The liver helps regulate blood glucose levels and produces urea. Glucose and other monosaccharides absorbed during digestion are delivered to the liver via the **hepatic portal vein**. Glucose-rich blood is processed by the liver, which converts excess glucose to glycogen for storage. If the blood has a low glucose concentration, the liver converts glycogen into glucose and releases it into the blood, restoring blood glucose levels to normal. In addition, the liver synthesises glucose from noncarbohydrate precursors via the process of **gluconeogenesis**. Glycogen metabolism is under both hormonal and nervous control.

The liver is also responsible for the processing of nitrogenous wastes. Excess amino acids are absorbed in the small intestine and transported to the liver via the hepatic portal vein. There the amino acids undergo a process called **deamination**, in which the amino group is removed from the amino acid and converted into ammonia, a highly toxic compound. In a complex biochemical process, the liver combines ammonia with carbon dioxide to form urea, a relatively nontoxic compound, which is released into the blood and eventually excreted by the kidneys.

The liver is also responsible for:

- detoxification of toxins
- storage of iron and vitamin B_{12}
- destruction of old erythrocytes
- synthesis of bile
- synthesis of various blood proteins
- defence against various antigens
- beta-oxidation of fatty acids to ketones
- interconversion of carbohydrates, fats and amino acids

The Large Intestine

The large intestine absorbs water and sodium not previously absorbed in the small intestine. However, the large intestine also functions as an excretory organ for excess salts. Excess calcium, iron and other salts are excreted into the colon and then eliminated with the faeces.

The Skin

The skin is the largest organ of the body, comprising an average of 16% of total body weight. The two major layers of the skin are the **epidermis** and the **dermis**, beneath which lies subcutaneous tissue, sometimes called the **hypodermis**.

The epidermis is the outermost epithelial layer and is composed of five cellular layers: the **stratum basalis (or stratum germinativum)**, the **stratum spinosum**, the **stratum granulosum**, the **stratum lucidum** and the **stratum corneum**. The deepest layer, the stratum basalis, continuously proliferates, pushing older epidermal cells outward. As the older cells reach the outermost layer (stratum corneum), they die, lose their nuclei and transform into squames (scales) of keratin. The keratinised cells of the stratum corneum are tightly packed, serving as a protective barrier against microbial attack. Hair projects above the surface of the epithelium; sweat pores open to the surface.

The dermis can be subdivided into a layer of loose connective tissue known as the **papillary layer**, and a layer of dense connective tissue known as the **reticular layer**. Within the dermis are the sweat glands, the sense organs, blood vessels and the bulbs of hair follicles. The **hypodermis**, composed of loose connective tissue, is abundant in fat cells and binds the outer skin layers to the body.

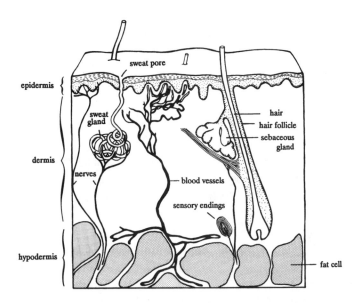

ENDOCRINE SYSTEM

The endocrine system acts as a means of internal communication, coordinating the activities of the organ systems. **Endocrine glands** synthesise and secrete chemical substances called **hormones** directly into the circulatory system. (In contrast, **exocrine glands**, such as the gall bladder, secrete substances that are transported by ducts.) Hormones regulate the function of **target organs** or tissues.

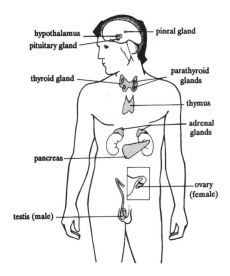

Endocrine Glands

Glands that synthesize and/or secrete hormones include the **pituitary**, **hypothalamus**, **thyroid**, **parathyroids**, **adrenals**, **pancreas**, **testes**, **ovaries**, **pineal**, **kidneys**, **gastrointestinal glands**, **heart** and **thymus**. Some hormones regulate a single type of cell or organ, while others have more widespread actions. The specificity of hormonal action is determined by the presence of specific receptors on or in the target cells.

NERVOUS SYSTEM

The nervous system enables organisms to receive and respond to **stimuli** from their external and internal environments. **Neurons** are the functional units of the nervous system. A neuron converts stimuli into electrochemical signals that are conducted through the nervous system.

Neuron Structure and Function

The neuron is an elongated cell consisting of **dendrites**, a **cell body** and an **axon**. Dendrites are cytoplasmic extensions that receive information and transmit it toward the cell body. The cell body (**soma**) contains the nucleus and controls the metabolic activity of the neuron. The **axon hillock** connects the cell body to the axon (nerve fibre), which is a long cellular process that transmits impulses away from the cell body. Most mammalian axons are ensheathed by an insulating substance known as **myelin**, which allows axons to conduct impulses faster. Myelin is produced by cells known as **glial cells**. (**Oligodendrocytes** produce myelin in the central nervous system, and **Schwann cells** produce myelin in the peripheral nervous system.) The gaps between segments of myelin are called **nodes of Ranvier**. Ultimately, the axons end as swellings known as **synaptic terminals** (sometimes also called synaptic boutons or knobs). Neurotransmitters are released from these terminals into the **synapse** (or **synaptic cleft**), which is the gap between the axon terminals of one cell and the dendrites of the next cell.

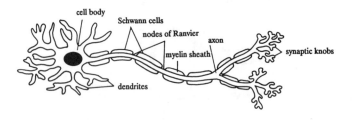

Central Nervous System

The central nervous system (CNS) consists of the **brain** and the **spinal cord**.

Brain

The brain is a jellylike mass of neurons that resides in the skull. Its functions include interpreting sensory information, forming motor plans and cognitive function (thinking). The brain consists of **grey matter** (cell bodies) and **white matter** (myelinated axons). The brain can be divided into the **forebrain**, **midbrain** and **hindbrain**.

Forebrain. The forebrain consists of the **telencephalon** and the **diencephalon**. The telencephalon consists of right and left hemispheres; each hemisphere can be divided into four different lobes: **frontal**, **parietal**, **temporal** and **occipital**. A major component of the telencephalon is the **cerebral cortex**, which is the highly convoluted grey matter that can be seen on the surface of the brain. The cortex processes and integrates sensory input and motor responses and is important for memory and creative thought. Right and left cerebral cortices communicate with each other through the **corpus callosum**.

The diencephalon contains the **thalamus** and **hypothalamus**. The thalamus is a relay and integration centre for the spinal cord and cerebral cortex. The hypothalamus controls visceral functions such as hunger, thirst, sex drive, water balance, blood pressure and temperature regulation. It also plays an important role in the control of the endocrine system.

Midbrain. The midbrain is a relay centre for visual and auditory impulses. It also plays an important role in motor control.

Hindbrain. The hindbrain is the posterior part of the brain and consists of the **cerebellum**, the **pons** and the **medulla**. The cerebellum helps to modulate motor impulses initiated by the motor cortex, and is important in the maintenance of balance, hand-eye coordination and the timing of rapid movements. One function of the pons is to act as a relay centre to allow the cortex to communicate with the cerebellum. The medulla (also called the medulla oblongata) controls many vital functions such as breathing, heart rate and gastrointestinal activity. Together, the midbrain, pons and medulla constitute the **brainstem**.

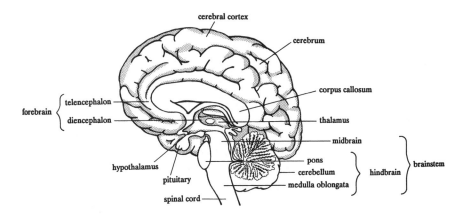

Spinal Cord

The spinal cord is an elongated structure continuous with the brainstem, that extends down the dorsal side of vertebrates. Nearly all nerves that innervate the viscera or muscles below the head pass through the spinal cord, and nearly all sensory information from below the head passes through the spinal cord on the way to the brain. The spinal cord can also integrate simple motor responses (e.g., reflexes) by itself. A cross-section of the spinal cord reveals an outer white matter area containing motor and sensory axons and an inner grey matter area containing nerve cell bodies. Sensory information enters the spinal cord dorsally; the cell bodies of these sensory neurons are located in the **dorsal root ganglia**. All motor information exits the spinal cord ventrally. Nerve branches entering and leaving the cord are called **roots**. The spinal cord is divided into four regions (going in order from the brainstem to the tail): **cervical**, **thoracic**, **lumbar** and **sacral**.

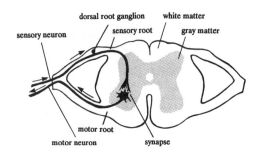

Special Senses

The body has three types of sensory receptors to monitor its internal and external environment: **interoceptors**, **proprioceptors** and **exteroceptors**.

Interoceptors monitor aspects of the internal environment such as blood pressure, the partial pressure of CO_2 in the blood and blood pH. Proprioceptors transmit information regarding the position of the body in space. These receptors are located in muscles and tendons to tell the brain where the limbs are in space, and are also located in the inner ear to tell the brain where the head is in space. Exteroceptors sense things in the external environment such as light, sound, taste, pain, touch and temperature.

The Eye

The eye detects light energy (as photons) and transmits information about intensity, colour and shape to the brain. The eyeball is covered by a thick, opaque layer known as the **sclera**, which is also known as the white of the eye. Beneath the sclera is the **choroid** layer, which helps to supply the retina with blood. The innermost layer of the eye is the **retina**, which contains the photoreceptors that sense the light. The transparent **cornea** at the front of the eye bends and focuses light rays. The rays then travel through an opening called the **pupil**, whose diameter is controlled by the pigmented, muscular **iris**. The iris responds to the intensity of light in the surroundings (light makes the pupil constrict). The light continues through the lens, which is suspended behind the pupil. The lens, the shape of which is controlled by the **ciliary muscles**, focuses the image onto the retina. In the retina are photoreceptors that **transduce** light into action potentials. There are two main types of photoreceptors: **cones** and **rods**. Cones respond to high-intensity illumination and are sensitive to colour, while rods detect low-intensity illumination and are important in night vision. The cones and rods contain various pigments that absorb specific wavelengths of light. The cones contain three different pigments that absorb red, green and blue wavelengths; the rod pigment, **rhodopsin**, absorbs one wavelength. The photoreceptor cells synapse onto **bipolar cells**, which in turn synapse onto **ganglion cells**. Axons of the ganglion cells bundle to form the right and left **optic nerves**, which conduct visual information to the brain. The point at which the optic nerve exits the eye is called the **blind spot** because photoreceptors are not present there. There is also a small area of the retina called the **fovea**, which is densely packed with cones, and is important for high acuity vision.

The eye also has its own circulation system. Near the base of the iris, the eye secretes aqueous humour, which travels to the anterior chamber of the eye from which it exits and eventually joins venous blood.

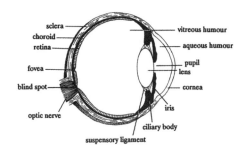

The Ear

The ear transduces sound energy (pressure waves) into impulses perceived by the brain as sound. The ear is also responsible for maintaining equilibrium (balance) in the body.

Sound waves pass through three regions as they enter the ear. First, they enter the **outer ear**, which consists of the **auricle** (pinna) and the **auditory canal**. At the end of the auditory canal is the **tympanic membrane (eardrum)** of the **middle ear**, which vibrates at the same frequency as the incoming sound. Next, the three bones, or **ossicles** (**malleus**, **incus** and **stapes**), amplify the stimulus, and transmit it through the **oval window**, which leads to the fluid-filled **inner ear**. The inner ear consists of the **cochlea** and the **semicircular canals**. The cochlea contains the **organ of Corti**, which has specialized sensory cells called hair cells. Vibration of the ossicles exerts pressure on the fluid in the cochlea, stimulating the hair cells to transduce the pressure into action potentials, which travel via the **auditory (cochlear) nerve** to the brain for processing.

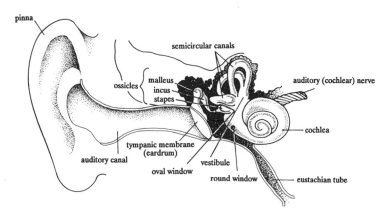

The three semicircular canals are each perpendicular to the other two and filled with a fluid called **endolymph**. At the base of each canal is a chamber with sensory hair cells; rotation of the head displaces endolymph in one of the canals, putting pressure on the hair cells in it. This changes the nature of impulses sent by the vestibular nerve to the brain. The brain interprets this information to determine the position of the head.

The Chemical Senses

The chemical senses are taste and smell. These senses transduce chemical changes in the environment, specifically in the mouth and nose, into **gustatory** and **olfactory** sensory impulses, which are interpreted by the nervous system.

Taste

Taste receptors, or **taste buds**, are located on the tongue, the soft palate, and the epiglottis. Taste buds are composed of approximately 40 epithelial cells. The outer surface of a taste bud contains a **taste pore**, from which microvilli, or **taste hairs**, protrude. The receptor surfaces for taste are on the taste hairs. Interwoven around the taste buds is a network of nerve fibres that are stimulated by the taste buds. These neurons transmit gustatory information to the brainstem via three cranial nerves. There are four kinds of taste sensations: sour, salty, sweet and bitter. Although most taste buds will respond to all four stimuli, they respond preferentially, i.e., at a lower threshold, to one or two of them.

Smell

Olfactory receptors are found in the olfactory membrane, which lies in the upper part of the nostrils over a total area of about 5 cm^2. The receptors are specialised neurons from which **olfactory hairs**, or **cilia**, project. These cilia form a dense mat in the nasal mucosa. When odourous substances enter the nasal cavity, they bind to receptors in the cilia, depolarising the olfactory receptors. Axons from the olfactory receptors join to form the **olfactory nerves.** The olfactory nerves project directly to the **olfactory bulbs** in the base of the brain.

REVIEW QUESTIONS

1. Which of the following is a normal pathway of blood flow?

    (A) right ventricle to aorta
    (B) pulmonary veins to left atrium
    (C) inferior vena cava to left atrium
    (D) pulmonary veins to left ventricle

2. Which of the following associations of brain structure and function is false?

    (A) hypothalamus: appetite
    (B) cerebellum: motor coordination
    (C) cerebral cortex: higher intellectual function
    (D) reticular activating system: sensory processing
    (E) medulla: basic emotional drives

3. Which statement about the respiratory system is NOT true?

    (A) Ciliated nasal membranes warm, moisten and filter inspired air.
    (B) Contraction of the diaphragm enlarges the thoracic cavity.
    (C) When the thoracic cavity enlarges, the pressure of air within the lungs falls.
    (D) When the pressure of air within the lungs is less than the atmospheric pressure, air will flow out of the lungs.
    (E) The respiratory process consists of inspiratory and expiratory acts following one another.

4. Which are correctly related?

   (A) white blood cell: no nucleus

   (B) smooth muscle cell: multinuclear

   (C) smooth muscle: voluntary action

   (D) cardiac muscle: involuntary action

   (E) smooth muscle: striations

5. The rate of breathing is controlled by involuntary centers in the

   (A) cerebrum

   (B) cerebellum

   (C) medulla oblongata

   (D) spinal cord

   (E) hypothalamus

6. The absorption of oxygen from the atmosphere into the blood takes place in the

   (A) pulmonary artery

   (B) pulmonary vein

   (C) alveoli

   (D) trachea

Answers and Explanations

1. B

Blood travelling from the left ventricle flows into the aorta, then goes to all areas of the body except the lungs. For example, blood in the brachiocephalic artery travels to the head and the shoulders, while blood in the renal artery travels to the kidney to be filtered. Blood flows from these arteries into arterioles, then into capillaries, where food, waste and energy will be exchanged. Next, the blood continues into venules and collects in veins, which then transport this blood to the superior and inferior vena cavas. This process is known as systemic circulation. In pulmonary circulation, the blood enters the right atrium and flows into the right ventricle. It is then transported to the lungs via the pulmonary artery, where capillary beds surround the alveoli so that gas exchange can occur. At this point, the pulmonary veins bring the blood back to the left atrium to start the process all over again.

2. E

The medulla monitors blood carbon dioxide levels and pH and adjusts breathing, temperature and heart rate. It is also the centre for reflex activities such as coughing, sneezing and swallowing, and is not associated with emotional drives. The other answer choices are true: The hypothalamus (A) is the centre that controls thirst, hunger, sleep, blood pressure and water balance; (B) the cerebellum controls muscle coordination and tone and maintains posture; (C) the cerebral cortex is the center for vision, hearing, smell, voluntary movement and memory; and (D) the reticular activating system receives and sorts sensory input.

3. D

There is low pressure inside the thoracic cavity due to expansion of the thoracic volume when the diaphragm contracts (as in (B) and (C)). When this pressure drops, air rushes in, and (A) the ciliated membrane warms, moistens and filters the inspired air. Air then travels through the bronchi, into the bronchioles and finally into the alveoli, where diffusion occurs to oxygenate the blood and release CO_2 carried back from the tissue. (D) is incorrect because when the pressure of air within the lungs is less than the atmospheric pressure, air actually rushes into the lungs rather than flowing out of them.

4. D

Cardiac cells have intercalated disc connections joining the cytoplasm between adjoining cardiac muscle cells. Although they have some striations, they are not voluntary. Smooth muscle, on the other hand, has no striations, is mononuclear and is involuntary. White blood cells have nuclei. In adult humans, red blood cells lack nuclei, in order to make room for as much haemoglobin as possible.

5. C

The breathing centre in the medulla oblongata monitors the increase in CO_2 through its sensory cells. It will also detect a decrease in pH in the blood, which is indicative of an increase of CO_2 levels in the blood. A decrease in O_2 is monitored peripherally by chemoreceptors, located in the carotid bodies in the carotid arteries and in the aortic bodies in the aorta. In (A), the cerebrum is involved in sensory interpretation, memory and thought, while the cerebellum (B) is involved in fine motor coordination, balance and equilibrium. Finally, the spinal cord (D) relays sensory and motor information to and from the brain, and the hypothalamus (E) regulates hunger, thirst, body temperature, sex drive and emotion.

6. C

Alveoli are thin air sacs that act as the sites of air exchange between the environment and the blood via passive diffusion. The trachea (D) is the region of the air intake pathway located between the glottis and the bronchi. It is also known as the windpipe.

Chapter 9: **Genetics and Evolution**

This chapter covers four main topics: molecular genetics, classical genetics and the genetic basis of evolution. Each of these will be discussed in detail and at the end of the chapter you will find practice questions to test your knowledge of these subjects.

DNA

Genes are composed of **DNA** (**deoxyribonucleic acid**), which contains information coded in the sequence of its base pairs, providing the cell with a blueprint for protein synthesis. Furthermore, DNA has the ability to self-replicate, which is crucial for cell division, and hence for organismal reproduction. DNA is the basis of heredity; self-replication ensures that its coded sequence will be passed on to successive generations. This is the central dogma of molecular genetics and it is summarised in the following figure.

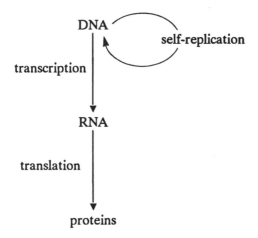

DNA Structure

DNA is a polymer built from simple building blocks called **nucleotides**, of which there are four types: **adenine** (A), **guanine** (G), **thymine** (T) and **cytosine** (C). Each nucleotide contains three parts, a five-carbon sugar (deoxyribose), a phosphate group and a nitrogenous base that distinguishes each of the four nucleotides (A, G, T or C). There are two types of bases: **purines** and **pyrimidines.** The purines are larger, with two rings in each base, and include adenine and guanine. The pyrimidines have one ring and in DNA are thymine and cytosine. The size of the bases is important, since this affects the way the bases fit together to make DNA.

To make DNA, nucleotides are polymerised, joined together in long regular strands of nucleotide building blocks. The phosphate group on one nucleotide forms a covalent bond to the sugar group on the next nucleotide to make a phosphate-sugar backbone in the polymer with the base groups projecting to one side, exposed. When a chain of nucleotides is polymerised, it always proceeds from the 5' toward the 3' end with new nucleotides added onto the 3' end, where 5' and 3' (pronounced "5 prime" and "3 prime") refers to the numbering of the sugar ring. On the 5' end of a DNA strand, the 5' OH group on the last deoxyribose sugar in the chain is free, while the 3' OH group is free on the last sugar at the other end of the strand. One polymer strand alone forms half of a DNA double helix—the other half is another strand oriented in the opposite direction (antiparallel). The two strands bind together to form the familiar DNA **double helix** with two strands wrapped around each other.

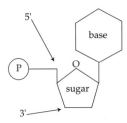

The binding of two DNA strands to each other requires that the base pairs in each strand hydrogen bond, or **base pair**, to the other strand in a very specific and restricted manner. An A in one strand can only bind to a T in the other.

(A-T) and G in one strand only bind to C in the other strand (G-C). This specificity is determined by the way that the base pairs hydrogen-bond with each other, with A and T forming two hydrogen bonds and G-C forming three. Also, each base pair must include one purine (big—two rings) and one pyrimidine (small—one ring) to fit in the space allowed inside the double helix. When the bases in two strands match correctly, the bases stack like plates one on top of the other on the inside of the double helix, with each strand wrapped around the other, and the phosphate-sugar backbones facing outward. The two complementary strands of DNA are always oriented in opposite directions in the double helix, with one strand oriented 5' to 3' and the complementary strand pointing in the other direction. The two strands for this reason are said to be **antiparallel**.

DNA Replication (Eukaryotic)

During replication the DNA helix unwinds and each strand acts as a template for complementary base-pairing in the synthesis of two new daughter helices. Each new daughter helix contains an intact strand from the parent helix and a newly synthesized strand; thus DNA replication is **semiconservative**. The daughter DNA helices are identical in composition to each other and to the parent DNA.

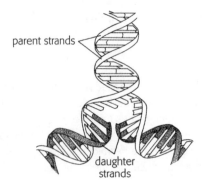

parent strands

daughter strands

DNA Repair

The DNA in the genome encodes all of the information cells and organisms need to function. Every enzyme in the cell is encoded in the genome, each with its own coding gene. If there are mistakes in the genome, then defective enzymes will be made and the cell or organism may not be able to function normally. DNA replication would introduce errors in the genome if the process were not tremendously accurate. Exposure to certain chemicals, UV light and radiation can also alter DNA and introduce these harmful mistakes into the genome. During the growth and life of an organism, cells will go through many rounds of cell division, making it all the more important that mistakes are not created in the genome during DNA replication.

The structure of DNA provides a way to keep the genome free of mistakes during DNA replication. If a mistake is made during DNA replication, base pairs will not fit properly into the normal double helical structure of DNA. DNA polymerase detects and fix these mistakes, proofreading DNA as it replicates DNA and correcting the mistakes to form the correct base pairing once again. Various mechanisms also repair DNA damage caused by chemicals and radiation, but occasional mistakes still occur, resulting in changes in the genome called mutations. Before mutations are discussed, first review information about ribonucleic acid (RNA).

RNA

In the central dogma, ribonucleic acid (RNA) is produced by reading genes from DNA. Like DNA, RNA is a polymer of nucleotides. Both DNA and RNA are nucleic acids and the structure of RNA is very similar to single-stranded DNA.

During RNA synthesis, the nucleotides in RNA are matched to base pair with the DNA template similar to the base-pairing of DNA with DNA during DNA replication. There are, however, a number of important differences. These differences include the use of the sugar ribose in the RNA backbone rather than deoxyribose, the presence of the base uracil in RNA rather than thymine and the fact that RNA is usually single-stranded, while DNA is usually double-stranded. Also, RNA is not proofread when it is made, unlike DNA.

There are three types of RNA with distinct functions: **messenger** RNA (mRNA), **ribosomal** RNA (rRNA) and **transfer** RNA (tRNA). mRNA encodes gene messages that are to be decoded in protein synthesis to form proteins. rRNA is a part of the structure of ribosomes and is involved in translation (protein synthesis). tRNAs also play a role in protein synthesis, with an anticodon that recognises one of the three base pair codons in mRNA and brings the amino acid that matches that codon to the translation process. tRNAs are relatively short, do not encode any proteins, have a compact, complex three-dimensional structure, including base pairing within the molecule, and have one end specialised to be bound to amino acids. The central role of RNAs in key cellular processes is believed by some to support the idea that life originated as an RNA-centered form that later evolved to use protein enzymes and DNA genomes.

Transcription and RNA Processing

Each gene in DNA has the information to make a protein, but DNA does not do this directly. First genes are read to make RNA. **Transcription** is the process in which genes in the DNA genome are used as templates to produce mRNA messages for proteins. The enzyme that synthesizes RNA in transcription, RNA polymerase, uses single-stranded DNA as a template to read the gene, matching base pairs as it synthesises new RNA from the DNA template (G matching with C and uracil matching with A). RNA is synthesised like DNA in one direction only, from the 5' end of the polymer to the 3' end. The messenger RNA is not proofread as it is produced, however, unlike DNA synthesis.

There are probably about 30,000 genes in the human genome, but not all of these are expressed in every tissue. Genes can be turned on or off by regulating gene transcription according to the needs of the cell and the organism. Transcription is turned on or off by regions of DNA near the start of genes called **promoters**. Promoters are short sequences of DNA that bind proteins called **transcription factors** that regulate transcription of genes by RNA polymerase. Transcription factors bind to specific sequences of DNA in promoters to turn genes on and off in response to hormones or other signalling mechanisms perceived by the cell.

In eukaryotic cells, mRNA is produced in the nucleus and is translated into proteins in the cytoplasm. Before the mRNA is translated, however, it is usually modified in the nucleus. The modifications include the addition of a special cap to the 5' end of the mRNA, the addition of poly A tail to the 3' end and the removal of RNA sections that do not encode a protein, a process called **splicing**. The part of the RNA molecule that encodes the protein message is called an **exon** and the part between coding blocks, the part that is removed, is called the **intron**. Splicing removes introns from mRNA and connects the exons together. Once splicing and processing are complete, the mRNA can be exported from the nucleus through the nuclear pores and is ready for translation to make proteins from the message.

Prokaryotic genes do not have introns and do not go through splicing. In fact, since there is no nucleus in prokaryotes, transcription and translation occur in the same compartment at the same time, with ribosomes translating an RNA before transcription is even complete. Prokaryotic genes are often found with several related genes next to each other in the genome and are even transcribed together in the same RNA molecule. These prokaryotic genes are **polycistronic** while eukaryotic genes are **monocistronic**, with only one gene per RNA message.

THE GENETIC CODE

The language of DNA consists of four "letters": A, T, C and G. The language of proteins consists of 20 "words": the 20 amino acids. The DNA language must be translated by mRNA in such a way as to produce the 20 words in the amino acid language; hence, the **triplet code**. (A two-letter [doublet] code would not suffice; with only four letters in the DNA alphabet, there would be only $4^2 = 16$ words possible—not enough to code for all 20 amino acids.) The base sequence of mRNA is translated as a series of triplets, otherwise known as **codons**. A sequence of three consecutive bases codes for a particular amino acid; e.g., the codon GGC specifies glycine, and the codon GUG specifies valine. The genetic code is universal for almost all organisms.

Given that there are 4^3, or 64, different codons possible based on the triplet code, and there are only 20 amino acids that need to be coded for, the code must contain synonyms. Most amino acids have more than one codon specifying them. This property is referred to as the **degeneracy** or **redundancy** of the genetic code.

PROTEIN TRANSLATION

Protein translation is the process in which the genetic code in mRNA is used to assemble amino acids in the correct sequence to make a protein. Translation occurs in the cytoplasm. After mRNA is processed and spliced in the nucleus and is ready to be translated, it is exported through a nuclear pore to the cytoplasm. To initiate translation, the mRNA is bound by a ribosome at the site on the mRNA where protein synthesis will begin. The start site of translation is the start codon AUG in the mRNA module, which codes for the amino acid methionine. Since all proteins have AUG as the start codon, all proteins have methionine as the first (or N-terminal) amino acid.

In the processed mRNA, each three-base pair codon codes for a specific amino acid that will be included in the protein amino acid chain. How do ribosomes match amino acids up to the correct codons? There are intermediary molecules, tRNAs, that match each amino acid up to its codons in mRNA. Each tRNA is activated to have a specific amino acid bound covalently at one end. At the other end, the tRNA has a three-base pair region called the **anticodon** that will match up and hybridise to the correct codon in mRNA, base-pairing with the mRNA during translation.

Enzymes called aminoacyl-tRNA synthetases attach amino acids to the correct tRNAs in a very accurate manner. If a tRNA has the wrong amino acid attached, the wrong amino acid will be built into a protein and the wrong protein sequence will be made. This could make the resulting protein unable to do its normal job, in the same manner as a mutation in a gene. There is proofreading in the production of activated tRNAs, but not in protein synthesis once an amino acid is built into a protein chain.

After the ribosome recognises the first codon, the start codon methionine, it matches up the next codon in the mRNA to the tRNA with the correct anticodon. If the mRNA has the three base-pair code GAU for aspartate, then the tRNA for aspartate, with CUA in its anticodon and aspartate bound to the other end, will match up to the codon on the ribosome. The ribosome will then join aspartate to the end of the growing protein chain, move down the mRNA one codon, and start again to match up another tRNA to the next codon in the mRNA. Once the next tRNA is bound to the ribosome, with its anticodon matching the mRNA codon, the next amino acid will be transferred from the bound tRNA to the end of the protein chain.

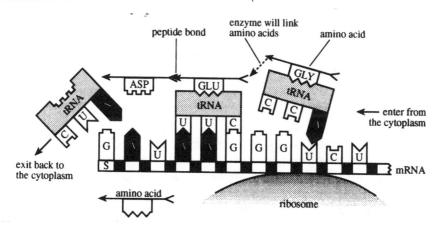

With each step in protein synthesis, the ribosome matches another tRNA to the correct mRNA codon, adds the next amino acid to the end of the protein chain, forms a peptide bond in the growing polymer, and releases the used tRNA to go back to the cytoplasm. The used tRNA will be recycled by the addition of the correct amino acid once again. When the ribosome reaches a stop codon in the mRNA, it stops translation and releases the mRNA. The mRNA can then be translated again or chewed into pieces by enzymes that degrade mRNA in the cell.

In eukaryotes, translation can occur either on ribosomes in the cytoplasm or on ribosomes bound to the rough endoplasmic reticulum, depending on where signals on the newly forming protein direct it to go. Proteins that will live in the cytoplasm are translated by ribosomes in the cytoplasm. Proteins that are destined for the endoplasmic reticulum (ER), Golgi or the plasma membrane, or that are to be secreted from the cell, are synthesised by ribosomes bound to the rough ER. When the protein is synthesised, it is inserted into the ER through the ER membrane. The protein sequence tells the ER where to send the protein. From the ER, the newly synthesised proteins are packaged into small spheres of membrane called **vesicles**. These vesicles move from the ER to the Golgi, where the proteins are further modified, then on to the plasma membrane where they are either secreted or remain as transmembrane proteins.

GENE MUTATIONS

A mutation is a change in the base sequence of DNA that may be inherited by offspring. The common types of mutations are **base-pair substitutions**, **base-pair insertions** and **base-pair deletions**.

Point Mutations

A point mutation occurs when a single nucleotide base is substituted by another. If the substitution occurs in a noncoding region, or if the substitution is transcribed into a codon that codes for the same amino acid, there will be no change in the amino acid sequence (a "silent" mutation). If the substitution changes the sequence, the result can range from insignificant to lethal, depending on the effect the substitution has on the protein. Sickle-cell anaemia most commonly results from a single base-pair substitution; sickle-cell haemoglobin has a valine (codon GUG) where normal haemoglobin has a glutamic acid (codon GAG).

Frame Shift Mutations

Base-pair insertions and deletions involve the addition or loss of nucleotides, respectively. Such mutations usually have more serious effects on the protein coded for, since nucleotides are read as a series of triplets. The addition or loss of a nucleotide(s) (except in multiples of three) will change the **reading frame** of the mRNA, and is known as a **frameshift mutation**. The protein, if synthesized at all, will most likely be nonfunctional.

Mutagenesis

Mutagenesis is the creation of mutations; it can be caused by internal genetic "mistakes" or by external cancer-causing agents called **mutagens**. Internal mistakes can occur during DNA replication, resulting in gene mutations and dysfunctional proteins. Physical mutagens such as X-rays and ultraviolet radiation, and chemical mutagens such as base analogs all result in mutations. Furthermore, DNA itself can act as a mutagen; mobile pieces of DNA called **transposon**s can insert themselves in genes and cause mutation.

MENDELIAN GENETICS

Around 1865, based on his observations of seven characteristics of the garden pea, Gregor Mendel developed the basic principles of genetics—**dominance, segregation** and **independent assortment**. Although Mendel formulated these principles, he was unable to propose any mechanism for hereditary patterns, since he knew nothing about chromosomes or genes. Hence his work was largely ignored until the early 1900s.

After Mendel's work was rediscovered, Thomas H. Morgan tied the principles of genetics to the chromosome theory. He linked specific traits to regions of specific chromosomes visible in the salivary glands of *Drosophila melanogaster*, the fruit fly. Morgan brought to light the giant chromosomes, at least 100 times the size of normal chromosomes, that are found in the fruit fly's salivary glands. These chromosomes are banded, and the bands coincide with gene locations, allowing geneticists to visibly follow major changes in the fly genome. Morgan also described sex-linked genes.

The fruit fly is a highly suitable organism for genetic research. With its short life cycle, it reproduces often and in large numbers, providing large sample sizes. It is easy to grow in the laboratory, but has a fairly complex body structure. Its chromosomes are large and easily recognisable in size and shape. They are also few in number (eight chromosomes/four pairs of chromosomes).

Finally, mutations occur relatively frequently in this organism, allowing genes for the affected traits to be studied. Some of the basic rules of gene transmission and expression are:

- **Genes** are elements of DNA that are responsible for observed traits.

- In eukaryotes, genes are found in large linear chromosomes, and each chromosome is a very long continuous DNA double helix. Humans have twenty-three different chromosomes, with two copies of each chromosome in most cells.

- Each chromosome contains a specific sequence of genes arranged along its length.

- Each gene has a specific location on a chromosome.

- Diploid organisms have two copies of each chromosome and therefore two copies of each gene (except for the *X* and *Y* chromosomes in males).

- The two copies of each gene can have a different sequence in an organism and a gene can have several different sequences in a population. These different versions of a gene are called **alleles**.

- The type of alleles an organism has, its genetic composition, is called the **genotype**.

- The appearance and physical expression of genes in an organism is called the **phenotype**.

- Types of alleles include dominant and recessive alleles. A dominant allele is expressed in an organism regardless of the second allele in the organism. A recessive allele will not be expressed if the other allele for the gene an organism carries is a dominant one.

- A **homozygous** individual has two copies (two alleles) of a gene that are identical and a **heterozygous** individual has two different alleles for a gene.

- The phenotype of an individual is determined by the genotype.

Dominant vs. Recessive

If two members of a pure-breeding strain are mated, their offspring will always have the same phenotype as the parents since they are all homozygous for the same allele. What happens if two different pure-breeding strains that are homozygous for two different alleles are crossed? In an example such as two different alleles for flower colour, what often occurs is that all of the offspring of the cross match the phenotype of one parent and not the other. For example, if a pure-breeding red strain is crossed with a pure-breeding white one, perhaps all of the offspring are red. Where did the allele coding for the white trait go? Did it disappear from the offspring?

If it is true that both parents contribute one copy of a gene to each of their offspring, then the allele cannot disappear. The offspring must all contain both a white allele and a red allele. Despite having both alleles, however, they only express one—the red allele. Red is then a **dominant allele** and white a **recessive allele**, since it is not expressed in heterozygotes such as the offspring in this cross of two pure-breeding strains.

Every human has two copies of each of their 23 chromosomes, with the exception of the *X* and *Y* chromosome in men. Thus, each gene is present in two copies that can either be the same, or different. For example, a gene for eye colour could have two alleles: *B* or *b*. *B* is a dominant allele for brown eye colour and *b* is a recessive allele for blue eye colour. There are three potential genotypes: *BB*, *Bb* or *bb*. *BB* individuals and *Bb* individuals have brown eyes, and only *bb* homozygous people have blue eyes. *Bb* people have brown eyes since the *B* allele is dominant and the recessive *b* allele is not expressed in the heterozygote.

Test Crosses

Often, a geneticist will study the transmission of a trait in a species such as flies or pea plants by performing crosses (matings) between organisms with defined traits. For example, an investigator may identify two possible phenotypes for flower colour in pea plants: pink and white. Pink plants bred together always produce pink offspring and white plants bred together always produce offspring with white flowers. It is likely that the differences in flower colour are caused by different alleles in a gene that controls flower colour. Which of these traits is determined by a recessive or dominant allele however? You cannot tell based on the colour alone which trait will be dominant or recessive. Either pink or white could be dominant, or neither.

The way to determine the dominant or recessive nature of each allele is by performing a test cross. Since the pink plants always produce pink plants and the white plants always produce white plants, these are both termed "pure-breeding" plants and are each homozygous for either the P allele (PP genotype has a pink phenotype) or for the p allele (pp genotype has a white phenotype).

Punnett Square

When performing a test cross, a useful tool is called a **Punnett Square**. To perform a Punnett Square, first determine the possible gametes each parent in the cross can produce. In the previous example, a PP parent can make gametes with either of the two P alleles and the pp parent can only make gametes with the p allele:

   PP parent: Gametes have either one P allele or the other P allele.

   pp parent: Gametes have either one p allele or the other p allele.

The next step is to examine all of the ways that these gametes could combine if these two parents were mated together in a test cross. This is where the Punnett Square comes in. On one side of the square, align the gametes from one parent, and on the other side of the square align the gametes from the other parent. At the intersection of each potential gamete pairing, fill in the square with the diploid zygote produced by matching the alleles. In this example, all of the offspring of this cross are going to be heterozygous.

If all of the offspring are pink, what does this reveal about the nature of these alleles? If the heterozygous Pp plant has the same phenotype as the homozygous PP plant, then the P allele is dominant over the p allele. If the p allele is not expressed in the heterozygote, the p allele is recessive and the P allele is dominant. The offspring of this cross (shown within the box) can be called the F_1 generation.

A Cross Between Two Pure-Breeding Strains (F_1 generation):

	P	P
p	Pp	Pp
p	Pp	Pp

The F_1 offspring all have the Pp genotype and the pink phenotype. What will occur if two of these F_1 plants are crossed? A Punnett Square can be used again to predict the genotypes in the F_2 generation.

   Parent 1: P and p gametes are produced

   Parent 2: P and p gametes are produced

F$_2$ Generation Punnett Square:

	P	p
P	PP	Pp
p	Pp	pp

Since we know that the *P* allele for pink is dominant, we can use the genotypes to predict phenotypes of the F$_2$ generation. *PP* homozygotes will be pink, and *Pp* heterozygotes will also be pink since *P* is dominant. *pp* plants will be white like the original pure-breeding white plants. Filling in the square with these phenotypes:

	P	p
P	PP (pink)	Pp (pink)
p	Pp (pink)	pp (white)

The ratios of the different genotypes and phenotypes in the Punnett Square should match the statistical probability of producing these in real life by a cross of this type. For example, if two heterozygous *Pp* plants are crossed, 75 percent of the offspring will be pink and 25 percent white. This is predicted from the Punnett Square based on the ratio of 3:1 for phenotypes that will produce pink (3) to white (1).

The behaviour of different pea plant traits helped Mendel to formulate two fundamental laws of Mendelian genetics, the Law of Segregation and the Law of Independent Assortment. Mendel derived these rules based purely on his knowledge of the transmission of traits, without knowing anything about the molecular basis for his observations in the mechanisms of meiosis.

Law of Segregation

The Law of Segregation states that if there are two alleles in an individual that determine a trait, these two alleles will separate during gamete formation and can act independently. For example, when a heterozygous *Pp* plant is forming gametes, the *P* and the *p* alleles can separate into different gametes and act independently during a cross. If this was not the case, and the *P* and *p* alleles could not separate, then all of the offspring would remain *Pp* and all of the F$_2$ would be pink still. The fact that white offspring are produced indicates that alleles do indeed segregate into gametes independently. The molecular basis for this observation is that during meiosis, each homologous chromosome carrying the two different alleles will end up in a different haploid gamete.

Law of Independent Assortment

The Law of Independent Assortment describes the relation between different genes. If the gene that determines plant height is on a different chromosome than the gene for flower colour, then these traits will act independently during test crosses. The two alleles for tallness are the dominant allele *T* for tall plants and the recessive *t* allele for short plants. The two alleles for colour are the dominant *Y* allele for yellow and the recessive *y* allele for white. When plants are crossed, the alleles for the tall gene act independently of the alleles for the colour gene. Example of a dihybrid cross in which tall and yellow are both hybrids:

	TY	Ty	tY	ty
TY	TTYY	TTYy	TtYY	TtYy
Ty	TTYy	Ttyy	TtYy	Ttyy
tY	TtYY	TtYy	ttYY	ttYy
ty	TtYy	Ttyy	ttYy	ttyy

Results of the cross:

Phenotype ratio:

9 tall yellow $\left(\dfrac{9}{16}\right)$: 3 tall green $\left(\dfrac{3}{16}\right)$: 3 short yellow $\left(\dfrac{3}{16}\right)$: 1 short green $\left(\dfrac{1}{16}\right)$

The simplest approach to an independent assortment problem is to consider each of the genes separately, determine the predicted Mendelian ratios for each of the traits alone, and then use the laws of probability to combine these. For example, in the previous cross, the predicted Mendelian phenotype ratios are $\dfrac{3}{4}$ for tall and $\dfrac{1}{4}$ for green. The probability of observing these phenotypes together is the product of their independent probabilities—that is, $\dfrac{3}{4} \times \dfrac{1}{4}$ or $\dfrac{3}{16}$. A significant variation from this ratio indicates linkage and a failure to assort independently.

NON-MENDELIAN INHERITANCE PATTERNS

While Mendel's laws hold true in many cases, these laws cannot explain the results of certain crosses. Sometimes an allele is only incompletely dominant or, perhaps, codominant. The genetics that enable the human species to have two genders would also not be possible under Mendel's laws.

Incomplete Dominance

Incomplete dominance is a blending of the effects of contrasting alleles. Both alleles are expressed partially, neither dominating the other.

An example of incomplete dominance is found in the four-o'clock plant and in the snapdragon flower. When a red flower (*RR*) is crossed with a white flower (*WW*), a pink blend (*RW*) is created. When two pink flowers are crossed, the yield is 25 percent red, 50 percent pink, and 25 percent white (phenotypic and genotypic ratio 1:2:1).

Codominance

In codominance, both alleles are fully expressed without one allele dominant over the other. An example is blood types. Blood type is determined by the expression of antigen proteins on the surface of red blood cells. The *A* allele and the *B* allele are codominant if both are present and combine to produce AB blood.

The allele for blood type A, I_A, and the allele for blood type B, I_B, are both dominant to the third allele, *i*. I_A and I_B may appear together to form blood type AB; however, when both are absent, blood type O results.

To summarise:

- I_A = gene for producing antigen A on the red blood cell
- I_B = gene for producing antigen B on the red blood cell
- i = recessive gene; does not produce either antigen

And these genes combine in various ways to form the following possible genotypes and blood types (phenotypes):

- I_AI_A or I_Ai = Type A blood
- I_BI_B or I_Bi = Type B blood
- I_AI_B = Type AB blood, with A and B alleles codominant
- ii = Type O blood

Sex Determination

Most organisms have two types of chromosomes: **autosomes**, which determine most of the organism's body characteristics, and **sex chromosomes**, which determine the sex of the organism. Humans have 22 pairs of autosomes and one pair of sex chromosomes. The sex chromosomes are known as X or Y. In humans, XX is present in females and XY in males. The Y chromosome carries very few genes. Sex is determined at the time of fertilization by the type of sperm fertilising the egg, since all eggs contain X chromosomes only. If the sperm carries an X chromosome, the offspring will be female (XX); if the sperm carries a Y chromosome, the offspring will be male (XY).

This process is illustrated in the Punnett Square that follows:

	X	Y	*(From the father)*
X	XX	XY	
X	XX	XY	

(From the mother)

The ratio of the sex of the offspring is 1:1.

Sex Linkage

Genes for certain traits, such as colour blindness or haemophilia, are located on the X chromosomes. Hence these genes are linked with the genes controlling sex determination. These genes seem to have no corresponding allele on the Y chromosome, with the result that the X chromosome contributed by the mother is the sole determinant of these traits in males.

Genes determining haemophilia and red-green colour blindness are sex-linked (on the X chromosome). They are recessive, implying that they can be hidden by a dominant normal allele on the other X-chromosome in a female. For this reason, the female with two X chromosomes may carry, but will rarely exhibit, these afflictions. The male, on the other hand, with his Y chromosome, has no dominant allele to mask the recessive gene on his X chromosome. As a consequence of having a single copy of X-linked genes, males exhibit sex-linked traits much more frequently than females do.

Cross 1: This is what happens when a haemophilia-carrying female and a normal male are crossed:

$XX_h \times XY$:

	X	X_h
X	XX	XX_h
X	XY	X_hY

The ratio of the sex of the offspring is 1:1.

Results of the cross:

XX = healthy female

XX_h = carrier but healthy female

XY = healthy male

X_hY = haemophiliac male

There are no male carriers of this trait since all males that have the haemophilia allele express it.

Cross 2: Here is a cross between a carrier female and a male haemophiliac:

$XX_h \times X_hY$:

	X	X_h
X_h	XX_h	X_hX_h
X	XY	X_hY

The ratio of the sex of the offspring is 1:1.

Results of the cross:

X_hX_h = haemophiliac female (very rare)

XX_h = carrier but healthy female

XY = healthy male

X_hY = haemophiliac male

Mutations

Mutations can create new alleles, the raw material that drives evolution via natural selection. Mutations are changes in the genes that are inherited. To be transmitted to the succeeding generation, mutations must occur in sex cells—eggs and sperm—rather than somatic cells (body cells). Mutations in nonsex cells are called somatic cell mutations and affect only the individual involved, not subsequent generations. A somatic mutation can cause cancer, but will have no effect on offspring since it is not present in gametes. Most mutations are recessive and harmful. Because they are recessive, these mutations can be masked or hidden by the dominant normal genes.

Chromosomal Mutations

These mutations result in changes in chromosome structure or abnormal chromosome duplication. In crossing over, segments of chromosomes switch positions during meiotic synapsis. This process breaks linkage patterns normally observed when the genes are on the same chromosome. A **translocation** is an event in which a piece of a chromosome breaks off and rejoins a different chromosome. **Nondisjunction** is the failure of some homologous pairs of chromosomes to separate following meiotic synapsis. The result is an extra chromosome or a missing chromosome for a given pair. For example, Down's syndrome is due to an extra chromosome #21 (Trisomy 21). The number of chromosomes in a case of single nondisjunction is $2n + 1$ or $2n - 1$. In Trisomy 21, the individual has 47 chromosomes instead of the usual 46.

Polyploidy ($3n$ or $4n$) involves a failure of meiosis during the formation of the gametes. The resulting gametes are $2n$. Fertilization can then be either $n + 2n = 3n$ or $2n + 2n = 4n$. Polyploidy is always lethal in humans although it is often found in fish and plants. Finally, **chromosome breakage** might be induced by environmental factors or other mutagens.

Gene Mutations

As discussed earlier in this chapter, there might be changes in the base sequence of DNA that result in changes in single genes, changing one or more base pairs and the protein produced by reading the gene.

GENETIC BASIS OF EVOLUTION

Genetic variation functions as the raw material for natural selection. Sources of genetic variation include inheritable mutations and recombination. Mutations are random changes in the nucleotide sequence of DNA. Recombination refers to novel genetic combinations resulting from sexual reproduction and crossing over.

The Hardy-Weinberg Equilibrium

Evolution can be viewed as a result of changing **gene frequencies** within a population. Gene frequency is the relative frequency of a particular allele. When the gene frequencies of a population are not changing, the gene pool is stable, and the population is not evolving. However, this is true only in ideal situations in which the following conditions are met:

1. The population is very large.
2. There are no mutations that affect the gene pool.
3. Mating between individuals in the population is random.
4. There is no net migration of individuals into or out of the population.
5. The genes in the population are all equally successful at reproducing.

Under these idealized conditions, a certain equilibrium will exist between all of the genes in a gene pool, which is described by the **Hardy-Weinberg equation**.

For a gene locus with only two alleles, T and t, **p** = the frequency of allele T and **q** = the frequency of allele t. By definition, for a given gene locus, **p + q = 1,** since the combined frequencies of the alleles must total 100%.

Thus $(p + q)^2 = (1)^2$ and

$p^2 + 2pq + q^2 = 1$

where p^2 = frequency of TT (dominant homozygotes)
$2pq$ = frequency of Tt (heterozygotes)
q^2 = frequency of tt (recessive homozygotes)

The Hardy-Weinberg equation may be used to determine gene frequencies in a large population in the absence of microevolutionary change (defined by the five conditions previously given). For example, individuals from a non-evolving population can be randomly crossed to demonstrate that the gene frequencies remain constant from generation to generation. Assume that in the original gene pool the gene frequency of the dominant gene for tallness, T, is .80, and the gene frequency of the recessive gene for shortness, t, is .20. Thus, $p = .80$ and $q = .20$. In a cross between two heterozygotes, the resulting F_1 genotype frequencies are: 64% TT, 16% + 16% = 32% Tt, and 4% tt (see the following Punnett Square).

Cross 1: This is what happens when a haemophilia-carrying female and a normal male are crossed:

	$p = .80$ (T)	$q = .20$ (t)
$p = .80$ (T)	($p^2 = .64$) TT = 64%	($pq = .16$) Tt = 16%
$q = .20$ (t)	($pq = .16$) Tt = 16%	($q^2 = .04$) tt = 4%

The gene frequencies of the F_1 generation can be calculated as follows:

64% TT = 64% T allele + 0% t allele

32% Tt = 16% T allele + 16% t allele

4% tt = 0% T allele + 4% t allele

Gene frequencies = 80% T allele + 20% t allele

Thus, $p = .80$ and $q = .20$. These frequencies are the same as those in the parent generation, thus demonstrating Hardy-Weinberg equilibrium in a non-evolving population.

Microevolution (Disruption of Hardy-Weinberg Equilibrium in Evolution)

No population can be represented indefinitely by the Hardy-Weinberg equilibrium because such idealized conditions do not exist in nature. Real populations have unstable gene pools and migrating populations. The agents of microevolutionary change—**natural selection, mutation, assortive mating, genetic drift** and **gene flow**—are all deviations from the five conditions of a Hardy-Weinberg population.

Natural Selection

Within a population of organisms, individuals are non-identical. Mutation is a source of new alleles, and sexual reproduction leads to constant shuffling of alleles in new genotypes. The variety of genotypes created in a population in this way creates a variety of phenotypes. If individuals have different phenotypes, then these individuals probably interact with their environment with differing degrees of success in escaping predators, finding food, avoiding disease and reproducing. The differential survival and reproduction of individuals based on inherited traits is **natural selection** as described first by Charles Darwin.

Fitness is a quantitative measure of the ability to contribute alleles and traits to offspring and future generations. The key to fitness is reproduction and survival of offspring. Avoiding predators, finding food, resistance to disease and other factors that improve survival are likely to improve fitness but only to the extent that they lead to more offspring and more of the alleles involved in the future gene pool. Finding a mate, mating, successful fertilization and caring for offspring are factors that can improve fitness as well. There are different strategies for improving fitness. For example, some animals have lots of offspring but provide little parental care, while other animals have few offspring but provide lots of care for each of them.

None of the other factors that alter Hardy-Weinberg equilibrium alter it in a directed fashion. Genetic drift, mutation and migration are all random in their effects on the gene pool. Natural selection, however, increases the prevalence of alleles in a population that increase survival and reproduction. Alleles that increase fitness will over time increase in their allele frequency in the gene pool, and increase the abundance of the associated phenotype as well. This effect will change the population in a directed manner over many generations, creating a population that is better adapted to its environment.

Different types of natural selection can occur, including **stabilizing selection**, **disruptive selection** and **directional selection**. Traits in a population such as the height of humans are often distributed according to a bell-shaped curve. The type of selection that occurs can affect the average value for the trait or it can alter the shape of the curve around the average. **Stabilizing selection** does not change the average, but makes the curve around the average sharper, so that values in the population lie closer to the average. For example, if both very small fish and very large fish tend to get eaten, then stabilizing selection may not alter the average fish size, but is likely to cause future generations to be closer to average.

Disruptive selection is the opposite, in which the peak value is selected against, selecting for either extreme in a trait, so that a single peak for a trait in a population tends to be split into two peaks. **Directional selection** alters the average value for a trait, such as selecting for dark wings in a population of moths in an industrial area.

Natural selection acts on an individual and its direct descendants. In some cases natural selection can also act on closely related organisms that share many of the same alleles. This type of natural selection, called **kin selection**, occurs in organisms that display social behavior. The key to fitness is that an organism's alleles are contributed to the next generation. Contribution of alleles can happen by an individual or by close relatives like siblings, aunts, uncles, etc., who share many of the same alleles. The evolution of social organisms is the result of the increased fitness that social behavior provides. Described cases of altruistic behavior in animals is probably the result of kin selection at work, in which an animal might sacrifice its own safety to allow relatives to survive, thereby increasing the fitness of itself and the whole social group it shares alleles with.

SPECIATION

A species is a group of organisms that is able to successfully interbreed with each other and not with other organisms. The key to defining a species is not external appearance. Within a species, there can be great phenotypic variation, as in the domestic dog. What defines a species is reproductive isolation, an inability to interbreed and create fertile offspring. Actual interbreeding is not necessary to make organisms the same species. Two groups of animals may live in different locations and never contact each other to interbreed, but if a researcher transports some of the animals and they create fertile offspring, they are part of the same species. Horses and donkey can interbreed and create offspring, the mule. The mule, however, is sterile, meaning the horses and donkeys are two different species.

Speciation, the creation of a new species, occurs when the gene pool for a group of organisms becomes reproductively isolated. At this point, evolution can act on that group that shares a gene pool separately from others. Two species can be derived from a single common ancestor species when two populations of a species are separated geographically through a process known as **allopatric speciation**.

Separation of a widely distributed population by emerging geographic barriers causes each population to evolve specific adaptations for the environment in which it lives, in addition to the accumulation of neutral (random, non-adaptive) changes. These adaptations will remain unique to the population in which they evolve, provided that interbreeding is prevented by the barrier. In time, genetic differences will reach the point where interbreeding becomes impossible and reproductive isolation would be maintained if the barrier were removed. In this manner, geographic barriers promote evolution.

Adaptive radiation is the production of a number of different species from a single ancestral species. Radiation refers to a branching out; adaptive refers to the hereditary change that allows a species to be more successful in its environment or to be successful in a new environment. Whenever two or more closely related populations occur together, natural selection favours evolution of different living habits. This results in the occupation of different niches by each population (this process is discussed in detail in chapter 10). This divergent evolution through adaptive radiation has been an extremely frequent occurrence.

REVIEW QUESTIONS

1. A factor that tends to keep the gene pool constant is

     I. nonrandom mating
     II. freedom to migrate
     III. no net mutations
     IV. large populations

   (A) I and II

   (B) III and IV

   (C) I, III, and IV

   (D) II, III, and IV

   (E) I, II, III, and IV

2. Which of the following statements regarding evolution is true?

   (A) Certain phenotypes are more fit in certain environments than others.

   (B) Natural selection creates new alleles.

   (C) Genotype, not phenotype, influences fitness.

   (D) Mutations always affect the fitness of an organism.

   (E) all of the above

3. The gene for colour blindness is *X*-linked. If normal parents have a colour-blind son, what is the probability that he inherited the gene for colour blindness from his mother?

    (A) 0%

    (B) 25%

    (C) 50%

    (D) 75%

    (E) 100%

4. The genes encoding for eukaryotic protein sequences are passed from one generation to the next in

    (A) other proteins

    (B) rRNA

    (C) tRNA

    (D) mRNA

    (E) DNA

5. Green (*Y*) is dominant over yellow (*y*) in peas, and the smooth allele (*W*) is dominant over wrinkled (*w*). Which cross must produce all green, smooth peas?

    (A) *YyWw* × *YyWw*

    (B) *Yyww* × *YYWw*

    (C) *YyWW* × *yyWW*

    (D) *YyWw* × *YYWW*

6. If one parent is homozygous dominant and the other is homozygous recessive, which of the following might appear in an F_2 generation, but not in an F_1 generation?

        I. heterozygous genotype
       II. dominant phenotype
      III. recessive phenotype

    (A) I only

    (B) II only

    (C) III only

    (D) I and II

    (E) II and III

Answers and Explanations

1. B

The Hardy-Weinberg Law states that gene ratios and allelic frequencies remain constant through the generations in a non-evolving population. Five criteria must be met in order for this to occur: random mating, a large population, no migration into or out of the population, no natural selection, and a lack of mutation. If all five of these criteria are met, gene frequencies will remain constant. Any time these five are not met, gene frequencies will change and evolution may occur.

2. A

In Darwin's theory of natural selection, some organisms in a species have variations in traits that give them an advantage over other members of the species. These adaptations enable these organisms and their offspring to survive in greater numbers than organisms that lack them, giving them greater fitness.

3. E

A female has two X chromosomes, one inherited from her mother and one inherited from her father, while a given male has one X chromosome inherited from his mother and one Y chromosome inherited from his father. If a male expresses an X-linked trait, he must have inherited it from his mother. If normal parents have a colour-blind son, he *must* have inherited the colour-blind gene, which is X-linked, from his mother. His mother *must* be a carrier of the colour-blind allele. The probability that a colour-blind son inherited the gene for colour-blindness from his mother is 100 percent.

4. E

DNA is the genetic material for all prokaryotes and eukaryotes.

5. D

Both green and smooth are dominant phenotypes. The goal in this question is to produce only green, smooth peas, so we want only dominant phenotype offspring. Therefore, we must avoid any crossing that may result in the mating or combining of two recessive alleles. In (A), crossing Yy and Yy could result in approximately one quarter of the offspring turning out yellow. Similarly, in choice (B), ww crossed with Ww would produce offspring of which approximately half would possess a wrinkled phenotype. In choice (C), Yy crossed with yy is likely to produce offspring which are approximately half yellow. Choice (D) is correct because one of the parents is a double dominant, meaning that all offspring will have the dominant phenotype, regardless of the genotype of the other parent.

6. C

In the $AA \times aa$ cross, the F_1 generation will be 100% Aa, a heterozygous genotype with a dominant phenotype. In the F_2 generation, there will be a 1:2:1 ratio of $AA:Aa:aa$. Therefore, the F_1 generation is entirely dominant heterozygous. Choices I and II can be eliminated, leaving only III.

Chapter 10: **Ecology**

This chapter and its corresponding practice questions review how organisms live. To understand how organisms live, biologists study molecules, cells, tissues and organs, breaking organisms down into their fundamental units. Organisms from bacteria to humans do not live on Earth in an isolated state, however. All organisms, including humans, live by interacting with other organisms and with the non-living (**abiotic**) environment. Life on Earth is a network of interacting organisms that depend on each other for survival. Ecology is the study of the interactions between organisms and their environment and how these shape both the organisms and the environments in which they live.

POPULATIONS IN THE ENVIRONMENT

Since ecology seeks to understand life at a broader level than the organism, it is the population rather than the individual that is the basic unit of study in this discipline. A **population** is a group of individuals that interbreed and share the same gene pool, the same definition used in population genetics. Every environment will include many different interacting populations. There are properties of populations that are not present in individuals, such as population growth and maximal population size. These distinct properties of populations are important for ecosystems.

Patterns of Population Growth

One of the key characteristics of a population is its rate of **population growth**. At any given time a population can grow, stay the same or shrink in size. The birth rate, the death rate and the population size determine the rate of growth, with the birth rate and death rate influenced by the environment. If the birth rate is high and the death rate is low, as in an environment where resources are unlimited, a population will grow rapidly. If a population of mice starts with a male and female mouse, and breeds once every three months, producing six male and female offspring in each generation, the population will have over two million mice in two years. A single bacterium reproducing by binary fission every thirty minutes can produce 8 million bacteria in 12 hours. This form of population growth produces a curve with rapidly increasing slope and is termed **exponential growth**, since every generation increases the population size in an exponential manner.

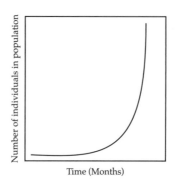

Exponential Population Growth

In nature, this rapid population growth may be observed when a population first encounters a favourable new environment, such as a rich growth medium inoculated with a small number of bacteria, or a fertile empty field invaded by a weed. Exponential growth cannot be maintained forever, though. A population of mice growing exponentially in a field of wheat will soon eat so much of the available food that starvation will occur; growth will slow and then halt. Bacteria reproducing without check would in a few days weigh more than the mass of the Earth. Limitations of the environment prevent exponential growth from proceeding indefinitely. Reasons for a slowdown in the growth rate include a lack of food, competition for other resources, predation, disease, accumulation of waste or lack of space, all acting more strongly to slow growth as the population becomes denser. Under these conditions, the growth curve may appear sigmoidal or logistic, as in the figure on the next page, with rapid exponential growth at first, followed by a slowing and levelling off of growth. In this curve, the population size at the point where the growth curve is flat is the maximum sustainable number of individuals, called the **carrying capacity**, and is observed when the birth rate and death rate are equal.

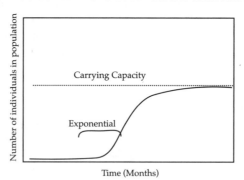

Logistic Population Growth

In natural populations, the environment is constantly changing, and the carrying capacity varies with it. For example, the carrying capacity for rabbits in a grassy plain will be greater in a year of plentiful rain and lush vegetation growth than in a year of drought. Populations often have regular fluctuations in size, suggesting that the carrying capacity changes in a periodic manner. If a population of rabbits consumes all available vegetation, the carrying capacity will be reduced and the population size will fall until the vegetation regrows and the carrying capacity for rabbits is increased once again. An example that is often used is the size of hare and lynx populations in Canada. In this environment, the primary food of the lynx is the hare. The hare population size regularly cycles up and then crashes, perhaps due to the rapid spread of disease in crowded conditions. The lynx population size cycles along with that of the hare, crashing in size after the hare population crashes, then building in size once again after the hare population rebounds.

The Role of the Abiotic Environment in Population Growth

The size and growth of a population are affected both by the biotic (living) and abiotic (non-living) portions of the environment. The abiotic portions include the air, water, soil, light and temperature that living organisms require. Not only are organisms dependent on the abiotic environment, but they in turn modify it. Plants create shade that alters the light environment for other plants, preserve water in the soil, consume carbon dioxide and produce oxygen. The modifications of the environment by a population affect the types of species the population lives in.

Chemical Cycles

Also included in the abiotic environment are inorganic chemicals required for life such as carbon and nitrogen. The movement of these essential elements between the biotic and abiotic environment forms cycles that are central to all life on Earth. Some organisms take the simple inorganic starting chemicals up from the soil and air and convert them into a biologically useful form. After material passes through the biological community, respiration and decay organisms return these chemicals to their inorganic state to begin the cycle again. If the following concepts are unclear, refer to chapter 11, Biochemistry for more information.

Carbon Cycle

The carbon cycle commences as gaseous CO_2 enters the living world when plants take it in and use it to produce glucose via photosynthesis. Plants use energy stored in glucose to make starch, proteins and fat.

Next, animals eat plants and use the digested nutrients to form carbohydrates, fats and proteins. Part of these organic compounds is used as fuel in respiration in plants and animals, releasing CO_2 into the air. Aside from expelled wastes, the rest of the organic carbon remains locked within an organism until its death, at which time decaying processes return the CO_2 to the air.

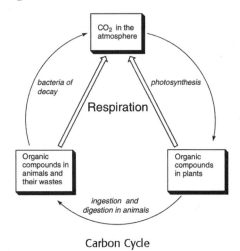

Carbon Cycle

Nitrogen Cycle

Nitrogen is an essential element of amino acids and nucleic acids, which are the building blocks for all living things. Since there is a finite amount of nitrogen on the Earth, it is important that it be recovered and reused.

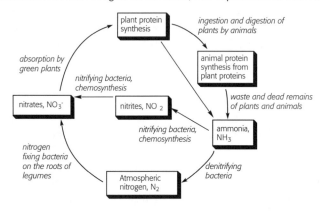

Nitrogen Cycle

The following bullets refer to the previous figure of the nitrogen cycle.

- Elemental (free) nitrogen, at the bottom of the figure, is chemically inert and cannot be used by most organisms. Lightning and nitrogen-fixing bacteria in the roots of legumes change the nitrogen to usable, soluble nitrates.

- The nitrates are absorbed by plants and are used to synthesise nucleic acids and plant proteins.

- Animals eat the plants and synthesise specific animal proteins from the plant proteins. Both plants and animals give off wastes and, eventually, die.

- The nitrogen locked up in the wastes and dead tissue is released by the process of decay, which converts the proteins into ammonia.

- Two fates await the ammonia (NH_3): part of it is nitrified to nitrites by chemosynthetic bacteria and then to usable nitrates by nitrifying bacteria. The rest of the ammonia is denitrified. This means that the ammonia is broken down to release free nitrogen, which returns us to the beginning of the cycle.

- Note that there are four kinds of bacteria: decaying, nitrifying, denitrifying and nitrogen-fixing. The bacteria have no use for the excretory ammonia, nitrites, nitrates and nitrogen they produce. These materials are essential, however, for the existence of other living organisms.

POPULATIONS IN COMMUNITIES AND ECOSYSTEMS

The next level of biological organization beyond a population is a **community**, which is all the interacting populations living together in an environment. The populations within a community interact with each other in a variety of ways, including **predation**, **competition** or **symbiosis**. These interactions affect the number of individuals in each population in the community and the number of different species in the community. The living community combined with the abiotic environment, the interactions between populations and the flow of energy and molecules within the system define an **ecosystem**.

Predation

Predation is the consumption of one organism by another, usually resulting in the death of the organism that is eaten. Both carnivores that consume meat, and herbivores, consuming plants only, are types of predators. Predation includes a zebra eating grass, a lion eating a zebra, a whale eating plankton, a paramecium eating yeast or a Venus flytrap eating a housefly. Predators often select weak or sick members of the prey population, removing alleles with poor fitness, and driving evolution in the prey towards more effective means of escaping predation. Predator and prey often coevolve, with the predator evolving to become more effective as the prey evolves to escape predation. Predator-prey relationships between populations in a community can influence the carrying capacity of prey populations involved and tend to achieve a balance such that the predator is effective enough to maintain its own population without decimating the prey it is dependent on. Predation can cause a community to maintain a greater diversity of species—without predation, one prey species will often predominate.

Competition and the Niche

A competitive relationship between populations in a community exists when different populations in the same location use a limiting resource. Competition can be **interspecific** (between species) or **intraspecific** (between organisms of the same species). Integral in understanding interspecific competition is the idea of the ecological **niche**. If the habitat is the physical environment in which the population lives, the niche is the way it lives within the habitat, including what it eats, where it lives, how it reproduces and all other aspects of the species that define the role it plays in the ecosystem. The niche occupied by each species is unique to that species and can, in part, define that species. Another way to understand the niche is to say that if the habitat is the address of a population, the niche is its profession.

Interspecific Competition

When two populations have overlap in their niches, such as by eating the same insects or occupying the same nesting sites, there is competition between the populations. The more the niches overlap, the greater the competition. Generally, when two populations compete, one will compete more effectively than the other and grow more rapidly. Competition can drive the less efficient population out of the community, with the "winner" occupying the niche on its own. Another result of competition for a niche can be that evolution drives the two populations to occupy niches that overlap less, reducing the competition. For example, if two species of related birds compete for the same nesting site, then they may evolve to reduce competition by using different nesting sites (see the following figure). Even in an environment with several different herbivores, their niches are unique since they evolve to have different heights, different sizes, different teeth and digestive tracts to avoid competition for the same plants. Several closely-related species of birds can live in the same tree and eat similar food, and yet occupy distinct niches by living in different part of the tree, with some near the crown, others in the middle and others still closer to the ground.

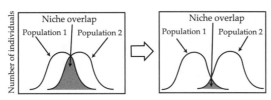

Evolution Drives Reduced Niche Overlap

Symbiosis

Symbionts live together in an intimate, often permanent association that may or may not be beneficial to them. Some symbiotic relationships are obligatory—that is, one or both organisms cannot survive without the other. Types of symbiotic relationships are generally classified according to the benefits the symbionts receive. Symbiotic relationships include commensalism, mutualism and parasitism.

Commensalism

In this relationship, one organism is benefited by the association and the other is not affected (this is symbolized as +/0). The host neither discourages nor fosters the relationship. The remora (sharksucker), for example, attaches itself to the underside of a shark. Through this association, the remora obtains the food the shark discards, wide geographic dispersal and protection from enemies. The shark is totally indifferent to the association. A similar association links the barnacle and the whale. The barnacle is a sessile crustacean that attaches to the whale and obtains wider feeding opportunities through its host's migrations.

Mutualism

This is a symbiotic relationship from which both organisms derive some benefit (+/+). In the instance of the tick bird and rhinoceros, the rhinoceros aids the bird through the provision of food in the form of parasites on its skin. The bird in its turn aids the rhinoceros by removing the parasites and by warning the rhinoceros of danger when it suddenly flies away.

Parasitism

A parasite takes from the host but gives nothing in return; thus, the parasite benefits at the expense of the host (+/−). Examples of parasites include leeches, ticks and sea lampreys. Parasitism exists when competition for food is most intense.

Intraspecific Competition

Competition is not restricted to interspecific interactions. Individuals belonging to the same species utilise the same resources; if a particular resource is limited, these organisms must compete with one another. Members of the same species compete, but they must also cooperate. Intraspecific cooperation may be extensive (as in the formation of societies in animal species) or may be nearly nonexistent. Hence, within a species, relationships between individuals are influenced by both disruptive and cohesive forces. Competition (for food or a mate, for example) is the chief disruptive force, while cohesive forces include reproduction and protection from predators and destructive weather.

COMMUNITY STRUCTURE

The populations within a community are organised in many different ways. Within the community, each population plays a different role depending on the source of energy for that population.

Producers

Producers are **autotrophs**, organisms that get energy from the environment (the sun or inorganic molecules) and use this energy along with simple molecules (carbon dioxide, water and minerals) to drive the biosynthesis of their own proteins, carbohydrates and lipids. The energy a producer such as a plant gets from the sun is stored in chemical bonds in the biological molecules it produces. Producers form the foundation of any community, passing on their energy to other organisms. In a terrestrial environment, green plants, photosynthetic bacteria or mosses are producers, using the energy of sunlight to produce biosynthetic energy through photosynthesis. In marine environments, green plants or algae are the main producers. There are even marine ecosystems at deep, dark ocean geothermal vents at which the entire community is based not on photosynthetic producers but on chemosynthetic bacteria that use the energy of inorganic molecules released from the volcanic vent to drive biosynthesis.

Consumers

Consumers get the energy to drive their own biosynthesis and to maintain life by ingesting and oxidising the complex molecules synthesised by other organisms. Since they get their energy by consuming other organisms, they are called **heterotrophs**. Herbivores (plant eaters), carnivores (meat eaters) and omnivores (eating both plants and animals) are all consumers. The adaptations of each consumer depend on the type of food it eats. Herbivores tend to have teeth for grinding and long digestive tracts that allow for the growth of symbiotic bacteria to digest cellulose found in plants. Carnivores are more likely to have pointed, fanglike teeth for catching and tearing prey and shorter digestive tracts than herbivores.

Primary consumers are animals that consume producers like green plants—for example, the cow, the grasshopper and the elephant. **Secondary consumers**, meanwhile, are carnivorous and consume primary consumers—for example, frogs, tigers and dragonflies. Finally, **tertiary consumers** feed on secondary consumers; examples include snakes that eat frogs.

Decay Organisms (Saprophytes)

Decay organisms, also called saprophytes or decomposers, are heterotrophs, since they derive their energy from oxidising complex biological molecules, but they do not consume living organisms. Decay organisms get energy from the biological organic molecules they encounter left as waste by producers and consumers, or the debris of dead organisms. They perform respiration to derive energy, and return carbon dioxide, nitrogen, phosphorus and other inorganic compounds to the environment to renew the cycles of these materials between the biotic and physical environments. Bacteria and fungi are the primary examples of decay organisms. Scavengers such as hyenas or vultures play a similar role, living on the stored chemical energy found in dead organisms.

THE FOOD WEB

The term **food chain** is often used to describe a community, depicting a simple linear relationship between a series of species, with one eating the other. For example, a food chain might contain grass as the producer, mice as the primary consumer, snakes as the secondary consumer and hawks as the tertiary consumer (see the following figure). The different levels in the food chain, such as producers and primary consumers, are sometimes called **trophic levels**. A more realistic depiction of the relationships within the community is a **food web,** in which every population interacts not with one other population, but several other populations. An animal in an ecosystem is often preyed on by several different predators, and predators commonly have a diet of several different prey, not just one. The greater the number of potential interactions in a community food web, the more stable the system will be, and the better able it will be to withstand and rebound from external pressures such as disease or weather.

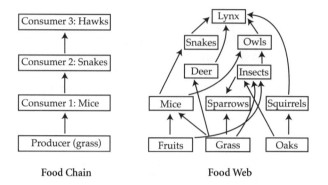

Food Chain   Food Web

ENERGY FLOW IN COMMUNITIES

Each trophic level in a food web contains different quantities of stored chemical energy in the populations it contains. When consumers eat producers and secondary consumers eat primary consumers, some energy is lost in each transfer from one level to another. As producers get energy from the sun, not all of the energy is converted into stored energy in chemical bonds. Some of the energy is lost at that level to the metabolic energy an organism requires to maintain its life. Plants consume some of the energy they produce in respiration to support their own metabolic activities. The total chemical energy generated by producers is **gross primary productivity**, and the total with losses to respiration subtracted is the **net primary productivity**.

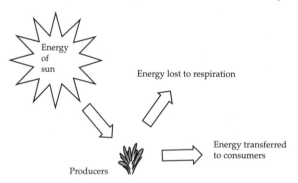

Energy Structure of a Community

At the next level of the energy pyramid, herbivores consume primary producers, incorporating about 10% of the energy consumed into their own stored chemical energy. The remainder is lost through respiration. Only about 10% of the stored chemical energy is present in the next higher trophic level at every stage (see the following figure). The energy contained in a community can be visualized as a **pyramid**, with the most energy in the producers and less energy at successive levels of consumers (see figure). The efficiency of energy transfer between levels can differ greatly from 10%, but the pyramid will always have the most energy in the producer level, with less in each level of consumers. A similar pyramid is observed if one compares the biomass or numbers of individuals in a community, with each successive level about 10% the size of the level beneath it. In terms of numbers, the shape of the pyramid can often vary, with a single large producer like a tree supporting a large number of primary consumers like birds or insects.

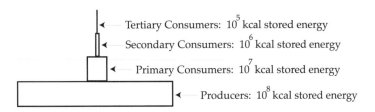

Food Pyramid

COMMUNITY DIVERSITY

The number of species within a community is termed the **community diversity**. The types of interactions between populations within a community affect the number of species in the community, as well as the physical environment. Predation has been observed as one factor that increases the diversity of species in a community, and competition may do the same through selective pressure driving populations into distinct niches. Warm environments like the tropics with very high productivity have the greatest diversity, and colder environments have less community diversity. Topographic diversity increases community diversity, perhaps by creating a greater number of niches in the environment. Larger land masses or ecosystems also have a greater community diversity.

Changes in Community over Time: Succession

Communities can change in composition over time, either as a result of a changing physical environment such as the climate or as the result of changes created by the populations that live in the community. When a population changes the environment it lives in, it may make the environment more favourable for some populations and less favourable for others, including itself. When a community changes as a result of organisms that live in the community, this is termed **succession**. For example, a grassland may provide abundant sunlight and rich soil that lead to colonisation by trees, followed by other trees that grow best in the shade of the pioneer trees. Successive communities are composed of populations best able to exist in each new set of conditions, both biotic and abiotic.

The community will continue to change until it arrives at a combination of populations that do not change the environment any further, leaving the community the same over time in what is called the **climax community**. The climax community is stable over time, with each generation leaving the environment it resides in the same, and it will remain in place unless it is disturbed by climate change, fire, humans or other catastrophes. If the climax community is disturbed, the series of community successions will begin again until a climax community is achieved once again. The type of climax community that is present in an environment depends on the abiotic factors of the ecosystem, including rainfall, temperature, soil and sunlight.

Here's an example of the progression of a climax community in an aquatic environment. This community starts with a pond:

- *Step 1—pond.* This pond contains plants such as algae and pondweed and animals such as protozoa, water insects and small fish.
- *Step 2—shallow water.* The pond begins to fill in with reeds, cattails and water lilies.
- *Step 3—moist land.* The former pond area is now filled with grass, herbs, shrubs, willow trees, frogs and snakes.
- *Step 4—woodland.* Pine or oak becomes the dominant tree of the climax community.

It is important to remember that the dominant species of the climax community is determined by such physical factors as temperature, nature of the soil and rainfall.

BIOMES

The conditions in a particular terrestrial and climatic region select plants and animals possessing suitable adaptations for that particular region. Each geographic region is inhabited by a distinct community called a **biome**.

Terrestrial Biomes

Land biomes are characterised and named according to the climax vegetation of the region in which they are found. The climax vegetation is the vegetation that becomes dominant and stable after years of evolutionary development. Since plants are important as food producers, they determine the nature of the inhabiting animal population; hence the climax vegetation determines the climax animal population. There are eight types of terrestrial biomes that can be formed as a result of all these factors:

- Tropical Forest
- Savanna
- Desert
- Temperate Deciduous Forest
- Northern Coniferous Forest
- Taiga
- Tundra
- Polar Region

Aquatic Biomes

In addition to the eight terrestrial biomes, there are aquatic biomes, each with its own characteristic plants and animals. More than 70% of the Earth's surface is covered by water, and most of the Earth's plant and animal life is found there. As much as 90% of the Earth's food and oxygen production (photosynthesis) takes place in the water. Aquatic biomes are classified according to criteria quite different from the criteria used to classify terrestrial biomes. Plants have little controlling influence in communities of aquatic biomes, as compared to their role in terrestrial biomes. Aquatic areas are also the most stable ecosystems on Earth. The conditions affecting temperature, amount of available oxygen and carbon dioxide and amount of suspended or dissolved materials are stable over very large areas, and show little tendency to change. For these reasons, aquatic food webs and aquatic communities tend to be balanced. There are two types of major aquatic biomes:

- Marine
- Freshwater

REVIEW QUESTIONS

1. A snake eats frogs, which eat grasshoppers. The snake is an example of a

    (A) primary consumer
    (B) secondary consumer
    (C) producer
    (D) tertiary consumer
    (E) decomposer

2. A stable ecosystem

    (A) requires a constant energy source
    (B) requires a living system
    (C) is self-sustaining
    (D) requires cycling of materials between the living system and the environment
    (E) all of the above

3. Mutualism is exemplified by

    (A) lichens
    (B) tapeworms
    (C) bread mould
    (D) nematodes

4. In an ecosystem, the greatest amount of stored chemical bond energy is generally found in

    (A) primary producers
    (B) secondary producers
    (C) primary consumers
    (D) secondary consumers
    (E) tertiary consumers

5. In a pond community, the greatest mass present would consist of

    (A) algae
    (B) insects
    (C) frogs
    (D) fish
    (E) fungi

6. A climax community

   (A) consists of only one species of life

   (B) is populated mainly by so-called pioneer organisms

   (C) is stable within a given climate

   (D) is independent of the environment

7. Living in a close nutritional relationship with another organism in which one organism benefits while the other is neither harmed nor benefited is best defined as

   (A) symbiosis

   (B) mutualism

   (C) commensalism

   (D) parasitism

8. Digestion of cellulose by protozoans found in a termite's gut is an example of

   (A) mutualism

   (B) parasitism

   (C) autotropism

   (D) commensalism

Answers and Explanations

1. D

Grasshoppers are primary consumers (they eat plants). The frog that eats these herbivorous insects is the secondary consumer, while the snake that eats the frogs is a tertiary consumer.

2. E

A stable ecosystem is self-sustaining and will therefore remain stable in the presence of a relatively stable physical environment (abiotic factors) and a relatively stable biotic community. A stable ecosystem requires a constant energy source, a living system incorporating this energy into organic compounds and a cycling of materials between the living system and the environment.

3. A

Mutualism is a close nutritional relationship between two species in which both benefit. Lichen is the result of a mutualistic relationship between fungi and algae. The algae attach to a rock via rootlets that the fungi produce. Through these rootlets, the fungus receives water, nutrients and an attachment, the lichen. The algae in its turn receives an attachment (lichen) to the rock, and can produce carbohydrates through photosynthetically utilising the water and nutrients from the fungus' rootlets. This is considered a +/+ situation. Tapeworms (B) are parasites. The tapeworm gets nutrition from the host as the host loses it, a +/− situation. Saprophytes, such as bread mould (C), are organisms that feed on dead and decaying material, while nematodes (D) are either free-living saprophytes or parasites.

4. A

In an ecosystem, the greatest amount of energy is always found among primary producers. Primary producers are either plants or photosynthetic bacteria. Energy is lost with each level in the pyramid, as it is utilised for maintenance of the organism, movement, and warmth. Only a fraction of the energy produced becomes new tissue that can be harvested by the next level up in the pyramid. Primary consumers are herbivores, while carnivores that ingest the herbivores are known as secondary consumers. They in their turn are preyed upon by tertiary consumers.

5. A

In an ecology pyramid, the primary producers (photosynthetic or chemosynthetic organisms, such as algae) are always the largest population. (B) and (E) are primary consumers, while (D) and (C) are secondary consumers.

6. C

A climax community is the final community in a particular biome's succession. (A) is incorrect because many species will live in a community. Meanwhile, pioneer species (B) are the species that colonise a biome, such as lichen on rocks, and are therefore the earliest species in a succession. (D) The climax community is dependent on the environment, especially the climate; factors such as type of soil and amount of rainfall will determine what organisms will survive and thrive there.

7. C

In a commensal relationship, which is a form of a symbiotic relationship, two organisms live in close association with each other. One benefits from this association, while the other is neither harmed nor benefited (in what is sometimes described as a "+/0" relationship). An example of a commensal relationship is the epiphyte plant, which lives on the branches of rainforest trees, gaining the advantage of being closer to sunlight.

8. A

Both the termite and the protozoans benefit. Termites cannot actually digest cellulose, but protozoans in their digestive systems can. In return, these tiny organisms receive a home and food and water. The terms mutualism, parasitism (B), autotropism (C) and commensalism (D) do not describe the example provided in the question.

Chapter 11: **Biochemistry**

This chapter reviews the essentials of biochemistry. It begins with a brief review of water, its properties and its importance. Other biological molecules including carbohydrates, lipids, proteins, enzymes and nucleic acids are also discussed. Finally, glycolysis, aerobic respiration, fermentation, the Krebs cycle and photosynthesis are explained in detail. Please note that some concepts from chemistry are mentioned here. For more information on chemistry, see Section V.

THE ROLE OF CARBON

At the elemental level, all life is composed primarily of carbon, hydrogen, oxygen, nitrogen, phosphorus and sulphur, with traces of other elements like iron, iodine, magnesium, and calcium that are also essential for life. Salts like sodium chloride are also essential components of life, but since they do not contain carbon they are known as **inorganic compounds.**

Chemicals that contain carbon are called **organic compounds**, and include the major types of biological molecules found in all organisms, including proteins, lipids, carbohydrates and nucleic acids. Before these molecules are discussed, first review a vastly important and seldom appreciated molecule of life: water.

WATER

Life is not possible without water. The presence of liquid water allowed life to evolve and to persist on Earth. The unique properties of water that allow it to play this role are based on the way the water molecule is put together. Each water molecule is composed of an atom of oxygen with two hydrogens attached at an angle. Oxygen draws the electrons in the molecule toward itself, giving itself a partial negative charge, while the hydrogens are partially positive. The water molecule as a whole is not charged but since the molecule is bent its unequal charge distribution makes one end positive and the other end negative. This unequal distribution of charge is called a **dipole moment**. When water molecules are together in a beaker, they interact with each other, with the partial positive and negative charges attracting each other, interactions called **hydrogen bonds**.

The strong hydrogen bonds between water molecules give water its many special properties. These bonds between water molecules that hold the molecules together give water structure and take a lot of energy to break. Hydrogen bonds give water a great deal of cohesion and surface tension compared to other liquids, allowing trees to transport water from their roots all the way to their leaves in a single long column of water. Bonds between water molecules also mean that it takes a great deal of energy to heat water and to make it boil compared to other liquids. Remember, heat in a liquid or gas is carried in the movement of the molecules: more heat means more rapid movement of molecules. When you add heat energy to water, the energy must break bonds between molecules before it can increase their movement to increase the temperature of the water. Liquid hydrocarbons, like octane, in contrast, have very low boiling points because the molecules in the liquid are held together very weakly and when heat is added the molecules easily move about rapidly (heat) and leave the liquid (boil). The great deal of energy that water requires to heat or boil means that our body temperature is stable and we can cool ourselves through evaporation using sweat. Water's ability to absorb heat also means that water remains liquid over a range of temperatures common on our planet.

Solutions in Water

In a solution, the substance that does the dissolving is called the **solvent**, and the molecules that are dissolved are called the **solute**. Since solutions and solutes are important in biology, we will talk a little more about measurements and calculations of solutions and about special classes of solutes called acids and bases.

Most biological reactions occur in water with solutes. Concentration is measured by **molarity**, which is the number of moles of solute in one litre. A **mole** is 6×10^{23} molecules of a substance, and has a specific weight called the molecular weight. For example, the molecular weight of salt, NaCl, is 28. Therefore, to obtain one mole of NaCl, 28 grams must be weighed out.

One mole of one substance has the same number of molecules as a mole of another substance even if it does not have the same weight. The unit of concentration used in chemistry and biology is **molar** (M). A 1 molar (1M) solution contains 1 mole of solute in 1 litre of solution. To make a one-litre solution with one mole of NaCl, we would weigh out 28 grams of NaCl and completely dissolve it in water. Then we would bring the total volume to one litre and this would be a one-molar (1M) solution of NaCl.

Acids and Bases

Acids and **bases** are particularly important types of solutes in biology. There are a few different ways that science defines acids and bases. For our purposes, an acid is defined as a proton donor and a base is a proton acceptor. A proton (H^+) is a hydrogen atom stripped of its single electron leaving a positively charged proton.

pH Scale

The concentration of hydrogen ions can be expressed as molar, but it can be hard to compare the acidity of solutions this way. Another common way to express the concentration of protons in a solution is by expressing them as a pH. The pH $= -\log[H^+]$, where $[H^+]$ is the concentration of hydrogen ions given in units of molarity. Thus, if the concentration of protons in solution is 10^{-8} M, then the pH $= 8$. The pH for acidic solutions is less than 7 and the pH of basic solutions is greater than 7. In the human body, the pH in the blood and tissues is about 7.4. This pH is carefully maintained and controlled since large changes in pH can harm cells and tissues.

OTHER BIOLOGICAL MOLECULES

There are a few other biological molecules you should be familiar with. These are carbohydrates, lipids, proteins, enzymes and nucleic acids. A description of each follows.

Carbohydrates

One of the main classes of biological molecules is **carbohydrates**, or sugars. Another name for carbohydrates is **saccharides**. The functions of carbohydrates include important roles in energy metabolism and storage, and structure of the cell and organisms. One carbohydrate, **cellulose**, provides the cell wall of plants, and is the singularly most abundant biological molecule on Earth. Carbohydrates are a short-term energy source due primarily to their structure.

Carbohydrates are built from simple building blocks, starting with simple sugars that have only a single sugar unit. Simple sugars are called **monosaccharides**, sugars with two subunits are called **disaccharides** and sugars with lots of subunits are called **polysaccharides**. All carbohydrates are composed of carbon, hydrogen and oxygen. Simple sugars have the general molecular formula $C_nH_{2n}O_n$.

Lipids (Fats and Oils)

Lipids are very nonpolar, or hydrophobic, molecules. They are composed mostly of nonpolar bonds, and tend to repel water. The structure of lipids allows them to play important roles in energy metabolism and in cellular membranes. Like carbohydrates, lipids are composed of carbon, hydrogen and oxygen, but lipids are very distinct from carbohydrates in their structure and function. Lipids have much lower oxygen content than carbohydrates and are less oxidised, storing more energy than carbohydrates.

Proteins

Carbohydrates and lipids provide energy and structure for cells. There is much more to life, however, than these functions. One of the characteristics of life is that it is very active, with cells continually carrying out a broad range of functions in order to grow, reproduce and survive. **Proteins** provide cells with the ability to carry out these functions, including the following:

Type of Protein	Functions	Examples
Hormonal	Chemical messengers	Insulin, glucagon
Transport	Transport of other substances	Haemoglobin, carrier proteins
Structural	Physical support	Collagen
Contractile	Movement	Actin/myosin
Antibodies	Immune defence	Immunoglobulins, interferons
Enzymes	Biological catalysts	Amylase, lipase, ATPase

The basic structure of proteins is formed by joining amino acids together in a chain with **peptide bonds**, creating a string of amino acids called a **polypeptide.**

Enzymes

Life uses chemistry to build, to generate energy, to move and to perform other functions. Many of these reactions would either occur very slowly or not at all on their own if the chemicals involved were simply mixed in a tube. **Enzymes** act as biological catalysts to speed up these reactions and make them useful for living organisms.

Nucleic Acids

Nucleic acids are another class of the essential biological molecules found in all living organisms, acting as informational molecules, including deoxyribonucleic acid (DNA) and ribonucleic acid (RNA). All organisms (except for some viruses) use DNA as their genome. The structure and function of nucleic acids is addressed in chapter 9, Genetics and Evolution.

HOW CELLS GET ENERGY TO MAKE ATP

Organisms eat carbohydrates and fats that contain chemical energy, digesting these molecules to trap their chemical energy in a molecule called ATP. ATP is then used in the cells to do most activities that require energy input to occur.

ATP, adenosine triphosphate, consists of adenosine, and three phosphate groups, a triphosphate. Each phosphate is negatively charged, and negative charges repel each other. Having three negative charges close together in the triphosphate stores a lot of energy, and when the triphosphate is split the energy is released, driving forward important cellular functions.

Cells in humans and other organisms use a common set of biochemical reactions to make ATP, pathways including **glycolysis**, the **Krebs cycle** and **electron transport**. It starts with glucose. In humans, glucose is present in the blood as a fuel for all cells. Cells take in glucose, which then enters the glycolytic pathway as the first step in the path to ATP.

GLYCOLYSIS

A metabolic pathway is a linked series of biochemical reactions that have a common purpose. **Glycolysis** is the first biochemical pathway in the capture of energy from glucose to make ATP. The glycolytic pathway consists of ten steps, each catalysed by an enzyme uniquely evolved to catalyse that reaction. (This chapter will not review all of the individual reactions or the individual enzymes, but being familiar with the idea of metabolic pathways and the function of glycolysis is a good idea.) Glycolysis takes glucose, a sugar molecule with six carbon atoms, and breaks it into two pyruvate molecules, each with three carbons, capturing energy in two different ways.

One way to capture energy is to directly produce ATP as part of the glycolytic pathway. At two different steps in the pathway, ATP is put into the reaction to drive the splitting of glucose, consuming 2 ATP molecules for each glucose molecule that enters the top of the pathway. Further along in the pathway 4 ATP are generated, for a net production of 2 ATP per glucose molecule.

This is not where most of the energy of glucose is extracted, however. In the burning of fuels to extract energy, the fuel molecules become more and more oxidised, and have less energy, releasing their energy to their surroundings. If you take a sugar cube and burn it, the sugar molecules are oxidised directly to carbon dioxide and release their energy rapidly as heat. In the body, the oxidation of glucose is more controlled, and the energy is transferred to other molecules that carry the energy and transfer it later in the process to make ATP. In glycolysis, glucose is oxidised to form pyruvate, and some of the energy is captured to make NADH, an energy carrier the cell uses to make ATP through electron transport, as we will see.

If you add up all of the reactions of glycolysis, the overall net reaction describing this whole reaction pathway becomes:

Glucose + 2Pi + 2ADP + 2NAD$^+$→

2 pyruvate + 2ATP + 2NADH + 2H$^+$ + 2H$_2$0

In eukaryotic cells, glycolysis occurs in the cytoplasm. In prokaryotes, where there are no organelles, all reactions occur in the same compartment.

Fermentation

Since NAD$^+$ is required for glycolysis, and it is converted to NADH as part of glycolysis, NAD$^+$ must be regenerated or glycolysis would run out of it and stop, halting ATP production. The NAD$^+$ is regenerated in one of two ways. In the first, NADH goes on to the electron transport chain and is used to produce more ATP, as described in the sections that follow, being converted back to NAD$^+$ in the process. The second way to regenerate NAD$^+$ occurs in the absence of oxygen or in anaerobic organisms that do not use oxidative metabolism. This alternate pathway is called **fermentation.**

Fermentation allows glycolysis to continue even in the absence of oxygen. In fermentation, NADH is regenerated back to NAD$^+$ in the absence of oxygen to allow glycolysis to continue to produce ATP, producing either ethanol or lactic acid as byproducts. **Ethanol fermentation** is carried out by yeast in the absence of oxygen and is used to make beer and wine. The first step in ethanol fermentation occurs when pyruvate is decarboxylated (loses a CO_2) to become the two-carbon molecule acetaldehyde. NADH from glycolysis then reduces acetaldehyde to ethanol and is itself oxidised back to NAD$^+$. The regenerated NAD$^+$ allows glycolysis to proceed and to continue ATP production. This process can continue until the alcohol level rises so high that it kills the organisms producing it.

Lactic acid fermentation occurs in some bacteria and fungi and in human muscles during strenuous exercise. Fermentation in muscle allows ATP production to continue when oxygen in the muscle is limited because it is consumed more rapidly than the blood stream can supply it. In lactic acid fermentation, pyruvate is reduced to lactic acid by NADH that is oxidised to regenerate NAD$^+$. The NAD$^+$ then allows glycolysis and ATP production to proceed. During exercise, the lactic acid produced can accumulate in muscle and cause pain as well as a drop in blood pH. After the exercise is complete, the lactic acid will be oxidised back to pyruvate to reenter oxidative metabolism pathways.

AEROBIC RESPIRATION

Although glycolysis produces two ATP and two NADH for every molecule of glucose, this is not where the eukaryotic cell extracts most of its energy from glucose. Glycolysis is only the beginning; aerobic respiration is the rest of the story. In aerobic respiration, glucose is fully burned by the cell as an energy source, going through the Krebs cycle and electron transport to trap energy ultimately used to make ATP.

The pyruvate left at the end of glycolysis still contains a great deal of energy that is extracted in **oxidative metabolism**. Oxidative metabolism of glucose produces a maximum total of 38 ATP in the complete oxidation of one glucose molecule, compared to two from glycolysis (or fermentation) alone (note that the actual total is 36 ATP/glucose in eukaryotes due to a slight energy cost for transport into the mitochondria). Oxidative respiration is a far more efficient energy production system than glycolysis or fermentation, so the ability to perform oxidative respiration gives organisms a competitive advantage in conditions where oxygen is available.

To accomplish this more efficient energy production, pyruvate from glycolysis is oxidised all the way to carbon dioxide in a pathway called the Krebs cycle. The Krebs cycle and the other steps of oxidative metabolism occur in mitochondria. As pyruvate is oxidised in the Krebs cycle, NADH and another high-energy electron carrier called FADH$_2$ are produced. In electron transport, the energy of these high-energy electron carriers creates a pH gradient by pumping protons (H$^+$ ions) out of the mitochondria. The energy of this pH gradient drives ATP synthesis, and this is the ultimate source of most of the ATP produced in the oxidative metabolism of glucose.

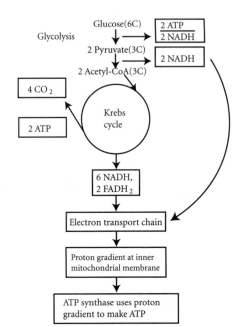

Aerobic Respiration

THE KREBS CYCLE

The **Krebs cycle**, also called the citric acid cycle or tricarboxylic acid cycle, is a series of reactions linked in a circle that extracts energy from the products of glycolysis to make the high-energy electron carriers NADH and $FADH_2$. In aerobic conditions, when oxygen is present, the pyruvate produced in the cytoplasm in glycolysis is transported through both mitochondrial membranes into the interior of the mitochondria. Here, pyruvate is converted into a two-carbon molecule called acetate, with the release of CO_2, linked to a large carrier molecule called coenzyme A, to make acetyl-coenzyme A. The oxidation of pyruvate to acetyl-CoA also produces more NADH that will go on to make ATP via the electron transport chain.

$$Pyruvate + CoA + NAD^+ \rightarrow acetyl\text{-}CoA + CO_2 + NADH$$

Acetyl-CoA is an important metabolic junction in the cell, and is involved in many different metabolic pathways. Acetyl-CoA enters the Krebs cycle by combining with a four-carbon intermediate to make the six-carbon citrate (or citric acid). In every complete loop of the Krebs cycle, two CO_2 molecules are produced and leave the cycle for every atom of acetyl-CoA that enters the cycle. This leaves the net level of intermediates in the cycle constant and regenerates the four-carbon intermediate that combines with another acetyl-CoA in the next round of the cycle. Every cycle also produces three NADH, one $FADH_2$ and one ATP. Since two acetyl-CoAs are produced from every glucose, the net result of the Krebs cycle is (for each glucose that enters glycolysis):

$$2\ Acetyl\text{-}CoA + 6NAD^+ + 2FAD + 2ADP + 2Pi + 4H_2O \rightarrow$$

$$4CO_2 + 6NADH + 2FADH_2 + 2ATP + 4H^+ + 2CoA$$

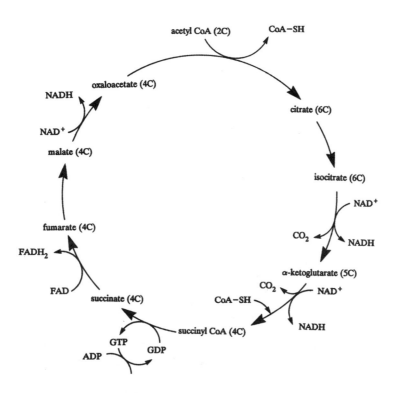

ELECTRON TRANSPORT

Glycolysis directly produces two ATP for every glucose, and the Krebs cycle directly produces two more ATP for every glucose. However, most of the energy of glucose is not extracted directly into ATP. The high-energy electron carriers NADH and $FADH_2$ contain much more of the energy that is extracted by the oxidation of glucose in glycolysis and the Krebs cycle.

Electron transport is the mechanism used to convert the energy held by these carriers into a more useful form that ultimately results in ATP production.

The electron transport chain is a series of proteins and electron carriers located in the inner mitochondrial membrane. NADH and $FADH_2$ transfer the high-energy electrons they carry to the chain and are oxidised back to NAD^+ and $FADH^+$, respectively. The high-energy electrons that enter the electron transport chain are transferred from one carrier to another, transferring energy to the carriers along the way. The carriers alternate between oxidised and reduced forms as they transfer electrons through the chain to the final electron acceptor at the end of the chain, oxygen, which is reduced to water. This oxygen is the oxygen needed for aerobic respiration and the oxygen we breathe and transport throughout the body. As electrons move through the series of oxidation-reduction reactions in the electron transport chain, their energy is used at three points in the chain to pump protons, hydrogen ions, out of the mitochondrial interior. The pumping of these H^+ ions out of mitochondria creates a pH gradient across the inner mitochondrial membrane, yet another form of energy conversion in the process of converting the energy in food into ATP. We still have not made ATP, but we are getting close. When anything is pumped against a concentration gradient, that concentration gradient contains energy. The inner mitochondrial membrane forms a tight seal that protons cannot leak through so once the protons are pumped out of mitochondria, their energy is stored. The next step is to take the energy and use it to make ATP.

A protein called **ATP synthase** found in the inner mitochondrial membrane harvests the energy of the pH gradient to produce the bulk of the ATP from oxidative glucose metabolism. ATP synthase allows the protons on the outside of the mitochondria to flow down their concentration gradient back into the mitochondria. Protons do not freely diffuse through the membrane, however. ATP synthase harnesses the energy of proton movement down the gradient through ATP synthase itself to make ATP, making three ATP for every NADH that enters electron transport and two ATP for every $FADH_2$ that enters electron transport.

The Krebs cycle, electron transport, production of the proton gradient and ATP production are all linked. If oxygen is removed, all of these processes stop, since they are all dependent on each other. If metabolic poisons allow protons to flow into mitochondria through the membrane, without going through ATP synthase, then the proton gradient will be destroyed. In this case, ATP production is said to be uncoupled from the Krebs cycle and electron transport, since ATP production would cease although the Krebs cycle and electron transport would increase their rate of activity. If metabolic needs of the cell increase, then all of these processes increase in rate. In this way the cell regulates ATP production and the associated pathways to meet its own needs.

PHOTOSYNTHESIS

Plants are **autotrophs**, or self-feeders, that generate their own chemical energy from the energy of the sun through photosynthesis. Photosynthesis occurs in plants in the **chloroplast**, an organelle that is specific to plants. In algae, a prokaryote, there are no chloroplasts, and photosynthesis occurs throughout the cytoplasm. Chloroplasts are found mainly in the cells of the **mesophyl**, the green tissue in the interior of the leaf. The leaf contains pores in its surface called **stomata** that allow carbon dioxide in and oxygen out to facilitate photosynthesis in the leaf. The chloroplast has an inner and outer membrane and within the inner membrane a fluid called the **stroma**. In addition, the interior of the chloroplast contains a series of membranes called the **thylakoid membranes** that form stacks called **grana**.

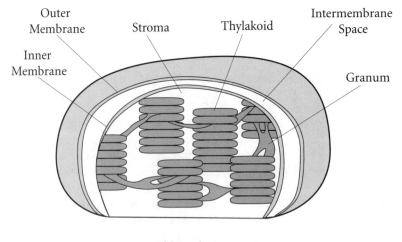

Chloroplast

Photosynthesis can be summarised with this equation:

$$6CO_2 + 12H_2O + light \rightarrow C_6H_{12}O_6 + 6O_2 + 6H_2O$$

Photosynthesis involves the reduction of CO_2 to a carbohydrate. It can be characterised as the reverse of respiration, in that reduction of CO_2 to produce glucose occurs instead of oxidation of glucose to make CO_2. One of the by-products of photosynthesis, oxygen, is of keen interest since it is the source of the oxygen that humans need to survive.

Photosythesis has two main parts, the **light reaction** and the **Calvin cycle**. The light reaction occurs in the interior of the thylakoid while the Calvin cycle occurs in the stroma. Plants are green because they reflect green color the most. The pigments involved in photosynthesis absorb the most strongly in the red and blue wavelengths.

Calvin Cycle

The Calvin cycle, also known as the "dark cycle", creates carbohydrates using the energy of ATP and the reducing power of NADPH produced in the light reactions. The carbon used in the creation of carbohydrates comes from atmospheric carbon dioxide, CO_2, so the process is sometimes called **carbon fixation**. CO_2 first combines with, or "is fixed to", ribulose bisphosphate, a five-carbon sugar with two phosphate groups attached. The resulting six-carbon compound is promptly split, resulting in the formation of two molecules of 3-phosphoglycerate, a three-carbon compound. The 3- phosphoglycerate is then phosphorylated by ATP and reduced by NADPH, which leads to the formation of glyceraldehyde 3-phosphate. This molecule can then be utilized as a starting point for the synthesis of glucose.

REVIEW QUESTIONS

1. Which of the following is NOT a biochemical reaction that makes ATP?

    (A) Krebs cycle
    (B) glycolyis
    (C) photosystem I
    (D) electron transport

2. Which is NOT a characteristic of proteins?

    (A) They contain genetic information.
    (B) They can act as hormones.
    (C) They can catalyze chemical reactions.
    (D) They act in cell membrane trafficking.
    (E) They can bind foreign materials.

3. Which of the following statements about the Krebs cycle is NOT true?

    (A) The Krebs cycle occurs in the matrix of the mitochondrion.
    (B) The Krebs cycle is linked to glycolysis by pyruvate.
    (C) The Krebs cycle is the single greatest direct source of ATP in the cell.
    (D) Citrate is an intermediate in the Krebs cycle.
    (E) The Krebs cycle produces nucleotides such as NADH and $FADH_2$.

4. The source of oxygen given off in photosynthesis is

   (A) water

   (B) carbon dioxide

   (C) glucose

   (D) starch

   (E) chlorophyll

5. Which of the following is NOT characteristic of fermentation?

   (A) It is anaerobic.

   (B) It requires glucose.

   (C) It produces energy.

   (D) It requires oxygen.

   (E) It produces ethanol.

6. Which part of cellular respiration directly produces a pH gradient during the oxidative metabolism of glucose?

   (A) glycolysis

   (B) anaerobic respiration

   (C) Krebs cycle

   (D) electron transport chain

Answers and Explanations

1. C

Photosystem I is not a biochemical reaction that makes ATP. Photosystem I is one of the systems of photosyntheses, but it is not itself a biochemical reaction.

2. A

Proteins may function as hormones (chemical messengers), enzymes (catalysts of chemical reactions), structural proteins (providers of physical support), transport proteins (carriers of important materials) and antibodies (binders of foreign particles). DNA is the only molecule in eukaryotes that contains genes.

3. C

The single greatest direct source of ATP in the cell is the proton gradient created by the electron transport chain, not the Krebs cycle. The Krebs cycle does occur in the matrix of the mitochondria (A), however, and oxidative phosphorylation (the electron transport chain) does occur in the inner membrane of the mitochondria known as the cristae. Citrate is an intermediate in this cycle (D). The Krebs cycle only forms two ATP directly; all of the other ATP that form during this cycle are produced when NADH and $FADH_2$ donate their electrons to the electron transport chain, which pumps protons so that ATP synthase can use the proton gradient to make ATP.

4. **A**

In the light reaction, light splits H_2O into excited electrons, H^+ and O_2. The excited electrons go on to form ATP and the H^+ electrons are incorporated into the carbohydrates produced during the dark reaction. O_2 is released into the environment as a waste product of this reaction. In choice (B), CO_2 donates the carbon and the oxygen required for carbohydrate formation in the dark reaction. Choices (C) and (D) are end products of photosynthesis, and choice (E), chlorophyll, is involved in the initial capture of sunlight.

5. **D**

Fermentation is a process that occurs during anaerobic respiration in organisms such as yeast. Glucose is converted to pyruvic acid, producing ATP. Then pyruvic acid is changed into ethyl alcohol, a waste product of the fermentation process. Fermentation produces energy but does not require oxygen. The oxygen-requiring reactions of respiration occur in aerobic respiration, not in fermentation, and they occur as NADH and $FADH_2$ molecules produced in the Krebs cycle are sent to the electron-transport chain for the production of ATPs. The final electron acceptor in these reactions is oxygen. In fermentation, there is no aerobic stage, and ATP is never produced through a Krebs cycle and electron transport chain mechanism.

6. **D**

The electron transport chain directly produces the pH gradient by pumping protons out of the mitochondrial matrix. This proton gradient is used to make ATP.

PART V

Essential Chemistry Review

Chapter 12: **Atomic Structure and Bonding**

This chapter details the structure of atoms and molecules. Topics include protons, neutrons, electrons and mass numbers, as well as the different types of bonding, such as chemical and covalent bonding. Practice questions at the end of the chapter will test your knowledge of these topics.

ATOMIC STRUCTURE

The **atom** is the basic building block of matter, representing the smallest unit of a chemical element. An atom in turn is composed of **subatomic particles** called protons, neutrons, and electrons. In 1911, Ernest Rutherford provided experimental evidence that an atom has a dense, positively charged nucleus that accounts for only a small portion of the volume of the atom. The protons and neutrons in an atom form the **nucleus**, the core of the atom. The electrons exist outside the nucleus in characteristic regions of space called **orbitals**. All atoms of an element show similar chemical properties and cannot be further broken down by chemical means.

Subatomic Particles

There are three kinds of particles found in a typical atom: **protons** and **neutrons**, which together make up the nucleus, and **electrons**, which are found in specific regions of space (orbitals) around the nucleus.

Protons

Protons carry a single positive charge and have a mass of approximately one **atomic mass unit** or **amu** (see following table). The **atomic number (Z)** of an element is equal to the number of protons found in an atom of that element. All atoms of a given element have the same atomic number; in other words, the number of protons an atom has defines what kind of element it is. The atomic number of an element can be found in the Periodic Table (see chapter 13) as an integer above the symbol for the element.

Neutrons

Neutrons carry no charge and have a mass only slightly larger than that of protons. The total number of neutrons and protons in an atom, known as the **mass number (A)**, determines its mass.

The convention $^A_Z X$ is used to show both the atomic number and mass number of an X atom, where Z is the atomic number and A is the mass number. Even though the number of protons must be the same for all atoms of an element, the number of neutrons, and hence the mass number, can be different. Atoms of the same element with different masses are known as **isotopes** of one another. Isotopes are referred to either by the convention previously described or, more commonly, by the name of the element followed by the mass number. For example, carbon-12 is a carbon atom with 6 protons and 6 neutrons, while carbon-14 is a carbon atom with 6 protons and 8 neutrons. Since isotopes have the same number of protons and electrons, they generally exhibit the same chemical properties.

Electrons

Electrons carry a charge equal in magnitude but opposite in sign to that of protons. An electron has a very small mass, approximately $\dfrac{1}{1837}$ the mass of a proton or neutron, which is negligible for most purposes. The electrons farthest from the nucleus are known as **valence electrons**. The farther the valence electrons are from the nucleus, the weaker the attractive force of the positively charged nucleus and the more likely the valence electrons are to be influenced by other atoms. Generally, the valence electrons and their activity determine the **reactivity** of an atom. In a neutral atom, the number of electrons is equal to the number of protons. A positive or negative charge on an atom is due to a loss or gain of electrons; the result is called an **ion**. A positively charged ion (one that has lost electrons) is known as a **cation**; a negatively charged ion (one that has gained electrons) is known as an **anion**. Some basic features of the three subatomic particles are summarised in the following table.

Subatomic Particle	Symbol	Relative Mass	Charge	Location
Proton	$^1_1 H$	1	+1	Nucleus
Neutron	$^1_0 N$	1	0	Nucleus
Electron	e^-	0	−1	Electron Orbitals

ATOMIC WEIGHTS AND ISOTOPES

To report the mass of something, one generally gives a number together with a unit such as kilograms (kg), grams (g), et cetera. Because the mass of an atom is so small, however, these units are not very convenient, and new ways have been devised to describe how much an atom weighs. A unit that can be used to report the mass of an atom is the previously mentioned atomic mass unit (amu). One amu is approximately the same as 1.66×10^{-24} g. How is this particular value chosen? The answer is that it is chosen so that a carbon-12 atom, with 6 protons and 6 neutrons, will have a mass of 12 amu. In other words, the amu is defined as one-twelfth the mass of the carbon-12 atom. It does not convert neatly to grams because the mass of a carbon-12 atom in grams is not a nice round number. In addition, since the mass of an electron is negligible, all the mass of the carbon-12 atom is considered to come from protons and neutrons.

Since the mass of a proton is about the same as that of a neutron, and there are 6 of each in the carbon-12 atom, protons and neutrons are considered to have a mass of $\frac{1}{12} \times 12$ amu $= 1$ amu each.

While it is necessary to have a way of describing the weight of an individual atom, in real life one generally works with a huge number of them at a time. The atomic weight is the mass in grams of **one mole (mol)** of atoms. Just like a pair corresponds to two, and a dozen corresponds to twelve, a mole corresponds to about 6.022×10^{23}. The atomic weight of an element, expressed in terms of g/mol, therefore, is the mass in grams of 6.022×10^{23} atoms of that element. This number, roughly 6.022×10^{23}, to which a mole corresponds, is known as **Avogadro's number**. Why this particular value and not something like 1.0×10^{-24}, for example? Once again, the answer lies in the carbon-12 atom: a mole of carbon-12 atoms weigh exactly 12 g. In other words, a mole is defined as the number of atoms in 12 g of carbon-12. A mole of atoms of an element heavier than carbon-12 (such as oxygen) would have an atomic weight higher than 12 g/mol, while a mole of atoms of an element lighter than carbon-12 (such as helium) would have an atomic weight less than 12 g/mol. Six g of carbon-12 would mean 3.011×10^{23} carbon-12 atoms, et cetera.

Avogadro's number serves as a conversion factor between one of something and a mole of something. Since 12 amu is the mass of 1 carbon-12 atom while 12 g is the mass of 1 mole of carbon-12 atoms, Avogadro's number also helps to convert between the mass units.

Specifically:

$$12 \text{ amu} \times (6.022 \times 10^{23}) = 12 \text{ g}$$

$$1 \text{ amu} = \frac{1 \text{g}}{6.022 \times 10^{23}} = 1.66 \times 10^{-24} \text{ g}$$

which is the conversion factor previously given. Note how this is derived from (or related to) the concept of the mole.

The **atomic weight** of an element is also found in the Periodic Table, as the number appearing below the symbol for the element. Notice, however, that these numbers are not whole numbers, which is odd considering that a proton and a neutron each have a mass of 1 amu and an atom can only have a whole number of these. Furthermore, even carbon, the element with which the standard is set, does not have a mass of 12.000 exactly. This is due to the presence of isotopes, as previously mentioned. The masses listed in the Periodic Table are weighted averages that account for the relative abundance of various isotopes. The word *weighted* is important: It is not simply the average of the masses of individual isotopes, but takes into account how frequently one encounters that isotope in a common sample of the element. There are, for example, 3 isotopes of hydrogen, with 0, 1 and 2 neutrons respectively. Together with the one proton that makes it hydrogen in the first place, the mass numbers for these isotopes are 1, 2 and 3. The atomic weight of hydrogen, however, is not simply 2 (the average of 1, 2 and 3) but about 1.008, that is, much closer to 1. This is because the isotope with no neutrons is so much more abundant that it counts much more heavily in calculating the average.

IMPORTANT TERMS TO REMEMBER

Atomic Number (Z)

Z is always an integer, and is equal to the number of protons in the nucleus. The number of protons is what defines an element: An atom or an ion or a nucleus is identified as carbon, for example, if and only if it has 6 protons. Each element has a unique number of protons. Z is used as a presubscript to the chemical symbol in isotopic notation, that is, it appears as a subscript before the chemical symbol. The chemical symbols and the atomic numbers of all the elements are given in the Periodic Table.

Mass Number (A)

A is an integer equal to the total number of nucleons (neutrons and protons) in a nucleus. Let N represent the number of neutrons in a nucleus. The equation relating A, N and Z is simply:

$A = N + Z$

In isotopic notation, A appears as a presuperscript to the chemical symbol: It appears as a superscript that comes before the chemical symbol. In general, then, a nucleus can be represented as

$$_Z^A X$$

where X is the chemical symbol for the element. This representation is sometimes referred to as a nuclide symbol. Note that since an element is defined by the atomic number, Z is technically redundant information if one has access to the Periodic Table. Often, then, this quantity is omitted.

Examples:

$_1^1 H$: a single proton; the nucleus of ordinary hydrogen.

Number of neutrons = presuperscript – presubscript = 1 – 1 = 0.

$_2^4 He$: the nucleus of ordinary helium, consisting of 2 protons and 2 neutrons. It is also known as an alpha particle (α -particle).

$_{92}^{235} U$: a fissionable form of uranium, consisting of 92 protons and 235 – 92 = 143 neutrons.

Atomic Mass and Atomic Mass Unit

Atomic mass is most commonly measured in atomic mass units (amu). By definition, 1 amu is exactly one-twelfth the mass of the neutral carbon-12 atom. In terms of more familiar mass units:

$1 \text{ amu} = 1.66 \times 10^{-27} \text{ kg} = 1.66 \times 10^{-24} \text{ g}$

Atomic Weight

Because isotopes exist, atoms of a given element can have different masses. The atomic weight refers to a weighted average of the masses of an element. The average is weighted according to the natural abundances of the various isotopic species of an element. The atomic weight can be measured in amu.

BOHR'S MODEL OF THE HYDROGEN ATOM

In his model of the structure of the hydrogen atom, Bohr postulated that an electron can exist only in certain fixed energy states; the energy of an electron is "quantised". According to this model, electrons revolve around the nucleus in **orbits**. The energy of the electron is related to the radius of its orbit: The smaller the radius, the lower the energy state of the electron. The smallest orbit (radius) an electron can have corresponds to the ground state of the hydrogen electron. At the **ground state level**, the electron is in its lowest energy state. The fact that only certain energy values are allowed means that only certain orbit sizes are allowed.

QUANTUM MECHANICAL MODEL OF ATOMS

While the concepts put forth by Bohr offered a reasonable explanation for the structure of the hydrogen atom and ions containing only one electron (such as He^+ and Li^{2+}), they did not explain the structures of atoms containing more than one electron. This is because Bohr's model does not take into consideration the repulsion between multiple electrons surrounding one nucleus. **Modern quantum mechanics** has led to a more rigourous and generalized study of the electronic structure of atoms. The most important difference between the Bohr model and modern quantum mechanical models is that Bohr's assumption that electrons follow a circular orbit at a fixed distance from the nucleus is no longer considered valid. Rather, electrons are described as being in a state of rapid motion within regions of space around the nucleus, called **orbitals**. An orbital is a representation of the probability of finding an electron within a given region. In the current quantum mechanical description of electrons, pinpointing the exact location of an electron at any given point in time is impossible. This idea is best described by the **Heisenberg uncertainty principle**, which states that it is impossible to determine, with perfect accuracy, the momentum and the position of an electron simultaneously. This means that if the momentum of the electron is being measured accurately, its position cannot be pinpointed, and vice versa.

ELECTRON CONFIGURATION AND ORBITAL FILLING

For a given atom or ion, the pattern by which orbitals are filled and the number of electrons within each principal level and subshell are designated by an **electron configuration**. In electron configuration notation, the first number denotes the principal energy level, the latter designates the subshell, and the superscript gives the number of electrons in that subshell. For example, $2p^4$ indicates that there are four electrons in the second (p) subshell of the second principal energy level.

When writing the electron configuration of an atom, remember the order in which subshells are filled. Subshells are filled from lowest to highest energy, and each subshell will fill completely before electrons begin to enter the next one. The **($n + l$) rule** is used to rank subshells by increasing energy. This rule states that the lower the values of the first and second quantum numbers, the lower the energy of the subshell. If two subshells possess the same ($n + l$) value, the subshell with the lower n value has a lower energy and will fill first. The order in which the subshells fill is shown in the following chart, which is arranged so that it is easily remembered: One simply lists the subshells in order, starting each shell with a new line. The order of filling them is found by crossing them with diagonal arrows.

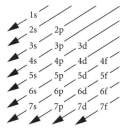

To determine which subshells are occupied, you must know the number of electrons in the atom. In the case of uncharged atoms, the number of electrons is equal to the atomic number. If the atom is charged, the number of electrons is equal to the atomic number plus the extra electrons if the atom is negative, or the atomic number minus the missing electrons if the atom is positive.

In subshells that contain more than one orbital, such as the $2p$ subshell with its 3 orbitals, the orbitals will fill according to **Hund's rule**. Hund's rule states that within a given subshell, orbitals are half-filled so that they each have one electron, all with parallel spins, before any orbital is fully occupied with two electrons of opposite spins. In other words, electrons would tend to avoid pairing as much as possible.

The presence of paired or unpaired electrons affects the chemical and magnetic properties of an atom or molecule. If the material has unpaired electrons, a magnetic field will align the spins of these electrons and weakly attract the atom. These materials are said to be **paramagnetic**. Materials that have no unpaired electrons and are slightly repelled by a magnetic field are said to be **diamagnetic**.

THE NUCLEUS OF AN ATOM

At the centre of an atom lies its **nucleus**, consisting of one or more nucleons (protons or neutrons) held together with considerably more energy than the energy needed to hold electrons in orbit around the nucleus. The radius of the nucleus is about 100,000 times smaller than the radius of the atom.

NUCLEAR REACTIONS AND DECAY

Nuclear reactions such as fusion, fission and radioactive decay involve either combining or splitting the nuclei of atoms. Since the binding energy per nucleon is greatest for intermediate-sized atoms, when small atoms combine or large atoms split a great amount of energy is released.

Fusion

Fusion occurs when small nuclei combine into a larger nucleus. As an example, many stars including the sun power themselves by fusing four hydrogen nuclei to make one helium nucleus. By this method, the sun produces 4×10^{26} J every second.

Fission

Fission is a process in which a large nucleus splits into smaller nuclei. Spontaneous fission rarely occurs. However, by the absorption of a low energy neutron, fission can be induced in certain nuclei. Of special interest are those fission reactions that release more neutrons, since these other neutrons will cause other atoms to undergo fission. This in turn releases more neutrons, creating a chain reaction. Such induced fission reactions power commercial nuclear electric-generating plants.

Some radioactive nuclei may be induced to fission via more than one decay channel or decay mode. For example, a different fission reaction may occur when uranium-235 absorbs a slow neutron and then immediately splits into barium-139, krypton-94 and three more neutrons with no intermediate state:

$$^{235}_{92}U + {}^{1}_{0}n \rightarrow {}^{236}_{92}U \rightarrow {}^{139}_{56}BA + {}^{94}_{36}Kr + 3\,{}^{1}_{0}n$$

Radioactive Decay

Radioactive decay is a naturally occurring, spontaneous decay of certain nuclei accompanied by the emission of specific particles. It could be classified as a certain type of fission.

CHEMICAL BONDING AND MOLECULAR STRUCTURE

The atoms of many elements can combine to form **molecules**. The atoms in most molecules are held together by strong attractive forces called **chemical bonds**. These bonds are formed via the interaction of the valence electrons of the combining atoms. The chemical and physical properties of the resulting molecules are often very different from those of their constituent elements.

In addition to the very strong forces within a molecule, there are weaker intermolecular forces between molecules. These intermolecular forces, although weaker than the intramolecular chemical bonds, are of considerable importance in understanding the physical properties of many substances.

Processes that involve the breaking and forming of chemical bonds are generally considered **chemical processes**, while those that only involve interactions between molecules are generally considered **physical processes**.

In the formation of chemical bonds, many molecules contain atoms bonded according to the **octet rule**, which states that an atom tends to bond with other atoms until it has eight electrons in its outermost shell, thereby forming a stable electron configuration similar to that of the noble gas elements (see chapter 15). Exceptions to this rule are as follows: hydrogen, which can have only two valence electrons (the configuration of He); lithium and beryllium, which bond to attain two and four valence electrons, respectively; boron, which bonds to attain six, and elements beyond the second row, such as phosphorus and sulphur, which can expand their octets to include more than eight electrons by incorporating d orbitals.

When classifying chemical bonds, it is helpful to introduce two distinct types: **ionic bonds** and **covalent bonds**. In ionic bonding, one or more electrons from an atom with a smaller ionisation energy are transferred to an atom with a great electron affinity, and the resulting ions are held together by **electrostatic forces**. In covalent bonding, an electron pair is shared between two atoms. In many cases, the bond is partially covalent and partially ionic; these bonds are called **polar covalent bonds**.

IONIC BONDS AND IONIC COMPOUNDS

Before reviewing the following topics, please note that they refer to topics such as elements, the Periodic Table, and chemical reactions that are covered in greater detail in chapters 13 and 14, respectively. If concepts or terms are unfamiliar, you can refer to these chapters for an explanation.

When two atoms with large differences in **electronegativity** (a measure of the attraction an atom has for electrons in a chemical bond) react, there is a complete transfer of electrons from the less electronegative atom to the more electronegative atom. The atom that loses electrons becomes a positively-charged ion, or cation, and the atom that gains electrons becomes a negatively charged ion, or anion. In general, the elements of Groups I and II (low electronegativities) bond ionically to elements of Group VII (high electronegativities). Elements of Groups I and II (metals) give up their electrons to form cations that have a noble gas configuration, while Group VII elements gain an electron to form anions with the noble gas configuration. For example, a neutral sodium atom has one valence electron in the $3s$ subshell, whereas a neutral chlorine atom has seven valence electrons. If sodium sheds itself of its valence electron, it will possess the same electronic configuration as neon, a noble or inert gas with a filled octet. Conversely, chlorine is one electron short of a stable octet: if it gains an extra electron, it will have the electronic configuration of argon. When the two come together, then, sodium loses an electron to chlorine:

$$Na + Cl \rightarrow Na^+ Cl^-$$

Since opposite charges attract, these two are now held together by electrostatic forces and form the compound (see Chapter 14) known as sodium chloride, or salt. This force of attraction between the charged ions is called an **ionic bond**.

As seen from the previous example, ionic compounds are formed by the interactions of cations and anions. The nomenclature, or naming, of ionic compounds is based on the names of the component ions. The following are some general guidelines:

1. The cationic species (usually metals) are usually named simply as the element, e.g., NaCl: *sodium* chloride, CaF_2: *calcium* fluoride. For elements that can form more than one positive ion, the charge is indicated by a Roman numeral in parentheses following the name of the element.

Fe^{2+} Iron (II) Cu^+ Copper (I)

Fe^{3+} Iron (III) Cu^{2+} Copper (II)

2. An older but still commonly used method is to add the endings –*ous* or –*ic* to the root of the Latin name of the element, to represent the ions with lesser or greater charge respectively.

Fe^{2+} Ferr*ous* Cu^+ Cupr*ous*

Fe^{3+} Ferr*ic* Cu^{2+} Cupr*ic*

3. **Monatomic anions** (single atom anions) are named by dropping the ending of the name of the element and adding –*ide*, as in the examples of sodium *chloride* and calcium *fluoride* given. Also:

H^-	Hydride
S^{2-}	Sulphide
N^{3-}	Nitride
O^{2-}	Oxide
P^{3-}	Phosphide

4. Many **polyatomic anions** contain oxygen and are called **oxyanions**. When an element forms two oxyanions, the name of the one with less oxygen ends in –*ite* and the one with more oxygen ends in –*ate*.

NO_2^-	Nitrite
SO_3^{2-}	Sulphite
NO_3^-	Nitrate
SO_4^{2-}	Sulphate

5. When the series of oxyanions contains four oxyanions, prefixes are also used. *Hypo*– and *per*– are used to indicate less oxygen and more oxygen, respectively. (Note that these prefixes are used only when there are more than two possibilities for the oxyanion.)

ClO^-	Hypochlorite
ClO_2^-	Chlorite
ClO_3^-	Chlorate
ClO_4^-	Perchlorate

6. Polyatomic anions often gain one or more H^+ ions to form anions of lower charge. The resulting ions are named by adding the word hydrogen or dihydrogen to the front of the anion's name. An older method uses the prefix *bi–* to indicate the addition of a single hydrogen ion.

HCO_3^-	Hydrogen carbonate or bicarbonate
HSO_4^-	Hydrogen sulphate or bisulfate
$H_2PO_4^-$	Dihydrogen phosphate

Using the previous rules, then, one can determine the names of ionic compounds such as the following:

$NaClO_4$	sodium perchlorate
$NaClO$	sodium hypochlorite
$NaNO_3$	sodium nitrate
KNO_2	potassium nitrite
Li_2SO_4	lithium sulphate
$MgSO_3$	magnesium sulphite

Note that the name itself does not explicitly tell how many ions of each there are; for example, the names lithium sulphite and calcium fluoride do not tell that there are two lithium ions and two fluoride ions in the respective compound—one must deduce that from knowing that the positive and negative charges have to balance each other to give a **neutral ionic compound**. Also, note that in a compound like lithium sulphate, both ionic and covalent bonds exist: the sulphur is bonded covalently to the oxygen atoms, while the sulphate anion as a whole interacts with lithium ions to form ionic bonds.

Metals, which are found in the left part of the Periodic Table, generally form positive ions, whereas non-metals, which are found in the right part of the Periodic Table, generally form negative ions. Note, however, the existence of anions that contain metallic elements, such as MnO_4^- (permanganate) and CrO_4^{2-} (chromate). All elements in a given group tend to form monatomic ions with the same charge. Thus ions of alkali metals (Group I) usually form cations with a single positive charge, the alkaline earth metals (Group II) form cations with a double positive charge, and the halides (Group VII) form anions with a single negative charge.

Ionic compounds have characteristic physical properties. They have high melting and boiling points due to the strong electrostatic forces between the ions. They can conduct electricity in the liquid and aqueous states, though not in the solid state. Ionic solids form crystal lattices consisting of infinite arrays of positive and negative ions in which the attractive forces between ions of opposite charge are maximised, while the repulsive forces between ions of like charge are minimised.

HYDROGEN BONDING

Hydrogen bonding is a specific, unusually strong form of dipole-dipole interaction (a type of intermolecular force). When hydrogen is bound to a highly electronegative atom such as fluorine, oxygen or nitrogen, the hydrogen atom carries little of the electron density of the covalent bond, most of which is shifted over to the electronegative atom. This positively charged hydrogen atom interacts with the partial negative charge located on the electronegative atoms of nearby molecules, causing the two molecules to experience an attraction for each other. Substances which display hydrogen bonding tend to have unusually high boiling points compared with compounds of similar molecular formula that do not participate in hydrogen bonding. The difference derives from the energy required to break the hydrogen bonds. Hydrogen bonding is particularly important in the behaviour of water, alcohols, amines and carboxylic acids. In fact, if it were not for the hydrogen bonding ability of water, life as we know it would not be possible on Earth.

COVALENT BONDS

When two or more atoms with similar electronegativities interact, they achieve a **noble gas electron configuration** by sharing electrons in what is known as a covalent bond. The binding force between the two atoms results from the attraction that each electron of the shared pair has for the two positive nuclei. This sharing of electrons is best envisioned by using dots to represent valence electrons as follows:

$$:\ddot{F}\cdot \;\; + \;\; \cdot\ddot{F}: \;\; \longrightarrow \;\; :\ddot{F}:\ddot{F}: \;\; \text{or} \;\; :\ddot{F}-\ddot{F}:$$

Each fluorine atom has seven valence electrons; they are both one short of a stable octet. Unlike the case of ionic bonding, however, there are no willing "electron donors" with low electronegativity around from which they can grab an electron. What they need to do is to each share one electron with its partner: The first structure drawn on the right hand side of the arrow shows how each F atom now has 8 valence electrons; the pair in the middle is shared by both. This pair of electrons is known as a bonding pair of electrons, as opposed to the unshared lone pairs, and is what constitutes the covalent bond between the two F atoms in the F_2 molecule. The bonding nature of these atoms is better indicated by the line between the atoms shown in the second structure.

Sometimes forming an octet requires sharing more than one electron from each atom. The oxygen molecule, O_2, and carbon monoxide, CO, for example, involve two and three pairs of bonding electrons, respectively:

$$\ddot{O}: \;\; + \;\; :\ddot{O} \;\; \longrightarrow \;\; \ddot{O}::\ddot{O} \;\; \text{or} \;\; \ddot{O}=\ddot{O}$$

$$\cdot\ddot{C}\cdot \;\; + \;\; :\ddot{O} \;\; \longrightarrow \;\; :C:::O: \;\; \text{or} \;\; :C\equiv O:$$

When two pairs of electrons are shared, the bond is known as a **double bond**. When three pairs of electrons are shared, the bond is known as a **triple bond**. The number of shared electron pairs between two atoms is called the **bond order**; hence a single bond (as in F_2) has a bond order of one, a double bond has a bond order of two, and a triple bond has a bond order of three.

TYPES OF COVALENT BONDING

The nature of a covalent bond depends on the relative electronegativities of the atoms sharing the electron pairs. Covalent bonds are considered to be **polar** or **non-polar** depending on the difference in electronegativities between the atoms.

Polar Covalent Bonds

Polar covalent bonding occurs between atoms with small differences in electronegativity. The bonding electron pair is not shared equally, but pulled more towards the element with the higher electronegativity. Yet the difference in electronegativity is not high enough for complete electron transfer (ionic bonding) to take place. As a result, the more electronegative atom acquires a partial negative charge, δ^- and the less electronegative atom acquires a partial positive charge, δ^+, giving the molecule partially ionic character. For instance, the covalent bond in HCl is polar because the two atoms have a small difference in electronegativity. Chlorine, the more electronegative atom, attains a partial negative charge and hydrogen attains a partial positive charge. This difference in charge between the atoms is indicated by an arrow crossed (like a plus sign) at the positive end pointing to the negative end, as shown in the following:

$$\overset{\delta+ \quad \delta-}{H - Cl}$$

This small separation of charge generates what is known as a **dipole moment**.

Non-polar Covalent Bonds

Non-polar covalent bonding occurs between atoms that have the same electronegativities.

The bonding electrons are shared equally, with no separation of charge across the bond. Not surprisingly, non-polar covalent bonds occur in diatomic molecules with the same atoms. Certain elements exist under normal conditions only as diatomic molecules: N_2, O_2, F_2, Cl_2, Br_2, I_2, H_2. Their positions in the Periodic Table form an inverted L-shape towards the top right, excluding the noble gases.

Coordinate Covalent Bonds

In a **coordinate covalent bond**, the shared electron pair comes from the lone pair of one of the atoms in the molecule. Once such a bond forms, it is indistinguishable from any other covalent bond. Distinguishing such a bond is useful only in keeping track of the valence electrons and formal charges. Coordinate bonds are typically found in Lewis acid-base compounds (see also chapter 14). A Lewis acid is a compound that can accept an electron pair to form a covalent bond; a Lewis base is a compound that can donate an electron pair to form a covalent bond. For example, in the reaction between boron trifluoride (BF_3) and ammonia (NH_3):

$$
\begin{array}{ccccc}
\overset{\textstyle F}{\underset{\textstyle F}{F-B}} & + & \overset{\textstyle H}{\underset{\textstyle H}{:N-H}} & \longrightarrow & \overset{\textstyle F \quad H}{\underset{\textstyle F \quad H}{F-B-N-H}} \\
\text{Lewis acid} & & \text{Lewis base} & & \text{Lewis acid-base compound}
\end{array}
$$

NH_3 donates a pair of electrons to form a coordinate covalent bond; thus, it acts as a Lewis base. BF_3 accepts this pair of electrons to form the coordinate covalent bond; thus, it acts as a Lewis acid.

GEOMETRY AND POLARITY OF COVALENT MOLECULES

The Lewis structure is not necessarily a good pictorial representation of the three-dimensional appearance of a molecule. The actual geometric arrangement of the bonds and different atoms is obtained by using the VSEPR theory described here. The shape of a molecule can affect its polarity.

The Valence Shell Electron-Pair Repulsion Theory

The **valence shell electron-pair repulsion (VSEPR) theory** uses Lewis structures to predict the molecular geometry of covalently-bonded molecules. It states that the three-dimensional arrangement of atoms surrounding a central atom is determined by the repulsions between the bonding and the non-bonding electron pairs in the valence shell of the central atom. These electron pairs arrange themselves as far apart as possible, thereby minimising repulsion.

The following steps are used to predict the geometrical structure of a molecule using the VSEPR theory.

- Draw the Lewis structure of the molecule.
- Count the total number of bonding and non-bonding electron pairs in the valence shell of the central atom.
- Arrange the electron pairs around the central atom so that they are as far apart from each other as possible. It is important not to forget to take into consideration non-bonding pairs.

Valence electron arrangements are summarised in the following table:

number of electrons	example	geometric arrangement of electron pairs around the central atom	shape	angle between electron pairs
2	$BeCl_2$	X — A — X	linear	180°
3	BH_3	(trigonal planar diagram)	trigonal planar	120°
4	CH_4	(tetrahedral diagram)	tetrahedral	109.5°
5	PCl_5	(trigonal bipyramidal diagram)	trigonal bipyramidal	90°,120°,180°
6	SF_6	(octahedral diagram)	octahedral	90°,180°

While the number of electron pairs dictates their overall arrangement around the central atom, it is only a starting point in arriving at the actual description of the geometry of the molecule. If one of the X's in the previous table is a lone pair of electrons rather than an actual atom or group of atoms, new terms need to be introduced to describe the spatial arrangement of the atoms.

In describing the shape of a molecule, only the arrangement of atoms (not electrons) is considered. Even though the electron pairs are arranged tetrahedrally, the shape of NH_3 is described as trigonal pyramidal. It is not trigonal planar because the lone pair repels the three bonding electron pairs, causing them to move as far away as possible.

The double bond behaves just like a single bond for purposes of predicting molecular shape. This compound has two groups of electrons around the carbon. According to the VSEPR theory, the two sets of electrons will orient themselves 180° apart, on opposite sides of the carbon atom, minimising electron repulsion. Therefore, the molecular structure of CO_2 is linear.

Polarity of Molecules

Earlier in this chapter, the concept of the dipole moment in a polar covalent bond was discussed. If a molecule has more than two atoms, there will be more than one bond. Each bond may or may not be a dipole, and in such cases one can talk about the polarity of the molecule as a whole. A molecule is polar if it has polar bonds and if the dipole moments of these bonds do not cancel one another (by pointing in opposite directions, for example). The **polarity** of a molecule, therefore, depends on the polarity of the constituent bonds and on the shape of the molecule. A molecule with only non-polar bonds is always non-polar; a molecule with polar bonds may be polar or non-polar, depending on the orientation of the bond dipoles. For instance, CCl_4 has four polar C–Cl bonds. According to the VSEPR theory, the shape of CCl_4 is tetrahedral. The four bond dipoles point to the vertices of the tetrahedron and cancel each other, resulting in a non-polar molecule.

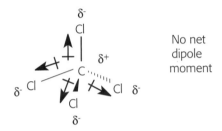

However, if the orientation of the bond dipoles is such that they do not cancel out, the molecules will have a net dipole moment and therefore be polar. For instance, H_2O has two polar O–H bonds. According to the VSEPR model, its shape is angular. The two dipoles add together to give a net dipole moment to the molecule, making the H_2O molecule polar.

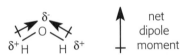

A molecule of two atoms bound by a polar bond must have a net dipole moment and therefore be polar. The two equal and opposite partial charges are localized at the ends of the molecule on the two atoms.

REVIEW QUESTIONS

1. An element with an atomic number of 26 has how many electrons in the $3d$ orbital?

   (A) 0
   (B) 2
   (C) 6
   (D) 8
   (E) 10

2. In going from $1s^2\, 2s^2\, 2p^6\, 3s^2\, 3p^6\, 4s^1$ to $1s^2\, 2s^2\, 2p^6\, 3s^2\, 3p^5\, 4s^2$, an electron would

   (A) absorb energy
   (B) emit energy
   (C) relax to the ground state
   (D) bind to another atom
   (E) undergo no change in energy

3. Which of the following orbitals has the lowest energy?

   (A) 2p

   (B) 3s

   (C) 3d

   (D) 4s

   (E) 3p

4. What is the formal charge on the nitrogen atom in HNO_3?

   (A) −1

   (B) +1

   (C) 0

   (D) +2

   (E) +3

Answers and Explanations

1. C

An element with an atomic number of 26 will have 6 electrons in its $3d$ subshell. This can be determined by writing the electron configuration for the element, $1s^2\ 2s^2\ 2p^6\ 3s^2\ 3p^6\ 3d^6\ 4s^2$. The number of electrons must equal 26; recall that the $4s$ subshell must be filled before the $3d$ because it has the lower energy. Thus, $3d$ will carry 6 electrons.

2. A

The difference between the first and second electron configurations is that in the second configuration one electron has moved from the $3p$ subshell to the $4s$ subshell. Although the $3p$ and $4s$ subshells have the same $(n + l)$ value, the $3p$ subshell fills first because it is slightly lower in energy. In order for an electron to move from the $3p$ subshell to the $4s$ subshell, it must absorb energy.

3. A

In order to determine which subshell has the lowest energy, the $(n + l)$ rule must be used. The values of the first and second quantum numbers are added together, and the subshell with the lowest $(n + l)$ value has the lowest energy. The sums of the five choices are $(2 + 1) = 3$, $(3 + 0) = 3$, $(3 + 2) = 5$, $(4 + 0) = 4$, $(3 + 1) = 4$. Choices A and B have the same $(n + l)$ value, so the subshell with the lower principal quantum number has the lower energy. This is the $2p$ subshell.

4. B

To answer this question, you need to write the Lewis dot diagrams and then use any one of several formulas to find the formal charge. One such formula is formal charge = valence electrons − [number of bonds + number of non-bonding electrons]. The Lewis dot structure of HNO_3 shows that nitrogen is double bonded to one oxygen, single bonded to another oxygen, and single bonded to another oxygen that is single bonded to a hydrogen—there are no lone electron pairs on the nitrogen. Using the formula, formal charge is equal to the valence electrons of nitrogen (5) minus the sum of the number of bonds and the number of non-bonding electrons, which in this case is 4. So, the formal charge on the nitrogen is 5 minus 4, or 1.

Chapter 13: **The Periodic Table and the Elements**

Chapter 13 offers an in-depth review of the Periodic Table, including its arrangement and the information it presents. Details about the types of elements and their properties and uses are also provided here. At the end of the chapter, answer the practice questions to reinforce what you just read.

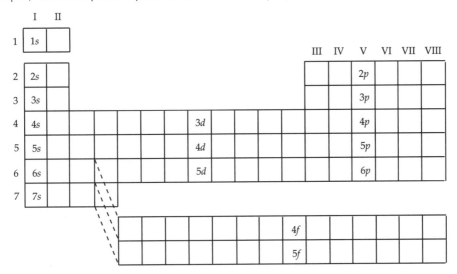

ABOUT THE PERIODIC TABLE

Each **element** is a class of atoms with the same number of protons in the nucleus. The Periodic Table arranges the elements in increasing atomic numbers. Its spatial layout is such that a lot of information about an element's properties can be deduced simply by examining its position. The vertical columns are called **groups**, while the horizontal rows are called **periods**. There are seven periods, representing the principal quantum numbers $n = 1$ to $n = 7$, and each period is filled more or less sequentially. The period an element is in tells the highest shell that is occupied, or the highest principal quantum number. Elements in the same group (same column) have the same electronic configuration in their valence, or outermost shell. For example, both magnesium (Mg) and calcium (Ca) are in the second column; they both have 2 electrons in the outermost s subshell, the only difference being that the principal quantum number is different for Ca ($n = 4$) than for Mg ($n = 3$). Because it is these outermost electrons, or valence electrons, that are involved in chemical bonding, they determine the chemical reactivity and properties of the element. In short, elements in the same group will tend to have similar chemical reactivities.

VALENCE ELECTRONS AND THE PERIODIC TABLE

The valence electrons of an atom are those electrons that are in its outer energy shell or that are available for bonding. The visual layout of the Periodic Table is convenient for determining the electron configuration of an atom (especially the valence electron configuration); this provides a quick alternative to the methods described in chapter 12.

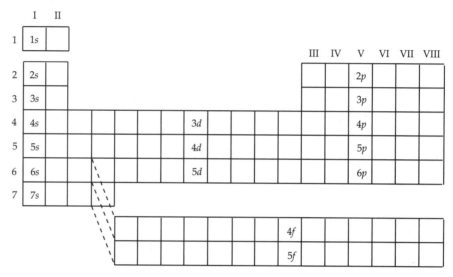

Elements in the leftmost column (Group 1 or IA) all have a single s electron in their valence shell; their electron configuration can therefore be represented as **[X]** ns^1, where [X] designates the electron configuration of the noble gas element (see the following) that immediately precedes it and is abbreviated this way because these electrons are core electrons that do not generally participate in chemical reactions, and are hence uninteresting from a chemical perspective. Elements in the second column (Group 2 or IIA) have electronic configurations **[X]** ns^2; their valence electrons are the two electrons in the outermost s subshell.

The next block of elements (elements in the next 10 columns, not including the 4f lanthanide and 5f actinide series) are all known as **transition elements** and have electrons in the d subshell; just how many they have depends on exactly which column they are in. Elements in the third column (Group 3 or IIIA), for example, have configurations **[X]** $ns^2 (n - 1)d^1$. (Note that the principal quantum number for the d subshell is one less than that for the s subshell—remember, for example, how after filling the 3p subshell, one fills the lower-energy 4s orbital first before "going back" to fill the 3d subshell.) Their valence electrons are those in the outermost s subshell and in the d subshell of the next-to-outermost energy shell. For the inner transition elements, the valence electrons are those in the s subshell of the outermost energy shell, the d subshell of the next-to-outermost energy shell, and the f subshell of the energy shell two levels below the outermost shell.

The last six columns of the Periodic Table contain elements with s and p valence electrons.

PERIODIC TRENDS OF THE ELEMENTS

The properties of the elements exhibit certain trends, which can be explained in terms of the position of the element in the Periodic Table, or in terms of the electron configuration of the element. Elements in general seek to gain or lose valence electrons so as to achieve the stable octet formation possessed by the **inert** or **noble gases** of Group VIII (last column of the Periodic Table). Two other important general trends exist. First, as one goes from left to right across a period, electrons are added one at a time; the electrons of the outermost shell experience an increasing amount of nuclear attraction, becoming closer and more tightly bound to the nucleus. Second, as one goes down a given column, the outermost electrons become less tightly bound to the nucleus. This is because the number of filled principal energy levels (which shield the outermost electrons from attraction by the nucleus) increases downward within each group. These trends help explain elemental properties such as atomic radius, ionisation potential, electron affinity, and electronegativity.

Atomic Radii

The **atomic radius** is an indication of the size of an atom. In general, the atomic radius decreases across a period from left to right and increases down a given group; the atoms with the largest atomic radii will therefore be found at the bottom of groups, and in Group I.

As one moves from left to right across a period, electrons are added one at a time to the outer energy shell. Electrons in the same shell cannot shield one another from the attractive pull of protons very efficiently. Therefore, since the number of protons is also increasing, producing a greater positive charge, the effective nuclear charge increases steadily across a period, meaning that the valence electrons feel a stronger and stronger attraction towards the nucleus. This causes the atomic radius to decrease.

As one moves down a group of the periodic table, the number of electrons and filled electron shells will increase, but the number of valence electrons will remain the same. Thus, the outermost electrons in a given group will feel the same amount of effective nuclear charge, but electrons will be found farther from the nucleus as the number of filled energy shells increases. Thus, the atomic radius will increase.

Ionisation Energy

The **ionisation energy (IE)**, or **ionisation potential**, is the energy required to completely remove an electron from an atom or ion. Removing an electron from an atom always requires an input of energy, since it is attracted to the positively-charged nucleus. The closer and more tightly bound an electron is to the nucleus, the more difficult it will be to remove, and the higher the ionisation energy will be. The first ionisation energy is the energy required to remove one valence electron from the parent atom; the second ionisation energy is the energy needed to remove a second valence electron from the ion with +1 charge to form the ion with +2 charge, and so on. Successive ionisation energies grow increasingly large; that is, the second ionisation energy is always greater than the first ionisation energy. For example:

$$Mg\ (g) \rightarrow Mg^+(g) + e^- \qquad \text{First Ionisation Energy} = 7.646\ eV$$

$$Mg^+\ (g) \rightarrow Mg^{2+}(g) + e^- \qquad \text{Second Ionisation Energy} = 15.035\ eV$$

Ionisation energy increases from left to right across a period as the atomic radius decreases. Moving down a group, the ionisation energy decreases as the atomic radius increases. Group I elements have low ionisation energies because the loss of an electron results in the formation of a stable octet.

Electron Affinity

Electron affinity is the energy that is released when an electron is added to a gaseous atom, and it represents the ease with which the atom can accept an electron. The stronger the attractive pull of the nucleus for electrons, the greater the electron affinity will be. A positive electron affinity value represents energy release when an electron is added to an atom.

Generalisations can be made about the electron affinities of particular groups in the Periodic Table. For example, the Group IIA elements, or **alkaline earths**, have low electron affinity values. These elements are relatively stable because their *s* subshell is filled: They do not particularly "care" to gain an extra electron, even though the process is still favourable. Group VIIA elements, or **halogens**, have high electron affinities because the addition of an electron to the atom results in a completely filled shell, which represents a stable electron configuration. Achieving the stable octet involves a release of energy, and the strong attraction of the nucleus for the electron leads to a high energy change. The Group VIII elements, or **noble gases**, have electron affinities on the order of zero since they already possess a stable octet: gaining an extra electron is really not that favourable and would not result in the release of much energy.

A layperson's way of describing the difference between ionisation energy and electron affinity is that the former tells how attached the atom is to the electrons it already has, while the latter tells how the atom feels about gaining another electron.

Electronegativity

Electronegativity is a measure of the attraction an atom has for electrons in a chemical bond. The greater the electronegativity of an atom, the greater its attraction for bonding electrons. It is related to ionisation energy and electron affinity: elements with low ionisation energies and low electron affinities will have low electronegativities because their nuclei do not attract electrons strongly, while elements with high ionisation energies and high electron affinities will have high electronegativities because of the strong pull the nucleus has on electrons. Therefore, electronegativity increases from left to right across periods. In any group, the electronegativity decreases as the atomic number increases, as a result of the increased distance between the valence electrons and the nucleus, i.e., greater atomic radius.

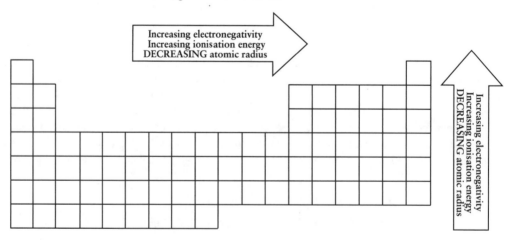

TYPES OF ELEMENTS

The **elements** of the periodic table may be classified into three categories: metals, located on the left side and in the middle of the periodic table; non-metals, located on the right side of the table; and metalloids (semi-metals), found along a diagonal line between the other two.

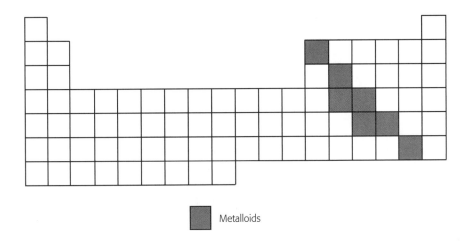

Metalloids

Metals

Metals are shiny solids at room temperature (except for mercury, which is a liquid), and generally have high melting points and densities. Metals have the characteristic ability to be deformed without breaking. The ability of a metal to be hammered into shapes is called **malleability** and the ability to be drawn into wires is called **ductility**. Many of the characteristic properties of metals, such as large atomic radius, low ionisation energy, and low electronegativity, are due to the fact that the few electrons in the valence shell of a metal atom can easily be removed. Because the valence electrons can move freely, metals are good **conductors** (mediums for transmitting) of heat and electricity. Group IA and IIA represent the most reactive metals. The transition elements are metals which have partially filled d orbitals.

Non-metals

Non-metals are generally brittle in the solid state and show little or no metallic lustre. They have high ionisation energies and electronegativities, and are usually poor conductors of heat and electricity. Most non-metals share the ability to gain electrons easily (i.e., they tend to form negative ions), but otherwise they display a wide range of chemical behaviours and reactivities. The non-metals are located on the upper right side of the periodic table; they are separated from the metals by a line cutting diagonally through the region of the periodic table containing elements with partially filled p orbitals.

Metalloids

The **metalloids**, or **semi-metals**, are found along the line between the metals and non-metals in the Periodic Table, and their properties vary considerably. Their densities, boiling points, and melting points fluctuate widely. The electronegativities and ionisation energies of metalloids lie between those of metals and non-metals; therefore, these elements possess characteristics of both those classes. For example, silicon has a metallic lustre, yet it is brittle and is not an efficient conductor. The reactivity of metalloids is dependent upon the element with which they are reacting. For example, boron (B) behaves as a non-metal when reacting with sodium (Na) and as a metal when reacting with fluorine (F). The elements classified as metalloids are **boron, silicon, germanium, arsenic, antimony** and **tellurium**.

THE CHEMISTRY OF GROUPS

Elements in the same group have the same number of valence electrons, and hence tend to have very similar chemical properties.

Alkali Metals

The **alkali metals** are the elements of Group IA. They possess most of the physical properties common to metals, yet their densities are lower than those of other metals. The alkali metals have only one loosely bound electron in their outermost shell, giving them the largest atomic radii of all the elements in their respective periods. Their metallic properties and high reactivity are determined by the fact that they have low ionisation energies; thus, they easily lose their valence electron to form **univalent cations** (cations with a +1 charge). Alkali metals have low electronegativities and react very readily with non-metals, especially halogens.

Alkaline Earth Metals

The **alkaline earth metals** are the elements of Group IIA. They also possess many characteristically metallic properties. Like the alkali metals, these properties are dependent upon the ease with which they lose electrons. The alkaline earths have two electrons in their outer shell and thus have smaller atomic radii than the alkali metals. However, the two valence electrons are not held very tightly by the nucleus, so they can be removed to form divalent cations. Alkaline earths have low electronegativities and low electron affinities.

Halogens

The **halogens**, Group VIIA (second to last column), are highly reactive non-metals with seven valence electrons (one short of the favoured octet configuration). Halogens are highly variable in their physical properties. For instance, the halogens range from gaseous (F_2 and Cl_2) to liquid (Br_2) to solid (I_2) at room temperature. Their chemical properties are more uniform: the electronegativities of halogens are very high, and they are particularly reactive towards alkali metals and alkaline earths, which "want" to donate electrons to the halogens to form stable ionic crystals.

Noble Gases

The **noble gases**, also called the inert gases, are found in Group VIII. They are fairly non-reactive because they have a complete valence shell, which is an energetically-favoured arrangement. They thus have high ionisation energies. They possess low boiling points and are all gases at room temperature.

Transition Elements

The **transition elements** are those that are found between the alkaline earth metals and those with valence p electrons (the last six columns). The numbering of the groups can get rather confusing because of the existence of two conventions, but you needn't be too concerned with this. These elements are metals and hence are also known as transition metals. They are very hard and have high melting and boiling points. As one moves across a period, the five d orbitals become progressively more filled. The d electrons are held only loosely by the nucleus and are relatively mobile, contributing to the malleability and high electrical conductivity of these elements. Chemically, transition elements have low ionisation energies and may exist in a variety of positively charged forms or oxidation states. This is because transition elements are capable of losing various numbers of electrons from the s and d orbitals of their valence shell. For instance, copper (Cu) can exist in either the +1 or the +2 oxidation state, and manganese (Mn) occurs in the +2, +3, +4, +6 or +7 state. Because of this ability to attain positive oxidation states, transition metals form many different ionic and partially ionic compounds. The dissolved ions can form complex ions either with molecules of water (hydration complexes) or with non-metals, forming highly-coloured solutions and compounds, such as $CuSO_4 \cdot 5H_2O$.

Complexes of transition metal ions, called **coordination complexes**, are an interesting class of species because many of them possess bright colours. This results from the fact that the formation of complexes causes the d orbitals (normally all of the same energy) to be split into two energy sublevels. Many of the complexes can thus absorb certain frequencies of light—those containing the precise amount of energy required to raise electrons from the lower to the higher d sublevel. The frequencies not absorbed give the complexes their characteristic colours.

REVIEW QUESTIONS

1. The modern Periodic Table is ordered on the basis of

    (A) atomic mass
    (B) atomic radius
    (C) atomic charge
    (D) atomic number
    (E) number of neutrons

2. The elements within each column of the Periodic Table

    (A) have similar valence electron configurations
    (B) have similar atomic radii
    (C) have the same principal quantum number
    (D) will react to form stable elements
    (E) have no similar chemical properties

3. Transition metal compounds generally exhibit bright colours because

    (A) the electrons in the partially filled d orbitals are easily promoted to excited states
    (B) the metals become complexed in water
    (C) the metals conduct electricity, producing coloured light
    (D) the electrons in the d orbitals emit energy as they relax

4. Which of the following elements is most electronegative?

    (A) S
    (B) Cl
    (C) Na
    (D) Mg
    (E) P

5. All halogens have similar reactivity because

   (A) they have the same number of protons
   (B) they have the same number of electrons
   (C) they have similar outer shell electron configurations
   (D) they have valence electrons with the same quantum numbers

6. Which of the following elements has the lowest electronegativity?

   (A) Caesium
   (B) Strontium
   (C) Calcium
   (D) Barium

7. Elements in a given period have the same

   (A) atomic weight
   (B) maximum azimuthal quantum number
   (C) maximum principal quantum number
   (D) valence electron structure
   (E) atomic number

8. All members of Group IA have similar reactivity because they have

   (A) the same number of protons
   (B) the same number of electrons
   (C) similar outer shell electron configurations
   (D) valence electrons with the same quantum numbers
   (E) the same number of neutrons

Answers and Explanations

1. D

When the Periodic Table was first being designed, it was thought that the periodicity of the elements could be explained on the basis of atomic mass. Dimitri Mendeleev, one of the creators of the Periodic Table, discovered that when the elements were arranged in order or increasing atomic mass, certain chemical properties were repeated at regular intervals. However, certain elements could not be fit into any group of a table based on increasing atomic mass. It was the discovery of the nucleus and its components that led scientists to order the elements by increasing atomic number, the number of protons.

2. A

You can determine the electron configuration of an atom by noting its placement in the Periodic Table. Elements in the leftmost column (Group 1 or IA) all have a single s electron in their valence shell. Elements in the second column (Group 2 or IIA) have their valence electrons as two electrons in the outermost s subshell. The next block of elements are transition elements and have electrons in the d subshell; just how many they have depends on exactly which column they are in. Elements in the third column (Group 3 or

IIIA), for example, have their valence electrons in the outermost *s* subshell and in the *d* subshell of the next-to-outermost energy shell. For the inner transition elements, the valence electrons are those in the *s* subshell of the outermost energy shell, the *d* subshell of the next-to-outermost energy shell, and the *f* subshell of the energy shell two levels below the outermost shell. The last six columns of the Periodic Table contain elements with *s* and *p* valence electrons.

3. A

The closely spaced split *d* orbitals allow for relatively low energy transitions; these transitions often occur in the visible region of the electromagnetic spectrum. The compound appears to have a colour that is complementary to the one that is absorbed. For example, if the transition occurs in the red region of the spectrum, the compound will appear green.

4. B

Chlorine has the greatest electronegativity because, out of all the choices, it lies farthest to the right and top of the Periodic Table. Chlorine has a great attraction for electrons in a chemical bond because it needs only one more electron to complete a stable octet formation. Therefore, it has a high electronegativity.

5. C

This question requires you to know something about the periodicity of the elements. Basically, all you are asked is why all the halogens behave so similarly in reactions. You know from studying the Periodic Table that there must be something that repeats or the table would not be periodic. What is it about the elements in a column that are the same? The number of valence electrons. Since the identity of the valence electrons is the same in each column, that is, columns in the *s* block have valence *s* electrons, columns in the *p* block have valence *s* and *p* electrons, and columns in the *d* block have valence *s* and *d* electrons, the only thing that can make them act similarly is the number of electrons in these shells. Furthermore, the number of electrons in the valence shell affects the reactivity and stability of the shell. The number of electrons affects the ionisation energy and electron affinity, whether the atom will form cations or anions and even the number of bonds the atom can participate in.

6. A

The least electronegative elements are located at the bottom left of the Periodic Table. Caesium has the lowest ionisation energy and, likewise, it is the least electronegative. Note that francium (Fr) would be lower still but is not a stable, naturally-occurring element.

7. C

The horizontal rows of the Periodic Table are called **periods**. The seven periods represent the principal quantum numbers $n = 1$ to $n = 7$; each period is filled more or less sequentially. The period an element is in tells the highest shell that is occupied, or the highest principal quantum number.

8. C

All members of Group IA have similar reactivities because they have a similar valence shell configuration (one loosely bound electron). They lose it easily to form univalent cations and react readily with non-metals, especially halogens.

Chapter 14: **Chemical Reactions**

This chapter provides essential review of acids and bases, compounds, chemical reactions, rates of reactions and dynamic equilibrium. If these topics are unfamiliar to you, be sure to review this important chapter carefully and reinforce these lessons by completing the practice questions found at the end.

ACIDS AND BASES

Many important reactions in chemical and biological systems involve two classes of compounds (see definition of compounds later in this chapter) called **acids** and **bases**. The presence of acids and bases can often be easily detected because they lead to colour changes in certain compounds called **indicators**, which may be in solution or on paper. A particular common indicator is **litmus paper**, which turns red in acidic solution and blue in basic solution.

Nomenclature of Acids

The name of an acid is related to the name of the parent anion (the anion that combines with H^+ to form the acid). Acids formed from anions whose names end in *-ide* have the prefix **hydro-** and the ending *-ic*.

F^-	Fluoride	HF	Hydrofluoric acid
Br^-	Bromide	HBr	Hydrobromic acid

Acids formed from oxyanions are called **oxyacids**. If the anion ends in *–ite* (less oxygen), then the acid will end with *-ous* acid. If the anion ends in *–ate* (more oxygen), then the acid will end with *-ic* acid. Prefixes in the names of the anions are retained. Some examples:

ClO^-	Hypochlorite	HClO	Hypochlorous acid
ClO_2^-	Chlorite	$HClO_2$	Chlorous acid
ClO_3^-	Chlorate	$HClO_3$	Chloric acid
ClO_4^-	Perchlorate	$HClO_4$	Perchloric acid
NO_2^-	Nitrite	HNO_2	Nitrous acid
NO_3^-	Nitrate	HNO_3	Nitric acid

Properties of Acids and Bases

The behaviour of acids and bases in solution is governed by equilibrium considerations. Some concepts you already may be familiar with will appear with new names in this context.

Hydrogen Ion Equilibria (pH and pOH)

Hydrogen ion or proton concentration, [H+], like concentrations of other particles, can of course be measured in the familiar units like molarity. However, it is more generally measured as pH, where:

$$pH = -\log [H^+] = \log \left(\frac{1}{[H^+]} \right)$$

where $[H^+]$ is its molarity and the logarithm is of base 10. (Log x) is the power to which 10 would be raised to obtain the number x, i.e.:

$$\log x = p \Leftrightarrow 10p = x$$

Likewise, hydroxide ion concentration, $[OH^-]$, can be measured as pOH where:

$$pOH = -\log [OH^-] = \log \left(\frac{1}{[OH^-]} \right)$$

It turns out, however, that pH and pOH are not totally independent of each other: knowing one would allow us to calculate the other. This is because in any aqueous solution, the H_2O solvent dissociates slightly:

$$H_2O(l) \Leftrightarrow H^+ (aq) + OH^- (aq)$$

This dissociation is an equilibrium reaction and is therefore described by an equilibrium constant, K_w, known as the water dissociation constant:

$$K_w = [H^+][OH^-] = 10^{-14} \text{ (at 25 °C)}$$

One can take the logarithm of both sides and manipulate the equation by using the properties of logarithms:

$$\log ([H^+][OH^-]) = \log (10^{-14})$$

$\log [H^+] + \log [OH^-]$	$= \log (10^{-14})$,	since $\log (xy) = \log x + \log y$
	$= -14$,	since $\log (10p) = p$
$-\log [H^+] - \log [OH^-]$	$= 14$,	where we have taken the negative of both sides
$\therefore pH + pOH = 14$		

In pure H_2O, $[H^+]$ is equal to $[OH^-]$, since equimolar amounts of H^+ and of OH^- are formed from the dissociation process. The pH and pOH would therefore also be equal, both having a value of 7. A solution with equal concentrations of H^+ and OH^- is neutral. A pH below 7 indicates a relative excess of H^+ ions, and therefore an acidic solution; a pH above 7 indicates a relative excess of OH^- ions, and therefore a basic solution.

It is important to realise that even when the pH deviates from the value of 7, the water dissociation equilibrium still holds. If an acid, for example HCl, dissociates in water at 25 °C and causes an increase in proton concentration such that the pH falls below 7, the hydroxide ion concentration will have to decrease so as to maintain the relation $K_w = [H^+][OH^-] = 10^{-14}$. Despite the higher concentration of H^+ relative to OH^-, the solution does not acquire a net positive charge because the conjugate base of the dissociated acid will be negatively charged (for example, Cl–) and thus will maintain charge neutrality.

It should also be pointed out that even though we have written acid-base reactions so far as involving protons, in aqueous solution the protons will interact with other water molecules, forming H_3O^+, known as the hydronium ion. The water dissociation reaction can therefore be written as

$$H_2O(l) + H_2O(l) \rightleftharpoons H_3O+ (aq) + OH^- (aq)$$

We shall be using H+ and H_3O+ interchangeably, unless otherwise stated.

STRONG AND WEAK ACIDS AND BASES

Strong acids and bases are those that completely dissociate into their component ions in aqueous solution. *Weak* acids and bases are those that only partially dissociate in aqueous solution.

Salt Formation

A **salt** is an ionic substance consisting of anions and cations, but not hydrogen or hydroxide ions. Any salt can be formed by the reaction of the appropriate acid and base. Acids and bases may react with each other, forming a **salt** and (often, but not always) water, in what is termed a **neutralisation reaction**. For example, a generic acid and a generic base react as follows:

$$HA + BOH \rightarrow BA + H_2O$$

The salt, BA, may precipitate out or remain ionised in solution, depending on its solubility and the amount produced. Neutralisation reactions generally go to completion. The **reverse reaction**, in which the salt ions react with water to give back the acid or base, is known as **hydrolysis**.

Four combinations of strong and weak acids and bases are possible:

1. strong acid + strong base: e.g., $HCl + NaOH \rightarrow NaCl + H_2O$
2. strong acid + weak base: e.g., $HCl + NH_3 \rightarrow NH_4Cl$
3. weak acid + strong base: e.g., $HClO + NaOH \rightarrow NaClO + H_2O$
4. weak acid + weak base: e.g., $HClO + NH_3 \rightarrow NH_4ClO$

The products of a reaction between equal concentrations of a strong acid and a strong base are a salt and water. The acid and base neutralise each other, so the resulting solution is neutral ($pH = 7$), and the ions formed in the reaction do not react with water. The product of a reaction between a strong acid and a weak base is also a salt but usually no water is formed since weak bases are usually not hydroxides; however, in this case, the cation of the salt will react with the water solvent, reforming the weak base. This reaction constitutes hydrolysis. For example:

$$HCl\ (aq) + NH_3\ (aq) \rightarrow NH_4^+\ (aq) + Cl^-\ (aq)\ \text{Reaction I}$$

$$NH_4^+\ (aq) + H_2O\ (aq) \rightarrow NH_3\ (aq) + H_3O^+\ (aq)\ \text{Reaction II}$$

NH_4^+ is the conjugate acid of a weak base (NH_3), and is therefore stronger than the conjugate base (Cl^-) of the strong acid HCl. NH_4^+ will thus react with OH^-, reducing the concentration of OH^-. There will thus be an excess of H^+, which will lower the pH of the solution.

On the other hand, when a weak acid reacts with a strong base the solution is basic, due to the hydrolysis of the salt to reform the acid, with the concurrent formation of hydroxide ion from the hydrolysed water molecules. The pH of a solution containing a weak acid and a weak base depends on the relative strengths of the reactants (the substances participating in the chemical reaction).

COMPOUNDS

A **compound** is a pure substance that is composed of two or more elements in a fixed proportion. Compounds can be broken down chemically to produce their constituent elements or other compounds. All elements, except for some of the noble gases, can react with other elements or compounds to form new compounds. These new compounds can react further to form yet different compounds.

MOLECULAR WEIGHT AND MOLAR MASS

A **molecule** is a combination of two or more atoms held together by covalent bonds. It is the smallest unit of a compound that displays the properties of that compound. Molecules may contain two atoms of the same element, as in N_2 and O_2, or may be comprised of two or more different atoms, as in CO_2 and $SOCl_2$.

Chapter 12 discussed the concept of atomic weight. Like atoms, molecules can also be characterised by their weight. The **molecular weight** is simply the sum of the weights of the atoms that make up the molecule.

> **Example:** What is the molecular weight of $SOCl_2$?

Solution: To find the molecular weight of $SOCl_2$, add together the atomic weights of each of the atoms.

1S =	1 × 32 amu =	32 amu
1O =	1 × 16 amu =	16 amu
2Cl =	2 × 35.5 amu =	71 amu
molecular weight =		119 amu

Ionic compounds do not form true molecules. In the solid state they can be considered to be a nearly infinite, three dimensional array of the charged particles of which the compound is composed. Since no actual molecule exists, molecular weight becomes meaningless, and the term **formula weight** is used in its place, although the calculation is the same: Simply add up the atomic masses of the elements in the compound's empirical formula (see the following). The formula weight of NaCl, for example, is the atomic weight of Na plus the atomic weight of Cl: (23 + 35.5) amu = 58.5 amu.

Remember that a mole of something is about 6.022×10^{23} of that thing. In addition, the atomic mass of an atom, reported in units of amu, is numerically the same as its mass in grams per mole. For example, one mole of an atom with atomic mass x amu has a mass of x grams. The same relationship holds for molecules: one mole of a compound has a mass in grams equal to the molecular weight of that compound in amu, and contains 6.022×10^{23} molecules of the compound. For example, the molecular weight of carbonic acid, H_2CO_3, is $(2 \times 1 \pm 12 + 3 \times 16) = 62$ amu. 62 g of H_2CO_3 represents one mole of carbonic acid and contains 6.022×10^{23} H_2CO_3 molecules. In other words, the molar mass of H_2CO_3 is 62 g/mol. This can also be arrived at by simply adding the molar atomic mass of the atoms in the compound: 1 mole of H_2CO_3 contains 2 moles of H atoms, 1 mole of C atoms, and 3 moles of O atoms.

Given the weight of a sample, one can determine the number of moles present with the following formula:

> number of moles = weight of sample (g) ÷ molar mass (g/mol)

> **Example:** How many moles are in 9.52 g of $MgCl_2$?

Solution: First, find the molar mass of $MgCl_2$.

$$1(24.31 \text{ g/mol}) + 2(35.45 \text{ g/mol}) = 95.21 \text{ g/mol}$$

Now, solve for the number of moles.

$$\frac{9.25 \text{g}}{95.21 \text{g/mol}} = 0.10 \text{ mol of } MgCl_2.$$

TYPES OF CHEMICAL REACTIONS

There are many ways in which elements and compounds can react to form other species; memorizing every reaction would be impossible, as well as unnecessary. However, nearly every inorganic reaction can be classified into at least one of four general categories.

Combination Reactions

Combination reactions are reactions in which two or more reactants form one product. The formation of sulphur dioxide by burning sulphur in air is an example of a combination reaction.

$$S\ (s) + O_2\ (g) \rightarrow SO_2\ (g)$$

The letters in parentheses designate the phase of the species: s for solid, g for gas, l for liquid, and aq for aqueous solution.

Decomposition Reactions

A **decomposition reaction** is defined as one in which a compound breaks down into two or more substances, usually as a result of heating. An example of a decomposition reaction is the breakdown of mercury (II) oxide (the sign Δ here represents the addition of heat).

$$2HgO(s) \xrightarrow{\ \Delta\ } 2Hg(l)O_2\ (g)$$

Single Displacement Reactions

Single displacement reactions occur when an atom (or ion) of one compound is replaced by an atom of another element. For example, zinc metal will displace copper ions in a copper sulphate solution to form zinc sulphate.

$$Zn\ (s) + CuSO_4\ (aq) \rightarrow Cu\ (s) + ZnSO_4\ (aq)$$

Single displacement reactions are often further classified as redox reactions. (These will be mentioned again later in this chapter.)

Double Displacement Reactions

In **double displacement reactions**, also called **metathesis reactions**, elements from two different compounds displace each other to form two new compounds. For example, when solutions of calcium chloride and silver nitrate are combined, insoluble silver chloride forms in a solution of calcium nitrate.

$$CaCl_2\ (aq) + 2\ AgNO_3\ (aq) \rightarrow Ca(NO_3)_2\ (aq) + 2\ AgCl\ (s)$$

Neutralisation reactions are a specific type of double displacements which occur when an acid reacts with a base to produce a solution of a salt and water. For example, hydrochloric acid and sodium hydroxide will react to form sodium chloride and water.

$$HCl\ (aq) + NaOH\ (aq) \rightarrow NaCl\ (aq) + H_2O\ (l)$$

NET IONIC EQUATIONS

Because reactions such as displacements often involve ions in solution, they can be written in ionic form. In the example where zinc is reacted with copper sulphate, the ionic equation would be:

$$Zn\ (s) + Cu^{2+}\ (aq) + SO_4{}^{2-}\ (aq) \rightarrow Cu\ (s) + Zn^{2+}\ (aq) + SO_4{}^{2-}\ (aq)$$

When displacement reactions occur, there are usually **spectator ions** that do not take part in the overall reaction but simply remain in solution throughout. The spectator ion in the previous equation is sulphate, which does not undergo any transformation during the reaction. A net ionic equation can be written showing only the species that actually participate in the reaction:

$$Zn\ (s) + Cu^{2+}\ (aq) \rightarrow Cu\ (s) + Zn^{2+}\ (aq)$$

Net ionic equations are important for demonstrating the actual reaction that occurs during a displacement reaction.

HEAT ENERGY AND CHEMICAL REACTIONS

Reactions that absorb heat energy are said to be *endothermic*, while those that release heat are said to be *exothermic*. An *adiabatic* process is one in which no heat exchange occurs (no heat goes into or out of the system). Melting and vaporisation are therefore endothermic, while freezing and condensation are exothermic processes. An *isothermal* process is one in which the temperature of the system remains constant.

OXIDATION REACTIONS AND REDUCTION

Redox chemistry involves the study of *redu*ction and *oxi*dation reactions: **reduction** refers to reactions in which a species gains electrons, while **oxidation** refers to those in which a species gives up or loses electrons. Since electrons can neither be created nor destroyed in normal chemical reactions (as opposed to nuclear reactions, discussed in Chapter 12), an isolated loss or gain of electrons cannot occur; in other words, neither oxidation nor reduction can occur all by itself. Each occurs simultaneously in a redox reaction, resulting in net electron transfer between the species. The electrons released during oxidation are taken up in the reduction process. The species undergoing reduction is said to be reduced when it gains electrons; a **reduced species** is also called an **oxidising agent** because it causes something else (the species giving up the electrons) to be oxidised. Similarly, a **reducing agent** causes another species to be reduced, and is itself oxidised. This is summarised here:

oxidising agent	reducing agent
reduced	oxidised
gains electrons	loses electrons

CHEMICAL KINETICS

Thermodynamics and the study of chemical equilibrium show whether the occurrence of a reaction is favourable and to what extent the reaction goes towards completion. Thermodynamics only reveals part of the story about chemical reactions. The inherent tendency of a reaction to occur does not necessarily have anything to do with how readily or quickly it takes place. Furthermore, thermodynamics does not provide a microscopic picture of how exactly a reaction is proceeding: how do the individual molecules interact with one another to lead to the end product? How many steps does the reaction have to go through? All these issues are investigated within the realm of **chemical kinetics**—the study of the rates of reactions, the effect of reaction conditions on these rates and the mechanisms implied by such observations.

REACTION RATES

The **rate of a reaction** is an indication of how rapidly it is occurring. First, you must have an exact, quantitative way of describing the rate. Then you can explore what the rate depends on.

Definition of Rate

Consider a reaction $2A + B \rightarrow C$, in which 1 mole of C is produced from every 2 moles of A and 1 mole of B. You want to come up with some quantitative way of describing just how fast the reaction has proceeded or is proceeding at any instant in time. The most natural way is to use either the disappearance of reactants over time, or the appearance of products over time. The faster either of these rates are, the faster the rate of reaction:

$$\text{rate} \quad \frac{\text{decrease in reactant concentration}}{\text{time}} \quad \frac{\text{increase in product concentration}}{\text{time}}$$

Because the concentration of a reactant decreases during the reaction while you want the rates to be positive numbers, a minus sign needs to be placed before a rate that is expressed in terms of reactants. For the reaction above, the rate of disappearance of A is $\frac{-\Delta[A]}{\Delta t}$, the rate of disappearance of B is $\frac{-\Delta[B]}{\Delta t}$, and the rate of disappearance of C is $\frac{-\Delta[C]}{\Delta t}$. In this particular reaction, the three rates are not equal. According to the stoichiometry of the reaction, A is used up twice as fast as B ($\frac{-\Delta[C]}{\Delta t} = -2 \times \frac{-\Delta[B]}{\Delta t}$), and A is consumed twice as fast as C is produced ($\frac{-\Delta[A]}{\Delta t} = 2 \times \frac{-\Delta[C]}{\Delta t}$). To show a standard rate of reaction in which the rates with respect to all substances are equal, the rate for each substance should be divided by its stoichiometric coefficient.

In this particular case, then:

$$\text{rate of reaction} = -\frac{1}{2}\frac{\Delta[A]}{\Delta t} = -\frac{-\Delta[B]}{\Delta t} = \frac{\Delta[C]}{\Delta t}$$

In general, for the reaction

$$a A + b B \rightarrow c C + d D,$$

$$\text{rate of reaction} = -\frac{1}{a}\frac{\Delta[A]}{\Delta t} = -\frac{1}{b}\frac{-\Delta[B]}{\Delta t} = \frac{1}{c}\frac{\Delta[C]}{\Delta t} = \frac{1}{d}\frac{\Delta[D]}{\Delta t}$$

Rate is expressed in units of concentration per unit time, most often moles per litre per second (mol/L x s), which is the same as molarity per second (molarity/s).

Rate Law

For nearly all forward, irreversible reactions, the rate is proportional to the product of all the concentrations of the reactants, each raised to some power.

For the general reaction:

$$a A + b B \rightarrow c C + d D$$

the rate is proportional to $[A]^x [B]^y$, that is:

$$\text{rate} = k [A]^x [B]^y.$$

This expression is the **rate law** for the previous general reaction, where k is known as the **rate constant**, and is different for different reactions and may also change depending on the reaction conditions. Multiplying the units of k by the concentration factors raised to the appropriate powers gives the rate in units of concentration/time. (The unit of k, therefore, depends on the values of x and y.) The exponents x and y are called the **orders of reaction**; x is the order of the reaction with respect to A and y is the order with respect to B. These exponents may be integers, fractions or zero, and must be determined experimentally. It is most important to realise that the exponents of the rate law are not necessarily equal to the **stoichiometric coefficients** (numbers used to indicate the number of moles of a given species involved in the reaction) in the overall reaction equation. It is generally *not* the case that $x = a$ and $y = b$, for example, unless if the reaction is a one-step process in which the stoichiometric equation is actually a microscopic description of how the molecules collide. (See Chapter 15, Quantitative Chemistry for more about stoichiometry.)

The overall order of a reaction (or the **reaction order**) is defined as the sum of the exponents, here equal to $x + y$.

FACTORS AFFECTING REACTION RATE

The rate of a chemical reaction as expressed in the applicable rate law involves both a rate constant and, except for zero order reactions, the concentration of reactants. The rate of a reaction, then, could be increased by either increasing the concentration of the reactants (which increases the number of effective collisions between the reactant molecules), or by altering the value of the rate constant. It has been noted already that the rate constant ultimately depends upon the energy difference between the reactants and the transition state. The smaller this activation energy is (the smaller the gap between the two energy levels), the larger the rate constant, and the faster the reaction will proceed. Two factors that most commonly affect the rate of a reaction are **temperature** and the presence of a **catalyst**.

For nearly all reactions, the reaction rate will increase as the temperature of the system increases. Since the **temperature** of a substance is generally a measure of the particles' average kinetic energy, increasing the temperature increases the average kinetic energy of the molecules. Consequently, the proportion of molecules having energies greater than E_a (thus capable of undergoing reaction) increases with higher temperature. Again, this is valid even for reactions that are exothermic because the activated complex is at a higher potential energy than the reactants. Raising the temperature of a system in which an exothermic reaction is occurring would shift the equilibrium in favour of the reactants, but the system would attain this equilibrium faster.

Catalysts are substances that increase the reaction rate without themselves being consumed; they do this by lowering the activation energy. Catalysts are important in biological systems and in industrial chemistry; **enzymes** are biological catalysts. Catalysts accomplish this lowering of activation energy by a variety of ways: they may, for example, increase the frequency of collision between the reactants, or change the relative orientation of the reactants making a higher percentage of collisions effective. The following figure compares the energy profiles of catalysed and uncatalysed reactions.

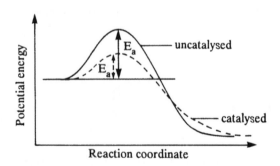

The energy barrier for the catalysed reaction is much lower than the energy barrier for the uncatalysed reaction. Note that the rates of both the forward and the reverse reactions are increased by catalysis, since E_a of the forward and reverse reactions are lowered by the same amount. Therefore, the presence of a catalyst causes the reaction to proceed more quickly towards equilibrium, without changing the position of the equilibrium, i.e., without changing the value of the equilibrium constant.

DYNAMIC EQUILIBRIUM

Although the kinetics of a reaction may override predictions based purely on thermodynamics, the two aspects are not totally separate. This is because one of the things that characterises equilibrium is that the forward and reverse reactions are occurring at the same rate: the relative rates of reactions set up a thermodynamic equilibrium in the system.

The ratio of the **forward rate constant** to the **reverse rate constant** is the **equilibrium constant** for that one-step process, i.e.:

$$A + B \underset{k_r}{\overset{k_f}{\rightleftarrows}} C$$

$$K_{eq} = \frac{k_f}{k_r}$$

where k_f is the rate constant of the forward reaction and k_r is the rate constant for the reverse reaction. The larger the value of k_f the faster the forward reaction occurs (relative to the reverse reaction); that is, products are formed more rapidly than they revert back to reactants, and so there will tend to be more products around at equilibrium, which is reflected in a large equilibrium constant.

It may now be more obvious why a catalyst does not affect the position of equilibrium: both k_f and k_r are increased by the same proportion, such that their ratio remains unchanged.

REVIEW QUESTIONS

1. Which of the following is most likely to increase the rate of a reaction?

    (A) decreasing the temperature
    (B) increasing the volume of the reaction vessel
    (C) reducing the activation energy
    (D) decreasing the concentration of the reactant in the reaction vessel

2. According to chemical kinetic theory, a reaction can occur

    (A) if the reactants collide with the proper orientation.
    (B) if the reactants possess sufficient energy of collision.
    (C) if the reactants are able to form a correct transition state.
    (D) All of the above.

3. At equilibrium

    (A) the forward reaction will continue.
    (B) a change in reaction conditions may shift the equilibrium.
    (C) the reverse reaction will not continue.
    (D) Both A and B.

4. All of the following are true statements concerning catalysts EXCEPT

(A) A catalyst will speed the rate-determining step.

(B) A catalyst will be used up in a reaction.

(C) A catalyst may induce steric strain in a molecule to make it react more readily.

(D) A catalyst will lower the activation energy of a reaction.

5. The reaction below is classified as a

$$CH_3CO_2Na + HClO_4 \rightarrow CH_3CO_2H + NaClO_4$$

(A) double displacement reaction.

(B) combination reaction.

(C) decomposition reaction.

(D) single displacement and decomposition reaction.

(E) combination and decomposition reaction.

Answers and Explanations

1. C

Reducing the activation energy makes it easier for molecules to overcome the barrier to reaction: at any temperature, there will now be more molecules that have sufficient energy to react. The rate of reaction will therefore be faster. All the other choices tend to decrease the reaction rate: lowering the temperature would mean decreasing the energy of the molecules; it will be more difficult for them to overcome the energy barrier. Increasing the volume of the reaction vessel, with all else remaining the same, would decrease the density (and hence concentration) of the reactant molecules, causing collisions among them to be less frequent.

2. D

In order for products to form, the reactant atoms or molecules need to collide at an orientation that allows them to react, and with sufficient energy to surmount the activation barrier as it goes through the transition state.

3. D

At equilibrium, both the forward and reverse reactions are proceeding. Any change in the equilibrium conditions will shift the equilibrium in order to alleviate the stress on the reaction.

4. B

The definition and properties of a catalyst are discussed in the section on factors affecting the reaction rate.

5. A

Since the only change is that the Na from CH_3CO_2Na exchanges with the H from $HClO_4$, this is a double displacement reaction. Alternatively, this reaction could be classified as a neutralisation, since it is an acid and a base that react.

Chapter 15: **Quantitative Chemistry**

This chapter covers quantitative chemistry. This includes topics such as balanced chemical equations and the yield of reactions. If you would like to test how much you have learned about these topics, answer the eight practice questions found at the end of the chapter.

BALANCING EQUATIONS

Chemical equations express how much and what type of reactants must be used to obtain a given quantity of product. From the **law of conservation of mass**, the mass of the reactants in a reaction must be equal to the mass of the products. More specifically, chemical equations must be balanced so that there are the same number of atoms of each element in the products as there are in the reactants. **Stoichiometry** is essentially the study of how the quantities of reactants and products are related in a chemical reaction. **Stoichiometric coefficients** are numbers used to indicate the number of moles of a given species involved in the reaction. For example, the reaction for the formation of water is:

$$2 H_2 (g) + O_2 (g) \rightarrow 2 H_2O (g)$$

The coefficients indicate that two moles of H_2 gas must be reacted with one mole of O_2 gas to produce two moles of water. In general, stoichiometric coefficients are given as whole numbers.

Given the identities of the compound participating in a reaction (the reactants and products), you need to balance the equation for the reaction before you can deduce any stoichiometric information from it. When balancing an equation, the important thing to realize is that you can only change the number in front of the compound, the one that tells you how many molecules (or moles) of that compound are needed for the reaction to occur. You may not change the subscripts—that would change the nature or the identity of the compound, and hence the reaction itself.

For example, in the previous reaction, if you are just given the information H_2 and O_2 react to form H_2O and are told to balance the equation to determine the molar relationships, you may *not* write $H_2 + O_2 \rightarrow H_2O_2$. Yes, all the elements are balanced, but the reaction has changed: you have written the formation of hydrogen peroxide instead of water.

> **Example:** Balance the following reaction.
>
> $$C_4H_{10} (l) + O_2 (g) \rightarrow CO_2 (g) + H_2O (l)$$

Solution: first, balance the carbons in reactants and products.

$$C_4H_{10} + O_2 \rightarrow 4 CO_2 + H_2O$$

Second, balance the hydrogens in reactants and products.

$$C_4H_{10} + O_2 \rightarrow 4\ CO_2 + 5\ H_2O$$

Third, balance the oxygens in the reactants and products.

$$2\ C_4H_{10} + 13\ O_2 \rightarrow 8\ CO_2 + 10\ H_2O$$

Finally, check that all of the elements, and the total charges, are balanced correctly. You could have balanced the elements in a different order, although in general it is easier to tackle the least represented atoms first.

Balancing Redox Reactions

In chapter 14, reduction and oxidation reactions were discussed; this is how you balance the equations for these reactions.

By assigning oxidation numbers to the reactants and products, one can determine how many moles of each species are required for conservation of charge and mass, which is necessary to balance the equation. In general, to balance a redox reaction, both the net charge and the number of atoms must be equal on both sides of the equation. The most common method for balancing redox equations is the **half-reaction method**, also known as the **ionelectron method**, in which the equation is separated into two half-reactions–the oxidation part and the reduction part. Each half-reaction is balanced separately, and they are then added to give a balanced overall reaction, in which electrons do not appear explicitly by convention. Consider a redox reaction between $KMnO_4$ and HI in an acidic solution:

$$MnO_4^- + I^- \rightarrow I_2 + Mn^{2+}$$

Step 1: separate the two half-reactions.

oxidation half-reaction: $MnO_4^- \rightarrow Mn^{2+}$

reduction half-reaction: $I^- \rightarrow I_2$

Step 2: balance the atoms of each half-reaction. First, balance all atoms except H and O. Next, in an acidic solution, add H_2O to balance the O atoms and then add H^+ to balance the H atoms. (In a basic solution, use OH^- and H_2O to balance the O's and H's.)

To balance the iodine atoms, place a coefficient of two before the I^- ion.

$$2\ I^- \rightarrow I_2$$

For the permanganate half-reaction, Mn is already balanced. Next, balance the oxygens by adding $4H_2O$ to the right side.

$$MnO_4^- \rightarrow Mn^{2+} + 4H_2O$$

Finally, add H^+ to the left side to balance the 4 H_2Os. These two half-reactions are now balanced in mass (but not in charge).

$$MnO_4^- + 8\ H^+ \rightarrow Mn^{2+} + 4H_2O$$

Step 3: Balance the charges of each half-reaction. The reduction half-reaction must consume the same number of electrons as are supplied by the oxidation half. For the oxidation reaction, add 2 electrons to the right side of the reaction:

$$2\ I^- \rightarrow I_2 + 2e^-$$

For the reduction reaction, a charge of +2 must exist on both sides. Add 5 electrons to the left side of the reaction to accomplish this:

$$5\,e^- + 8\,H^+ + MnO_4^- \rightarrow Mn^{2+} + 4H_2O$$

Step 4: Both half-reactions must have the same number of electrons so that they will cancel. Multiply the oxidation half by 5 and the reduction half by 2 and add the two:

$$5(2\,I^- \rightarrow I_2 + 2e^-)$$

$$2(5\,e^- + 8\,H^+ + MnO_4^- \rightarrow Mn^{2+} + 4H_2O)$$

The final equation is:

$$10\,I^- + 10\,e^- + 16\,H^+ + 2\,MnO_4^- \rightarrow 5\,I_2 + 2\,Mn^{2+} + 10\,e^- + 8\,H_2O$$

To get the overall equation, cancel out the electrons and any H_2Os, H^+s, OH^-s or e^-s that appear on both sides of the equation.

$$10\,I^- + 16\,H^+ + 2\,MnO_4^- \rightarrow 5\,I_2 + 2\,Mn^{2+} + 8\,H_2O$$

Step 5: Finally, confirm that mass and charge are balanced. There is a +4 net charge on each side of the reaction equation, and the atoms are stoichiometrically balanced.

As you may have noticed, balancing redox equations can be trickier and more involved than other types of reactions because often one needs to supply additional chemical species like water and protons to the equation, rather than simply playing with stoichiometric coefficients. The previous scheme is the most general one that can be applied; it may be that many intermediate steps can be omitted if the equation is simpler. For example, for the equation:

$$Zn\,(s) + HCl\,(aq) \rightarrow ZnCl_2\,(aq) + H_2\,(g)$$

one may balance it by just supplying coefficients.

APPLICATIONS OF STOICHIOMETRY

Once an equation has been balanced, the ratio of moles of reactant to moles of products is known, and that information can be used to solve many types of stoichiometry problems.

> **Example:** How many grams of calcium chloride are needed to prepare
> 72 g of silver chloride according to the following equation?

$$CaCl_2\,(aq) + 2AgNO_3\,(aq) \rightarrow Ca(NO_3)_2\,(aq) + 2AgCl\,(s)$$

Solution: Noting first that the equation is balanced, 1 mole of $CaCl_2$ yields 2 moles of AgCl when it is reacted with two moles of $AgNO_3$. The molar mass of $CaCl_2$ is 110 g, and the molar mass of AgCl is 144 g. As the first step, find out how many moles of AgCl are wanted:

$$\#mol\ AgCl = \frac{72g}{144\ g/mol} = 0.5mol$$

Based on the stoichiometric relationship between AgCl and $CaCl_2$, you know that you need 0.5/2 = 0.25 mol $CaCl_2$. The mass of $CaCl_2$ needed is therefore 0.25 mol × 110 g/mol = 27.5 g.

This line of reasoning can be quite time-consuming to go through. A powerful technique in handling such problems is that of **dimensional analysis**, in which you arrange the numbers and quantities so that the units cancel to give you the right one that you want. For this problem, the calculations could have been done in one step:

$$72 \text{ g AgCl} = \frac{1 \text{ mol AgCl}}{144 \text{ g AgCl}} \times \frac{1 \text{mol CaCl}_2}{2 \text{ mol AgCl}} \times \frac{110 \text{ g CaCl}_2}{1 \text{ mol CaCl}_2} = 27.5 \text{ g CaCl}_2$$

Note that you start with the value of 72 g AgCl given in the question and multiply it by three fractions that have in common the property that the numerator is equivalent to (or "corresponds to") the quantity in the denominator:

1 mol of AgCl is equivalent to 144 g of AgCl; 1 mol CaCl2 gives 2 mol AgCl in this reaction; 1 mol CaCl2 is equivalent to 110 g $CaCl_2$. Because of the equivalence between numerator and denominator, you can switch the two and not affect the fraction as a whole. The way you have decided which to use as numerator and which to use as denominator is dictated by which units you want to cancel. For example,, you want to get rid of the weight of AgCl and obtain the number of moles instead, and so you have chosen to put 144 g AgCl in the denominator to cancel the unit of (g AgCl) in the starting value:

$$72 \text{ g AgCl} = \frac{1 \text{ mol AgCl}}{144 \text{ g AgCl}} = \frac{72}{144} \text{ mol AgCl} = 0.5 \text{ g mol AgCl}$$

You can verify that all the units do cancel to yield at the end "g $CaCl_2$", which is what you want. The way the equation has to be set up to give the right unit tells how to manipulate the numbers, without having to spend too much time trying to recall, "Should I divide by the molar mass or multiply?"

LIMITING REACTANTS

When reactants are mixed, they are seldom added in the exact stoichiometric proportions as shown in the balanced equation. Therefore, in most reactions, one of the reactants will be used up first. This reactant is known as the **limiting reactant** (or **limiting reagent**) because it limits the amount of product that can be formed in the reaction. The reactant that remains after all of the limiting reactant is used up is called the **excess reactant**.

> **Example:** If 28 g of Fe react with 24 g of S to produce FeS, what would be the limiting reactant? How many grams of excess reactant would be present in the vessel at the end of the reaction?

Solution: first, the balanced equation needs to be determined. The question states that Fe and S come together to form FeS:

Fe + S → FeS

This is already balanced.

Next, the number of moles for each reactant must be determined.

$$28 \text{ g Fe} \times \frac{1 \text{mol Fe}}{56 \text{ g}} = 0.5 \text{ mol Fe}$$

$$24 \text{ g S} \times \frac{1 \text{mol S}}{32 \text{ g}} = 0.75 \text{ mol S}$$

Since one mole of Fe is needed to react with one mole of S, and there are 0.5 mol Fe versus 0.75 mol S, the limiting reagent is Fe. Thus, 0.5 mol Fe will react with 0.5 mol S, leaving an excess of 0.25 mol S in the vessel.

The mass of the excess reactant will be:

$$.25 \text{ mol S} \times \frac{32 \text{ g}}{1 \text{ mol S}} = 8 \text{ g S}$$

Note that the limiting reactant is not necessarily the one with the smallest mass. It depends also on the molecular (or atomic) weights of all the reactants and also the stoichiometric relationship. In the previous example, for example, there is a higher mass of Fe than S, yet Fe is the limiting reactant.

Yields

The **yield** of a reaction, which is the amount of product predicted or obtained when the reaction is carried out, can be determined or predicted from the balanced equation. There are three distinct ways of reporting yields. The **theoretical yield** is the amount of product that can be predicted from a balanced equation, assuming that all of the limiting reagent has been used, that no competing side reactions have occurred, and all of the product has been collected. The theoretical yield is seldom obtained; therefore, chemists speak of the **actual yield**, which is the amount of product that is isolated from the reaction experimentally.

The term **percent yield** is used to express the relationship between the actual yield and the theoretical yield, and is given by the following equation:

$$\text{percent yield} = \frac{\text{actual yield}}{\text{theoretical yield}} \times 100\%$$

> **Example:** What is the percent yield for a reaction in which 27 g of Cu is produced by reacting 32.5 g of Zn in excess $CuSO_4$ solution?

Solution: The balanced equation is as follows:

$$Zn \text{ (s)} + CuSO_4 \text{ (aq)} \rightarrow Cu \text{ (s)} + ZnSO_4 \text{ (aq)}$$

Calculate the theoretical yield for Cu. The question states that $CuSO_4$ is in excess, and so the theoretical yield will be dictated by the amount of Zn:

$$32.5 \text{ g Zn} \times \frac{1 \text{ mol Zn}}{65.4 \text{ g Zn}} \times \frac{1 \text{ mol Cu}}{1 \text{ mol Zn}} \times \frac{63.5 \text{ g Zn}}{1 \text{ mol Cu}} = 31.6 \text{ g Cu}$$

31.6 g Cu = theoretical yield

This is the most one can ever hope to get. The actual yield, as stated, is 27 g. The percent yield is therefore $\frac{27}{31.6} \times 100\% = 85\%$.

REVIEW QUESTIONS

1. What is the sum of the coefficients of the following equation when it is balanced?

$$C_6H_{12}O_6 + O_2 \rightarrow CO_2 + H_2O$$

(A) 20

(B) 38

(C) 21

(D) 19

(E) 18

2. Aspirin ($C_9H_8O_4$) is prepared by reacting salicylic acid ($C_7H_6O_3$) and acetic anhydride ($C_4H_6O_3$):

$$C_7H_6O_3 + C_4H_6O_3 \rightarrow C_9H_8O_4 + C_2H_4O_2$$

How many moles of salicylic acid should be used to prepare six 5-grain aspirin tablets?
($1\ g = 15.5$ grains)

(A) 0.01

(B) 0.1

(C) 1.0

(D) 2.0

(E) 31.0

3. What would be the stoichiometric coefficient of hydrochloric acid in the following equation?

$$....Cl_2 + ...H_2O \rightarrow ...HCl + ...HClO_3$$

(A) 1

(B) 3

(C) 5

(D) 10

4. Acetylene, used as a fuel in welding torches, is produced in a reaction between calcium carbide and water:

$$CaC_2 + 2\ H_2O \rightarrow Ca(OH)_2 + C_2H_2$$

How many grams of C_2H_2 are formed from 0.400 moles of CaC_2?

(A) 0.400

(B) 0.800

(C) 4.00

(D) 10.4

(E) 26.0

5. When the following reaction is balanced, what is the net ionic charge on the right side of the equation?

$$...H^+ + ...MnO_4^- + ...Fe^{2+} \rightarrow ...Mn^{2+} + ...Fe^{3+} + ...H_2O$$

(A) +5

(B) +7

(C) +10

(D) +17

6. What is the sum of the coefficients of the products for the following reaction, after balancing?

$$...K_2Cr_2O_7 + ...HCl \rightarrow ...KCl + ...CrCl_3 + ...H_2O + ...Cl_2$$

(A) 10

(B) 12

(C) 13

(D) 14

Questions 7–8 refer to the following equation.

$$...Ag(NH_3)_2{}^+ \rightarrow ...Ag^+ + ...NH_3$$

7. What is the sum of the coefficients once the equation is balanced?

    (A) 1
    (B) 2
    (C) 3
    (D) 4

8. How many moles of $Ag(NH_3)_2{}^+$ are required to produce 11 moles of ammonia?

    (A) 1
    (B) 2
    (C) 5.5
    (D) 11

Answers and Explanations

1. D

In order to answer this question, the equation must first be balanced. Starting with carbon, it can be seen that there are six carbons on the reactant side and only one on the product side, so a coefficient of six should be placed in front of the carbon dioxide. For the hydrogen, there are 12 atoms on the left and only two on the right; thus, a coefficient of six should go in front of water. Now, for oxygen, there are eight atoms on the left and 18 on the right. In order to balance the oxygen, ten more atoms of oxygen must be added to the left side. The best way to do this is to put a coefficient of six in front of oxygen, since putting a stoichiometric coefficient in front of the glucose molecule would unbalance the equation in terms of carbon and hydrogen. Therefore, the final balanced equation is: $C_6H_{12}O_6 + 6\ O_2 \rightarrow 6\ CO_2 + 6\ H_2O$

2. A

According to the balanced equation, one mole of salicylic acid will yield one mole of aspirin. Therefore, to solve this question, the number of moles of aspirin in six 5-grain tablets, or 30 grains of aspirin, must be determined, using the following relationship.

$$\frac{1\ g}{15.5\ grains} = \frac{x}{30\ grains}$$

$$x \approx 2g$$

Therefore, the weight of the aspirin produced is about 2 grams, which must be converted to moles. The molecular weight of aspirin is $9(C) + 8(H) + 4(O) = 9(12\ g/mol) + 8(1\ g/mol) + 4(16\ g/mol) = 180\ g/mol$. Then, the number of moles in two grams of aspirin is calculated.

$$\frac{2\ g}{180\ g/mol} = 0.01\ mol$$

3. C

To answer this question, you must balance the equation given to find the stoichiometric coefficient for hydrochloric acid. Start with oxygen since it's the only element that is present in only one compound on each side of the equation. Since there are three oxygens on the right side of the equation, you have to place a "3"

before the water molecule on the left. There are now six hydrogen atoms on the left side of the equation, so a "5" must be placed before the HCl on the right side for a total on six hydrogens on that side also. Before jumping right to the answer, balance the entire equation, since the answer might be five or some multiple of five, depending on the other compounds. There are six chlorines on the right, so you must place a "3" before the Cl_2 on the left. The equation is now fully balanced and it's clear that the answer is five.

4. D

According to the balanced equation, one mole of CaC_2 yields one mole of C_2H_2. Therefore, if 0.400 moles of CaC_2 were used, 0.400 moles of C_2H_2 would be produced. The molecular weight of C_2H_2 is 2(12 g/mol) + 2(1 g/mol) = 26 g/mol. Thus, the mass of C_2H_2 is 26 g/mol × 0.400 mol = 10.4 g.

5. D

The balanced equation looks like this:

$$8H^+ + MnO_4^- + 5Fe^{2+} \rightarrow Mn^{2+} + 5Fe^{3+} + 4H_2O.$$

One Mn^{2+} and five Fe^{3+} yield a total charge of +17.

6. D

$$1K_2Cr_2O_7 + 14HCl \rightarrow 2KCl + 2CrCl_3 + 7H_2O + 3Cl_2$$

$$2 + 2 + 7 + 3 = 14$$

7. D

The balanced equation looks like this:

$$1Ag(NH_3)_2{}^+ \rightarrow 1Ag^+ + 2NH_3$$

$$1 + 1 + 2 = 4$$

8. C

$$\frac{1Ag(NH_3)_2{}^+}{2NH_3} = \frac{X}{11NH_3}$$

$$X = \frac{11}{2}$$

5.5 moles

PART VI

Essential Physics Review

Chapter 16: **Electrostatics, Electricity, and Magnetism**

In this chapter we will present and summarise fundamental concepts pertaining to the behaviour of electrical charges. The first section will deal with static electric charges and the forces that they exert on each other. The second section will take a look at electric charges in motion, electric currents, and electrical circuits. In the final section we will look at some of the other effects of moving charges including magnetic phenomena.

CHARGE

The fundamental property of matter that is responsible for all electrical phenomena is called **charge**. There are two types of charge arbitrarily designated as either "positive" or "negative". The smallest possible charge is that carried by the electron, the particle-like entity found outside the nucleus of an atom. The charge of an electron is equal to -1.60×10^{-19} Coulomb (C), which is equal in magnitude to the charge on a proton but of the opposite sign. The proton, which is one of the constituents of the nucleus of the atom has a charge equal to $+1.60 \times 10^{-19}$ C. The other constituent of the nucleus is called the neutron which has no net charge. The behaviour of electric charge is such that like charges repel each other, and unlike charges attract.

> **Example:** Three charges A, B and C are located in a region of space. Charge A attracts Charge B, but repels Charge C. How will Charge B affect Charge C?

Solution: Since A attracts B they must be oppositely charged. Since A repels C, C must be the same type charge as A. Therefore B is opposite in sign to C and will attract it.

Charge may be transferred from one object to another; however, since the electron resides on the outside of the atom, it is much more mobile than the proton, and is the particle that is actually able to move from one atom to another. So charge transfer is accomplished primarily through the motion of electrons.

The Law of Conservation of Charge

While charge may be transferred from one location to another, the total amount of charge is constant. For example if an object gains 1 C of charge, this amount of charge must have come from another object or objects that have lost exactly the same amount.

Coulomb's Law

Coulomb's Law relates the electrostatic force between any two charges. If for example there are two charges q_1 and q_2 separated by a distance r, as shown in the figure below, then the force that each exerts on the other is given by:

$$F = \frac{kq_1q_2}{r^2}$$

Where k is called the Coulomb's Law constant. $k = 8.99 \times 10^9$ Nm^2/C^2.

Example: Two charges are separated by a distance r and exert forces on each other equal to F. If the distance is doubled between the charges, how much is the force between the charges reduced?

Solution: The new force is $\frac{1}{4}$ the original force. Since $F \propto \frac{1}{r^2}$, if r is doubled the force is reduced to $\frac{1}{4}$

$$F_1 = \frac{kq_1q_2}{r^2} \qquad F_2 = \frac{kq_1q_2}{(2r)^2} = \frac{kq_1q_2}{4r^2} = \frac{1}{4}F_1$$

This type of relationship where the force is proportional to the inverse square of the distance is called an **inverse square law**. In this type of situation the force falls off rapidly as a function of distance due to the r being squared in the denominator. The Gravitational force also obeys an inverse square law. A graph of force as a function of distance between objects that obey an inverse square law is shown in the figure below.

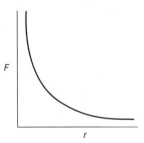

There may be more than two charges in a region in space. In this case, to calculate the total or net force acting on a given charge in the region, calculate the force on that charge due to each of the other charges separately, and then add these forces to determine the net force.

Example: Three positive charges each with a magnitude of 1×10^{-6} C are in a line as shown in the figure below. If $r = 0.10m$, determine the net electrostatic force on q_1.

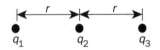

Solution: Calculate the forces that q_2 and q_3 exert on q_1 separately:

$$F \text{ of } q_2 \text{ on } q_1 \quad \frac{kq_1q_2}{r^2} = \frac{(9 \times 10^9 \ Nm^2 / C^2)(1 \times 10^{-6})(1 \times 10^{-6})}{(0.10m)^2} = 0.90N \text{ to the left.}$$

$$F \text{ of } q_3 \text{ on } q_1 \quad \frac{kq_1q_3}{r^2} = \frac{(9 \times 10^9 \ Nm^2 / C^2)(1 \times 10^{-6})(1 \times 10^{-6})}{(0.20m)^2} = 0.23N \text{ also to the left.}$$

The total force is the sum of these two forces $= 1.1N$ to the left.

Transfer of Charge

As mentioned above charge transfer is accomplished primarily by motion of electrons. An example of charge transfer is exhibited when a plastic rod is rubbed with a piece of silk. In this case electrons are removed from the glass, and stick to the silk giving it a net negative charge. Due to a net deficiency of electrons the rod is left with a net positive charge. If the charged rod and silk are then separated but held close together they will exert attractive forces on each other due to being oppositely charged.

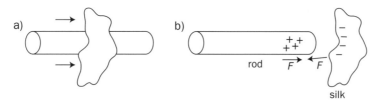

If the positively-charged rod is then held next to another material that has no net charge, and without touching it, it can still exert a force of attraction on the neutral material, a small piece of wood for example. This is because the electrons in the neutral material will redistribute themselves. Since the rod is positively charged, the electrons in the wood will be attracted to the rod resulting in the wood having a region of net negative charge closer to the rod, and net positive charge further away from the rod. The rod and wood will therefore exert attractive forces on each other.

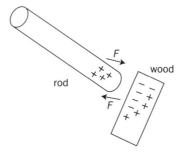

THE ELECTRIC FIELD

An **electric field** defines the region in space around a charge or charges in which another charge will feel a force if placed in that region. However the field exists even if no external charge is brought in to the region. In other words the field is said to exist in the empty space around any charge. The direction of the electric field at a point in space is defined to be in the direction of force that a very small positive "test charge" would feel if it happened to be placed at that point. Therefore the direction of the electric field in the space around positive charges would be directed away from those charges, and the field around negative charges would be directed towards them. The strength of the electric field is given by: $E = \dfrac{F}{q}$ where E is the field strength in Newtons per Coulomb of charge, and F is the force that a small positive test charge q would feel if it happened to be placed in the region.

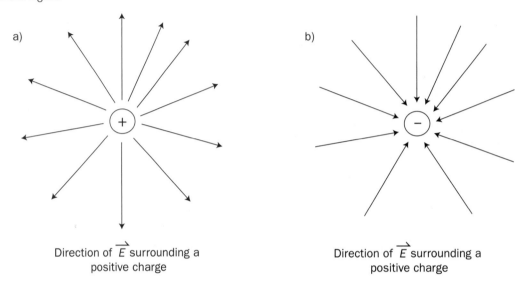

a)

Direction of $\overrightarrow{E}$ surrounding a
positive charge

b)

Direction of $\overrightarrow{E}$ surrounding a
positive charge

> **Example:** At a region in space surrounding a distribution of charges the electric field strength is measured to be $500N/C$ pointing in a direction due east. If a $.001\ C$ charge is brought into that region what magnitude and direction of force will this charge experience?

Solution: $F = qE = (.001C)(500N/C) = 5N$

ELECTRIC POTENTIAL (VOLTAGE)

The **electric potential V** is related to the amount of energy that is available to do work on electric charges in an electric field. The potential difference between two points is the amount of work it would take to move a charge q between those two points against the electric field, divided by the amount of the charge:

$$\Delta V = \frac{Work}{q}$$

The units of potential, and potential difference are $\dfrac{\text{Joules}}{\text{Coulomb}}$

$$1\frac{J}{C} = 1\ \text{Volt}(V)$$

ΔV is therefore proportional to the amount of energy that the charge has gained by having been moved a distance against the force of the electric field. The idea is similar to lifting a mass up in a gravitational field thus giving the object gravitational potential energy.

Electric potential is also called **voltage** and is an essential concept in analysing electric circuits.

ELECTRIC CIRCUITS

An **electric circuit** consists of a complete path of conducting material through which electric charges can flow. They require some means by which energy is supplied to the circuit (for example a battery) so that the charges will be able to flow. Usually there are various electrical components within the circuit, such as resistors, capacitors, diodes etc. that are designed to do work, or perform a specific task using the flow of electric charge as an energy source.

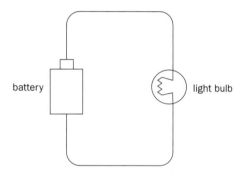

Conductors and Insulators

Conductors are materials through which electric charge can flow easily. Metals are particularly good conductors due to the fact that electrons in metals are extremely mobile, and move from atom to atom quite easily. Most wiring in electrical circuits is made of a metal core (copper is very common) surrounded by a thin layer of insulating material.

Insulators are materials that do not conduct electric charge easily, due to the relative immobility of their electrons. Good insulators include rubber, many plastics, polystyrene etc.

Current, Voltage and Resistance

Current (I) is defined as the rate at which charge flows through a conductor. The units of current are Coulombs/Second. $1 \ C/S = 1$ Ampere (A). Although for the most part it is electrons that are actually in motion in a circuit, by convention the direction of I is said to be in the direction that positive charge would flow through the circuit. For example in the circuit shown below, the battery has a positive and negative end. Although most of the charge flow in the circuit is actually electrons moving in the anticlockwise direction, we say that it is positive charge moving clockwise and thus give the current direction shown. When analysing the behaviour of circuits this presents no problem, as a positive charge flow in one direction is mathematically (and conceptually) equivalent to a negative charge flow in the other direction.

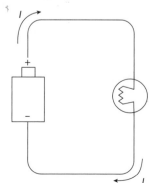

As discussed above voltage or electrical potential is proportional to how much energy is available to move charge through a circuit. Therefore a 9V battery provides more energy to the circuit than a 1.5V battery.

As charge moves through a circuit it encounters resistance to flow. **Resistance** is a measure of how severely the charge flow is impeded in its motion. Resistance is similar in concept to friction in mechanical systems. The wires, and all of the elements and devices in the circuit have resistance, although the resistance of the wires is usually neglected when there are other elements in the circuit, since it is usually very small relative to the other resistances. Many devices convert electrical energy to some other form of energy. For example a light bulb converts electrical energy to heat and light, and an electric fan converts electrical energy to mechanical energy. These devices create resistance to the current that flows through them and are called **resistors**. The unit of resistance is the Ohm (Ω). $1\ \Omega = 1\ J/C$. Schematic symbols used for battery voltage, resistance and current are summarised in the table below.

Quantity	Symbol	Unit	Schematic Symbol
Battery Voltage	V	Volts (V)	$-\mid\mid^+$
Current	I	Amps (A)	→
Resistance	R	Ohms (Ω)	—⋀⋀⋀—

Ohm's Law

As the voltage is increased in a circuit the resulting current also becomes larger. In many circuits there is a simple relationship between the voltage and the current as shown in the graph below.

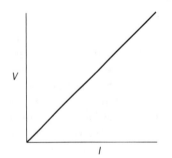
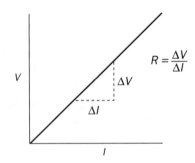

This linear relationship implies that current is directly proportional to voltage, or that the ratio of V to I is a constant. This ratio is equal to R, the Resistance of the circuit, expressed by **Ohm's Law**:

$$\frac{V}{I} = R$$

Although this is not a fundamental principle (like Newton's 2nd Law for example) and there are many circuits that do not obey this relationship, many simple circuits can be analysed using Ohm's Law.

Example: In the circuit below, the battery has a voltage equal to $3V$, and the resistor has a resistance of $1\,\Omega$. a) What is the current in the circuit? b) With what value resistor would you have to replace the 1Ω resistor to increase the current in the circuit to $12A$?

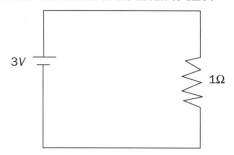

3V

1Ω

Solution: a) $I = \dfrac{V}{R} = \dfrac{3V}{1\Omega} = 3\,A$ b) $R = \dfrac{V}{I} = \dfrac{3V}{12A} = 0.25\,\Omega$

Electrical Power in Circuits

Power is defined as the rate at which work is done, or the rate at which energy is transferred from one form to another: $P = \dfrac{W}{t}$, or $P = \dfrac{E}{t}$. In an electric circuit power can be related to voltage, current and resistance as follows:

$$P = IV = \frac{V^2}{R} = I^2R$$

The units of power are Joules/Second (J/s), and $I\,J/s = 1$ Watt (W). A $60W$ light bulb means that the filament of the bulb converts $60J$ of electrical energy to heat and light energy every second.

> **Example:** For the circuit in the example above determine the power dissipated by the circuit for the situations described in a) and b).

Solution: a) $P = IV = (3A)(3V) = 9W$ (or $P = I^2R = (3A)^2(1\Omega) = 9W$)

b) $P = IV = (12A)(3V) = 36W$

Note that the circuit with lower resistance and more current uses energy at a much greater rate.

The kilowatt-hour

The **kilowatt-hour** (KWh) is actually a unit of energy. 1 KWh is the energy used by a circuit, or electrical device operating at a power of $1KW$ ($= 1000W = 1000J/s$), for a time of 1 hour. In Joules $1KWh = 1000J/s(1hr)(3600s/hr) = 3.6$ million Joules. The electrical meter outside a home measures the amount of energy used in units of KWh.

> **Example:** Over a one month period of time, the household electrical meter reads a total energy use of 120KWh. a) How much energy in Joules have been used in the month in question? b) The electricity company charges a rate of 20 cents per KWh. What will the electricity bill be for that month?

Solution: a) $E = 120\text{KWh}(1000\text{W/KW})(1\text{hr})(3600s/hr) = 4.3 \times 10^8\text{J}$

b) total cost $= 120\text{KWh}(20\text{cents/KWh}) = 2400$ cents $= \$24$

Circuits with Multiple Resistors

Resistors in a circuit can be placed in **series**, in **parallel** or in a combination of series and parallel arrangements.

Series Circuits

Resistors in series are all placed in the same path in the circuit (as shown below.)

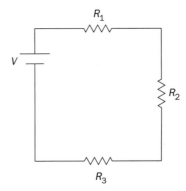

The current must therefore be the same through each resistor in the series arrangement.

The total resistance in a series circuit is the sum of the individual resistances:

$$R_{total} = R_1 + R_2 + R_3 + \dots$$

Example: For the circuit shown below determine: a) the total resistance of the circuit. b) the total current in the circuit. c) the amount of voltage dropped across each of the resistors. d) the power dissipated by the circuit.

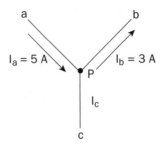

Solution:

a) $R_{total} = 3\Omega + 5\Omega + 7\Omega = 15\Omega$

b) $IR = \frac{1}{3}A(3\Omega) = 1V$

c) Use Ohm's Law for the individual section of the circuit

V across the 3Ω resistor $= IR = \dfrac{1}{3}A(3\Omega) = 1V$

$$V_{5\Omega} = \dfrac{1}{3}A(5\Omega) = \dfrac{5}{3}V$$

$$V_{7\Omega} = \dfrac{1}{3}A(7\Omega) = \dfrac{7}{3}V$$

The total of the individual voltage drops adds up to the 5V of the battery.

d) $P = IV = \dfrac{1}{3}A(5V) = \dfrac{5}{3}W$

Parallel circuits

Resistors in parallel are arranged in separate branches in the circuit as shown in the figure below.

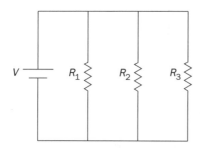

Because they are in separate branches, the current through each resistor may be different; however, the voltage drop across each resistor in parallel must be the same. When resistors are placed in parallel the total resistance of the circuit is actually less than any of the individual resistors, and the more resistors you add in parallel the lower the total resistance becomes, and the higher the total current.

$$\dfrac{1}{R_{total}} = \dfrac{1}{R_1} + \dfrac{1}{R_2} + \dfrac{1}{R_3} + \ldots$$

Example: For the circuit shown below determine: a) the total resistance. b) the voltage drop across each resistor. c) the current through each resistor d) the power dissipated by the circuit.

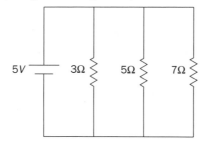

a) $\dfrac{1}{R_{total}} = \dfrac{1}{3}\Omega + \dfrac{1}{5}\Omega + \dfrac{1}{7}\Omega = 0.68$, therefore $R = \dfrac{1}{0.68} = 1.5\Omega$

$I_{total} = \dfrac{V_{battery}}{R_{total}} = \dfrac{5V}{1.5\Omega} = 3.33A$

b) Each resistor must have the same voltage drop as the battery, therefore $V_1 = V_2 = V_3 = 5V$

c) Use Ohm's Law individually for each R, such that $I_1 = \dfrac{V_1}{R_1} = \dfrac{5V}{3\Omega} = \dfrac{5}{3}A$, $I_2 = \dfrac{5V}{5\Omega} = 1A$, and

$I_3 = \dfrac{5V}{7\Omega} = \dfrac{5}{7}A$ with these three currents adding together to give the total current of $3.33A$.

d) $P = IV = 3.33A(5V) = 16.7W$

Notice that for the same three resistors, the parallel arrangement gives a much lower resistance, and a higher total current and power for the circuit.

It is easy to show that for resistors arranged in parallel, burning out one element in the circuit will leave the others unaffected. In a series arrangement, if one element in the line is broken the entire circuit will be disrupted. This is one of the reasons that household wiring is arranged in a parallel system.

Measuring voltage and current in circuits

An **ammeter** is used to measure current through a resistor. This must be placed in series with the resistor so that it receives the same current as that passing through the resistor. However, so as not to affect the current, the ammeter must have a very low resistance.

A **voltmeter** is used to measure voltage drop across a resistor. The voltmeter must be placed in parallel with the resistor so that it drops the same voltage as the resistor; however, it must have a very high resistance relative to the resistor so that very little current will want to flow through it.

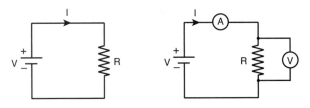

Other common circuit elements

Capacitors are devices that store charge and electric field in a circuit that can be used at a later time.

Diodes are devices that are used to regulate the voltage in circuits, and to make logic gates. A diode has a very high resistance in one direction, and therefore current can only flow the other way. LED's, or Light Emitting Diodes are commonly used for indicator lights in such devices as computers or televisions.

Thermistors are devices used as temperature sensors. Their resistance decreases with increasing temperature, so that the higher the temperature the more current will flow through them.

LDR's are "Light Dependent Resistors" and are used to detect light levels. Their resistance decreases as light intensity increases.

Direct current and alternating current

Direct current (or dc) is when the current in the circuit flows in only one direction. Batteries supply dc. In a dc circuit the voltage is a constant value, resulting in a constant value of current in the circuit.

Alternating current (or ac) is a current that constantly switches directions. This is the type of current supplied by the generators that supply power to large systems, like a house, city, etc. This current oscillates very rapidly, (60 times a second, or 60 Hz (hertz) in the U.S., and 50Hz in the U.K.). The alternating current is due to a rapidly changing voltage source. Therefore the voltage and current in this type of circuit are constantly changing; however, the oscillation is so rapid that circuit elements operate continuously.

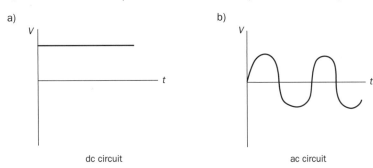

dc circuit   ac circuit

Household circuits and wiring

Household circuits are wired in parallel. Separate branches in a parallel circuit remain unaffected by the other branches. Therefore if an electrical appliance or device in the house breaks, for example if the filament of a light bulb burns out, then the other appliances will operate normally. Also appliances are designed to operate at a specific voltage and current. The only way to insure the proper voltage is for each appliance to be in its own separate branch in a parallel circuit.

Fuses and circuit breakers

As seen above, the more branches that are connected in parallel the smaller the total resistance, and therefore the larger the total current in a circuit. For example, the more appliances that are turned on simultaneously in a house the more parallel branches the circuit has, and therefore the higher total current in the circuit. When the current gets too high the wires may heat up to temperatures large enough to melt the surrounding insulation. This is a dangerous situation that can lead to an electrical fire. For this reason circuits are often protected from overheating. The idea is to break the circuit once the temperature gets beyond a certain level. One way to do this is to place a **fuse** in the circuit. A fuse contains a piece of wire or metal that melts easily. If the temperature gets too high the fuse will melt, thus breaking the circuit. Another way to protect the circuit is by using a **circuit breaker**. With a circuit breaker a spring-loaded switch is held closed by a spring loaded iron bolt. An electromagnet is set up so that if it receives sufficient current it can pull the bolt away from the switch, because the higher the current the stronger the electromagnet. A circuit breaker does not have to be replaced like a fuse, it simply needs to be reset once the wires cool down.

A **short circuit** occurs when for some reason the circuit is able to bypass the resistor. For example if a wire became frayed as shown in the figure below, the two wires could touch and the current would bypass the resistor. Since the total resistance of the circuit would become greatly reduced the current would become very high. A fuse or circuit breaker could protect the system if a short circuit occurred.

Grounding and electrical safety

Electrical circuits can also pose an electrocution danger in certain circumstances. Current above 100mA driven through a person is often fatal. The amount of current will depend on how high the voltage is, and the resistance of both the person, and the device or appliance to which the person is in contact. To receive an electric shock two parts of the body must be in contact with conductors at different potentials, since potential difference is a property of two points. In typical wiring one of the two wires is connected physically to the ground, this wire is said to be **grounded** or **earthed**. This arrangement prevents the wiring from reaching excessively high potentials; however, this means that if a person contacts the high voltage wire and any grounded conductor, including the ground itself, he or she will receive a shock. For example if a short circuit occurs within an appliance, the exterior of the appliance may be at high potential, and if a person were to be in contact with the appliance and the ground, a current will flow through them. To avoid this many appliances and power tools are equipped with three wire cords. The third wire runs from the exterior of the appliance to a grounded wire in the outlet. Normally no current flows through this wire; however, if a short circuit should occur this third wire provides a very low resistance path for the current to travel to ground, bypassing the person.

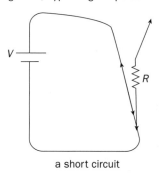

a short circuit

MAGNETIC FIELDS

A **magnetic field** (B) is defined as a region in space in which a magnet will experience a force, such that the north side of the magnet will feel a force in the direction of the field and the south side of the magnet will experience a force opposite to the field direction. Magnetic fields are seen to exist around permanent magnets like those shown in the figure below. The Earth itself has a magnetic field, and a magnet (such as the needle on a compass) will feel a force in the direction of the Earth's field as long as no other stronger fields wash out the effect of that of the Earth. The unit of magnetic field is the **Tesla** (T). $1T = N/C(m/s)$.

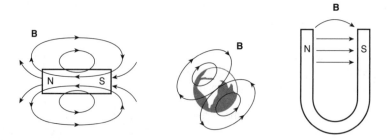

Permanent magnets like the bar magnet and horseshoe magnet shown above, are created when certain susceptible materials called **ferromagnetic** materials are placed in an external magnetic field. The ferromagnetic material then aligns itself at the atomic level such that it produces a net magnetic field in the same direction as the external field. The term ferromagnetic is derived from ferrous (iron bearing) because the element iron is the most highly susceptible material to being magnetised.

Ultimately, the source of all magnetic fields are moving charges. All materials have moving charge because electrons are in constant motion around the nuclei of atoms. Therefore each atom has its own magnetic field. The reason that most materials do not exhibit observable magnetic fields is because the fields of the individual atoms are oriented randomly such that on average they cancel out. When a ferromagnetic material is placed inside an external field, the electron motions within the material can align themselves in the same direction, giving a net magnetic field in the material in the same direction as the external field.

Magnetic field due to a current carrying wire

Since a current consists of moving charge, a current-carrying wire has a magnetic field around it. The direction of the magnetic field is in a circular pattern around the wire. The direction of the field can be determined by the **first right hand rule**. According to this rule, if you place the thumb of your right hand in the direction of current flow (using the convention that current is in the direction of positive charge flow), then your fingers will curl around your thumb in the direction of the field.

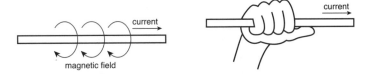

The **solenoid** is common electrical element in which the wire is wrapped into a stacked coil. If a straight wire was bent into a loop, the circular field would be such that the field inside the loop would be in one direction and the field outside the loop in the opposite direction. With several stacked loops, like in a solenoid, it can be seen that the net field looks exactly like the field due to a bar magnet.

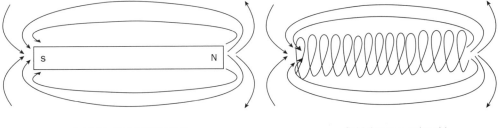

field due to a bar magnet   field due to a solenoid

If an iron core is placed inside the coils of a solenoid, the field lines are intensified, due to the fact that the field inside the iron core aligns itself in the direction of the solenoid's field. Such a device is called an **electromagnet**.

Moving charges in magnetic fields

Not only do moving charges create magnetic fields, but a charge moving through an external field may experience a force due its interacting with the external field. The way this happens is not so simple as an electric force on a charge in an electric field, where the force is always parallel to the field lines, and is independent of whether the charge is moving or not ($F = qE$). For there to be a magnetic force on an electric charge: 1) The charge must be in motion or there will be no force. 2) The charge must have at least some component of velocity **perpendicular** to the field lines. If the charge is in motion parallel to the magnetic field there will be no force. Mathematically, the magnetic force on a charge q moving through a magnetic field B with velocity v is given by

$$F = qvB\sin\theta$$

where θ is the angle between the field lines and the direction of the velocity as shown.

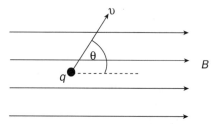

The direction of the force is neither in the direction of the field, nor in the direction of the velocity; rather it is perpendicular to both. The exact direction is given by the **second right hand rule**. For this rule place the thumb of your right hand in the direction of the motion of the charge, and your fingers in the direction of the magnetic field. The force on a positive charge will be in a direction coming out of your palm. The force on a negative charge will be exactly the opposite (out of the back of your hand.) Or you can use your left hand when determining the force on negative charges, such that the direction of force on the negative charge comes out of the palm of your left hand. The positive charge shown below is moving up the plane of the page. The field is oriented directly into the page, so the positive charge will experience a force to the left.

X	X	X	X	X
X	X		X	X
X	X		X	X
X	X	(p)	X	X
X	X	X	X	X

(a)

(b)

Example: For each of the following charges determine the magnitude and direction of the magnetic force acting on it. In each case $B = 0.50T$, the velocity of the charge $= 500m/s$, and the magnitude of the charge $= 1 \times 10^{-3}C$, although in part b) the charge is negative.

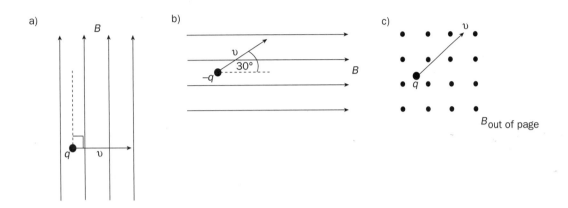

Solution: a) $F = qvB\sin\theta = (1 \times 10^{-3}\ C)\ (500m/s)(.5T)\sin(90) = 0.25\ N$ in a direction out of the page by the right hand rule.

b) $F = (-1 \times 10^{-3}\ C)(500m/s)(.5T)\sin(30) = 0.125N$ into the page

c) $F = (1 \times 10^{-3}\ C)(500m/s)(0.5T)\sin(90) = 0.25N$ down and to the right. (perpendicular to both v and B)

Force on a current carrying wire

Because a current in a wire is moving charge, these charges and therefore the wire itself may experience a force, under the same conditions as a single charge, if the wire is placed inside a magnetic field. In this case the force can be expressed in terms of current I, and length L of the wire that is immersed in the field.

$$F = ILB\sin\theta$$

The direction of force is given by the same right hand rule as for a single charge with the velocity of the charge replaced by the direction of the current.

Example: What force will be exerted on the 2.0m length of wire placed in the magnetic field of $3 \times 10^{-3}T$ shown below, if the current in the wire has a magnitude = 5.0A?

X	X		X	X
X	X		X	X
X	X	2 m X	X	
X	X		X	X
X	X		X	X

$i = 5\ A$

(a)

(b)

$F = ILB\sin\theta = (5A)(2m)(3 \times 10^{-3}T)\sin(90) = 0.03N$

The electric motor

An **electric motor** is a device that operates because of the force that a current-carrying wire experiences when immersed in a magnetic field. In a motor, a coil of wire is placed inside a magnetic field. A current is run through the coil and therefore the wires experience forces that cause the coil to spin. A simplified diagram of an electric motor is shown below. Also shown is a top view, and an edge on view of a single coil in the motor, illustrating how the forces on the wires produce a net torque, thus causing the loop to spin.

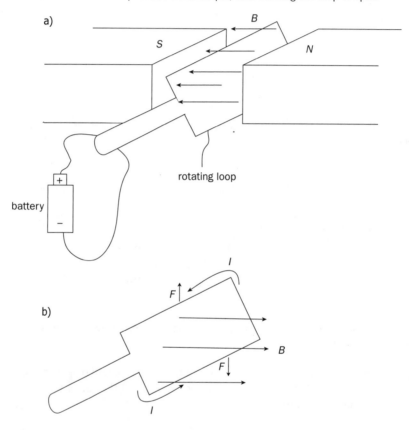

ELECTROMAGNETIC INDUCTION

Above we have shown that a current produces a magnetic field, but the reverse is also possible—a magnetic field can produce a current. This phenomenon is called **electromagnetic induction**. An electric current can be produced when a magnet is moved through a coil of wire, or, alternatively when a wire is moved through a magnetic field.

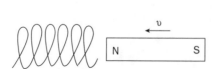

Moving the magnet near the solenoid induces a current in the solenoid

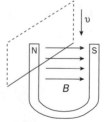

Moving a wire through a magnetic field induces a current in the wire

In the case where the wire is moved: we know that moving charges in a magnetic field can experience a magnetic force. So if the wire is moved through the magnetic field the charges within the wire may experience a force due to their interaction with the field in a direction perpendicular to both the velocity of the wire, and the field lines. For the wire shown above this force will be along the length of the wire, causing the charges to move through the wire, thus creating a current in the direction of the magnetic force. There is no apparent voltage source such as a battery, nevertheless an **induced voltage** is created in the wire, causing an **induced current** to flow.

In the case where the magnet is moved: the strength of the field within the coil of wire is constantly changing as the magnet is moved. If the magnet is just held stationary next to the coil, no induced current will flow; however, if the magnet is in motion, and therefore the field strength within the wire varies, an induced current will appear in the wire. Alternatively, the same effect can be generated by moving the coil instead of the magnet, changing the area inside the coil over a period of time say by constricting the wires, or changing the angle of the coil to the external magnetic field. In each of these cases the "amount" of field within the coil is varying over time, and it is this variation over time that creates the induced voltage, and current. The amount of voltage and current produced depends on the rate at which the field within the coil varies. The faster the rate of change, the greater the induced voltage.

The electromagnetic generator

The **electromagnetic generator** uses the principle of electromagnetic induction to produce a current. A generator in essence is an electric motor run in reverse. In an electric motor electrical energy is converted to mechanical energy by running a current through a wire that is immersed in a magnetic field. In a generator mechanical energy is converted to electrical energy. With a generator the coil of wire within the magnetic field is spun manually. Since the area within the loop of wire will therefore experience a changing amount of field over time, a voltage and current will be induced in the wire. The electrical energy that powers cities is produced by electromagnetic generators. For example, a hydroelectric plant uses the energy of falling water to spin a turbine inside a magnetic field, thus converting mechanical to electrical energy. The energy to spin the turbine could also be produced by the burning of fossil fuels, or in nuclear reactions. A nuclear power plant is a place where the energy released in nuclear fission reactions is used to ultimately spin a turbine and generate electricity. Most generators generate ac current because as the coil is spun inside the field the current is constantly reversing direction. In fact the frequency of the ac current depends directly on the rate at which the turbine is spun. A 50Hz ac current is generated by the coil in a generator being spun at a rate of 50 Hz.

Transformers

A **transformer** is a device that changes the voltage from an ac power supply using the principle of electromagnetic induction. A transformer can change a high voltage supply into a lower voltage (a step down transformer), or vice versa (a step up transformer.) Because more energy is lost to heat when current is higher, it is more economical to transmit electricity from the power stations at a high voltage, and a low current. For this reason step up transformers are used at the power station. However, these voltages are much too dangerous to use in the home so step down transformers are used locally to reduce voltages to safe levels. Transformers are essentially comprised of two solenoids placed in close proximity to each other. The primary coil is connected to an ac power supply. Because the current is constantly changing in the primary coil it produces a constantly changing magnetic field. This changing field in turn induces an ac current in the secondary coil. The primary coil and secondary coil contain a different number of loops, and the difference in voltage between the two coils is proportional to the difference in the number of loops. A step down transformer is when the primary coil has more loops than the secondary coil, and vice versa for a step up transformer.

REVIEW QUESTIONS

1. Two electric charges, located a distance d apart, experience an electrostatic force F. If the charges are moved to a distance of $\frac{1}{3}$ from each other what is the new electrostatic force?

   (A) 3F

   (B) 9F

   (C) $\frac{1}{3}$

   (D) $\frac{1}{9}$

2. Two equal positive charges are placed a distance d apart. They are fixed in place so that they cannot move. Where can a third charge be placed so that it experiences no electrostatic force?

   (A) It should be placed a distance d from either of the charges.

   (B) It depends on the sign of the third charge.

   (C) It should be placed exactly in the middle of the two charges.

   (D) There is nowhere that the third charge will experience no force.

3. An electric circuit has 10V battery and a single 5Ω resistor. The current in the circuit, and the power dissipated by the circuit are:

   (A) 2A, 10W

   (B) 2A, 20W

   (C) 5A, 5W

   (D) 10A, 5W

4. The concept of electric potential (or voltage) is most closely related to which of the following?

   (A) Electrical energy

   (B) Electrical power

   (C) Electric current

   (D) Force

5. In the circuit shown below $R_1 > R_2 > R_3$, which resistor has the greatest current flowing through it?

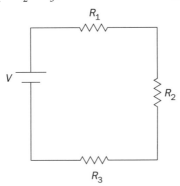

(A) R_1

(B) R_2

(C) R_3

(D) They all have equal current.

6. In the circuit shown below $R_1 > R_2 > R_3$, which resistor has the greatest current flowing through it?

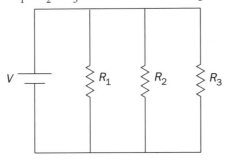

(A) R_1

(B) R_2

(C) R_3

(D) They all have equal current.

7. The Earth's magnetic field is oriented due north at a certain location. At this location a high energy electron is moving due east through the atmosphere. What direction of magnetic force will the electron experience?

(A) due east

(B) due north

(C) up (away from the Earth)

(D) down (towards the Earth)

8. A generator is a device that:

    (A) converts mechanical energy to electrical energy.

    (B) is like an electric motor run in reverse.

    (C) is found in nuclear power plants.

    (D) none of the above.

    (E) all of the above.

Answers and Explanations

1. **B**

$F = \dfrac{kq_1 q_2}{d^2}$. If the new distance is one third the original distance then the new force is nine times as great.

2. **C**

The third charge must be placed exactly in the middle. The forces that the two charges exert on the third charge must be equal in magnitude and opposite in direction such that they cancel out. The only place where this will be true is right in the middle. Also the sign of the third charge doesn't matter. If it is a positive charge then the other charges will both repel it, the forces cancelling, and if it is a negative charge the other charges will both attract it, the forces still cancelling.

3. **B**

$I = \dfrac{V}{R} = \dfrac{10V}{5\Omega} = 2A, \quad P = IV = (2A)(10V) = 20V$

4. **A**

Electric potential is directly proportional to electric potential energy. (It is equal to the electric potential energy per charge.)

5. **D**

Since the resistors are connected in series they all must have equal current flowing through them.

6. **C**

Since the resistors are connected in parallel, each resistor drops the same voltage. According to Ohm's Law $I = \dfrac{V}{R}$, therefore since each R has the same V, the R with the least resistance will have the greatest current flowing through it.

7. **D**

The electron is a negative charge and will therefore experience a force in the opposite direction as a positive charge. Using the right hand rule therefore the electron experiences a force straight downward.

8. **E**

Each of the statements (A) through (C) are true.

Chapter 17: **Forces and Motion**

In this chapter we will summarise and review the fundamental concepts of motion. The first section will address the study of **kinematics** which addresses *how* things move. Motion will be described quantitatively and visually, using position versus time and velocity versus time graphs. In the following section we review dynamics, the study of causes of motion, or more particularly the causes of changing motion, incapsulated in Newton's Three Laws of motion.

DISTANCE AND DISPLACEMENT

Distance and **displacement** are similar ideas in that they both represent a length that can be measured in feet, metres, miles or any other length unit.

Distance is defined as the total length travelled during some motion.

Distance does not depend on direction, or changes in direction. A quantity that does not depend on any particular direction is called a **scalar** quantity. For example mass is an example of a scalar quantity, as it would make no sense to talk of the property of mass having direction.

> **Example:** A bird flies 10 miles in a straight line due east then turns around and flies 5 miles back the way it came before landing in a tree. What is the distance the bird travels?

Solution: $d = 10$ miles $+ 5$ miles $= 15$ miles

Displacement can be contrasted to distance in that it has a direction associated with it.

Displacement is defined as the straight line distance from the beginning to the end of a motion. The direction of the displacement is given by an arrow pointing from the initial to the final position. Mathematically:

Displacement $=$ final position $-$ initial position $= x_f - x_i = \Delta x$ (assuming motion along a single axis or one dimensional motion.)

Quantities that have a particular direction associated with them are called **vector** quantities. A force is another example of a vector quantity. We speak of applying a force in a particular direction, and the effect of a force on an object will depend on the direction of that force.

> **Example:** For the motion of the bird described above find the displacement for the entire flight.

Solution: $\Delta x = x_{final} - x_{initial} = 5$ miles $- 0 = 5$ miles due east

Of if we call east the "positive" direction, then $\Delta x = + 5$ miles.

A way to look at the net displacement is that the bird has a displacement of 10 miles to the east followed by a displacement of 5 miles to the west giving a net displacement of 5 miles to the east. The above is an example of one dimensional motion. In one dimensional motion direction can be defined by a positive or negative direction; however, motion can also be in two or three dimensions. In 2 or 3-D, direction must be defined more specifically.

Example: You take your dog on a walk to the park. First you travel 1000 metres due east down Maple Street. You then turn north onto Elm street and travel another 800 metres to the park as shown in the diagram. What is the distance and the displacement of your walk?

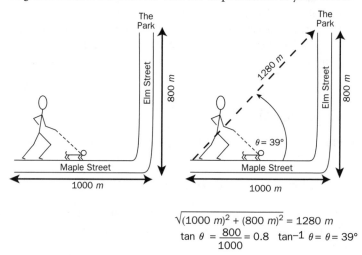

$$\sqrt{(1000\ m)^2 + (800\ m)^2} = 1280\ m$$
$$\tan \theta = \frac{800}{1000} = 0.8 \quad \tan^{-1} \theta = \theta = 39°$$

Solution: The total length of your walk is simply 1000 metres + 800 metres = 1800 metres. This is the *distance* that you have travelled.

Here displacement consists of both Δx and Δy since motion is in two dimensions.

$\Delta x = 1000m$, $\Delta y = 800m$, and the net displacement is the straight line distance between the initial and final position. Therefore as shown above the displacement is 1280m in a direction 39 degrees to the x axis (or 39 degrees north of due east)

SPEED AND VELOCITY

Average **speed** is defined as the total distance travelled during a motion divided by the time it took to complete the motion. Mathematically,

$$s = \frac{d}{\Delta t}. \text{ (Speed is a scalar.)}$$

Average **velocity** is defined as the displacement from the beginning to the end of a motion divided by the time it took to complete that motion.

$$v = \frac{\Delta x}{\Delta t} \text{ (in one dimension)}$$

(Velocity is a vector.)

> **Example:** For the bird described above it takes 30 minutes to fly the 10 miles to the east, and 15 minutes to fly the 5 miles back. a) What is the average speed of the bird? b) What is the average velocity of the bird?

Solution:

a)

$$s = \frac{d}{\Delta t} = \frac{15 \text{ miles}}{45 \text{ min}} = 0.33 \text{mi/min} = .33\text{mi/min} \times 60\text{min/hr} = 20\text{ mi /hr}$$

b) $v = \frac{\Delta x}{\Delta t} = +\frac{5 \text{ mi}}{45 \text{ min}} = +0.11 \text{ mi/min} = +6.7 \text{ mi/hr (or 6.7 mi/hr to the east.)}$ You can also think of a

velocity of +20*mi/hr* for half an hour followed by a velocity of −20*mi/hr* for a quarter hour, giving an average of +6.7 *mi/hr* for the motion.

ACCELERATION

If velocity and/or speed of an object are changing then the object is said to be accelerating.

Acceleration is the rate at which velocity is changing. Mathematically

$$a = \frac{\Delta v}{\Delta t} \text{ (acceleration is a vector.)}$$

In one dimension the rate of change of velocity is equivalent in amount to the rate of change of the speed, so in the following examples the terms velocity and speed will sometimes be used interchangeably.

> **Example:** A car is travelling driving the road at a constant speed of 20 m/s when it merges into faster traffic. The cars speed increases to 30 m/s during a 5 second interval of time, after which time it maintains a constant speed of 30 m/s.
>
> a) During the 5 second period when the car is speeding up, what is its acceleration?
>
> b) What is the acceleration after achieving a constant speed of 30 m/s?

Solution:

a) $a = \frac{\Delta v}{\Delta t} = (30\text{m/s} - 20\text{m/s})/5\text{s} = 2\text{m/s/s or } 2\text{m/s}^2.$

b) $a = 0$ since $\Delta v = 0$.

The units 2m/s/s or 2m/s² can be interpreted physically as follows. Since acceleration is equal to the rate of change in velocity or speed during a time interval, then the units 2 m/s² say that the speed changes by an amount of 2 metres per second every second, or 2 metres per second per second. For example if you begin with an initial speed of 20 m/s and you start accelerating at a rate of 2m/s^2, then after one second you are now travelling at 22 m/s, one second later you are travelling at 24 m/s etc. You speed up at a rate of 2 m/s each second.

> **Example:** You are riding your bicycle at a speed of 15 m/s when a car cuts in front of you. You have to apply your brakes quickly and you come to a stop in a time of 2 seconds; what is your acceleration?

Solution: In this case you are slowing down, and your final speed is less than your initial speed, so

$$a = \frac{\Delta v}{\Delta t} = \frac{(0 \text{ m/s} - 15 \text{ m/s})}{2\text{s}} = -7.5 \text{ m/s}^2 .$$

The negative sign means that if we assume the initial direction of motion is "positive" then the acceleration is opposite to that direction or "negative". We could just as easily have said that the initial velocity was in the negative direction and therefore the acceleration is positive. In either case you would be slowing down. Sometimes people call this a "deceleration". A deceleration means that the acceleration is opposite to the direction of the initial motion regardless of what direction you choose to call the positive direction.

> **Example:** You throw a ball into the air, and it falls back to your hand as shown.

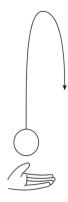

> During the time the ball is in the air, that is from just after you have released it to just before you catch it, what is the direction of its acceleration,
>
> a) on the way up?
>
> b) at the top?
>
> c) on the way down?

Solution: The acceleration is downward in each case. On the way up the ball is slowing down, therefore it must be accelerating in the downward direction. If it were accelerating upward it would have to be speeding up in the upward direction. ***Do not confuse the direction of motion with the direction of the acceleration. They are not necessarily the same although they may be***. In this case the ball is "decelerating" and the acceleration is opposite to the motion direction.

At the top the acceleration *does not* = 0 just because the velocity = 0. The acceleration is the *rate of change* of the velocity, and the ball's velocity is constantly changing. It spends no measurable amount of time at $v = 0$.

The ball just passes through 0 velocity just like it passes through any other instantaneous value of velocity. It is constantly changing and never constant, and therefore constantly accelerating. At the apex of the toss the ball is passing through the last moment of slowing down in the upward direction before it starts speeding up in the downward direction.

On the way down the ball is speeding up constantly in the downward direction, and the acceleration is still downward.

The Acceleration due to Gravity

The example above refers to the *acceleration due to gravity or free fall acceleration* of a body. Gravity is an attraction that exists between all objects that have mass. Gravity is actually a weak force compared to the other fundamental forces. For example the force of gravity between relatively small masses (on the order of the mass of a person or the mass of a rock) are so small that they are unnoticeable. However if at least one of the masses is large, for example the size of a planetary body, then the force between the objects becomes obvious. If an object is tossed up into the air or a person jumps off of a ledge they are pulled to the ground. This is due to the gravitational attraction between these objects and the mass of the Earth. Due to this force of attraction objects that are dropped above the ground will accelerate towards the Earth. In fact all objects when dropped near the surface of the Earth will have the same rate of gravitational acceleration as long as air resistance is not a major factor. For example drop a football and a marble together. They will hit the ground at the same time. The only reason that a feather will take longer to hit the ground is due to the fact that air resistance is affecting it more than the ball. If air was eliminated altogether the feather and the ball would fall together. In fact in a famous demonstration of this phenomenon the first astronauts on the Moon dropped a feather and a hammer together. They accelerated at exactly the same rate (although at a smaller rate than they would have on Earth due to the lesser gravity on the Moon) and hit the ground at the same time.

The rate of the acceleration due to gravity in the absence of air resistance at the surface of the Earth $= 9.8$ m/s^2 for all objects, regardless of mass. The next section will deal with the gravitational force in more detail, and the effect of air resistance on the free-fall acceleration.

GRAPHING MOTION

It can be very useful to represent motion in graphical form. This gives a visual representation of motion that can be interpreted at a glance.

We will look at two types of graphs, **distance-time** or **position-time** graphs, and **velocity-time** graphs.

Position-time graphs

Below are examples of three different position-time (*x-t*) graphs. The vertical axis represents the position of the object, and the horizontal axis represents the time. Therefore, each point on the graphs represents where an object is located at a particular time. The solid line that connects the points contains inferred points where we assume the object should have been located at those times based on the trend that we observe in the actual data.

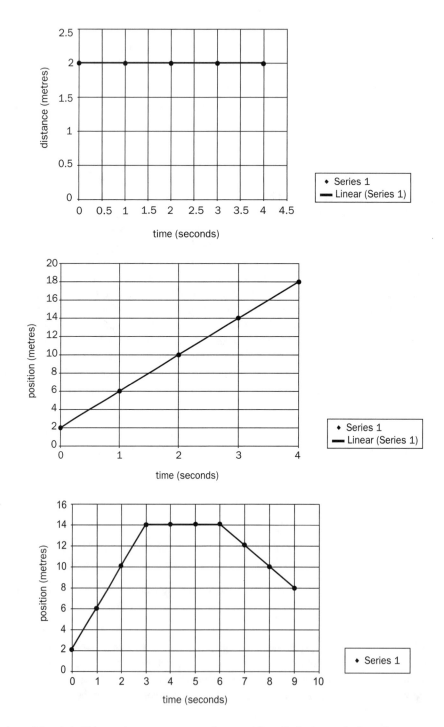

Interpretation of Graph A: This graph represents a stationary object. Each data point is at the exact same position, therefore the object hasn't gone anywhere, and the solid line that fits the trend in the data has a slope of zero representing no change in position.

Interpretation of Graph B: In this case the object is moving at a constant velocity. For each time increment an equal distance is covered. Here the object starts at a position of $x = 2$ m, one second later it is at $x = 6$ m, one second after that at $x = 10$ m. It covers a distance of 4 m each second. The slope of the line is equal to the change in the y axis/the change in the x axis. This is equal to 4, which corresponds physically to the velocity of the object. Therefore the slope of a position-time graph represents the velocity of the object.

Interpretation of Graph C: In this case the object starts off with the same motion as in graph B. The object moves at a constant 4 m/s for 3 seconds. The object then stops and stays at a position of 14 m from the origin until $t = 6$ s. For the last 3 seconds the object turns around and moves in the negative direction. The slope of the graph for this part of the motion is equal to -2m/s. And the final position at $t = 9$s, is $x = 8$m.

The x-t graphs below represent objects that are speeding up and slowing down respectively.

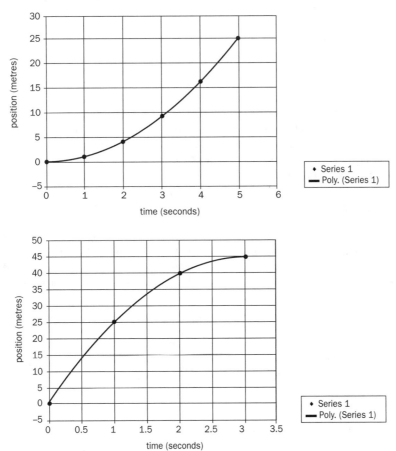

Example: Describe the motion of the object represented by the *x-t* graph shown below.

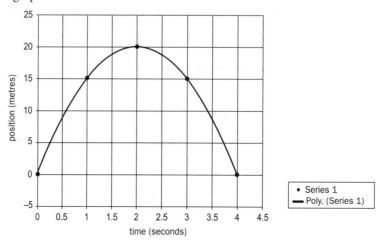

Solution: This object is moving at a relatively high velocity when the timer starts as represented by the steep slope just after $t = 0$. The object gradually slows until it instantaneously stops (represented by an instantaneously 0 slope at the peak of the graph), and then speeds up in the opposite direction. It has returned to its original starting point when the timer stops moving in the negative direction with about equal speed to its original motion in the positive direction.

Velocity-time graphs

While a position-time graph represents where an object is at any given time, a **velocity-time graph** or *v-t* graph represents how fast it is going at any given time. A velocity time graph for a particular motion could be derived from the position-time graph for that motion, by determining the slope of the *x-t* graph at a number of different times. These slopes are equal to the velocity at that time, which can then be plotted on a *v-t* graph. Some examples of *v-t* graphs are shown below.

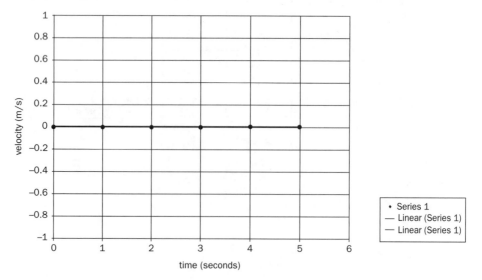

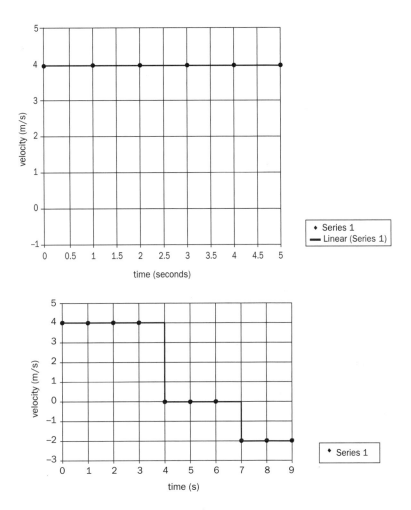

Interpretation of Graph I: In this graph the velocity at each time has a constant value of zero indicating no motion. This corresponds to the same motion represented by the position time Graph A shown above.

Interpretation of Graph II: Here the velocity at each time has a constant value of 4 m/s, corresponding to the motion represented by position-time Graph B shown above. A *v-t* graph can't say anything about the position where the object started; for example you can't know by looking at this graph that the object started at $x = 2$ or not. However you *can* determine how far the object moved from that moment on. Since the object is moving at a constant speed of 4 m/s, it must be true that from wherever it started it has traveled a distance of 4 m/s x the time elapsed from the starting point.

Interpretation of Graph III: The velocity is a constant 4 m/s for the first 3 seconds, 0 m/s for the next three seconds, and −2 m/s for the final 3 seconds which is the same motion described by the *x-t* Graph A above.

The three velocity-time graphs below represent velocities that are continuously changing over time.

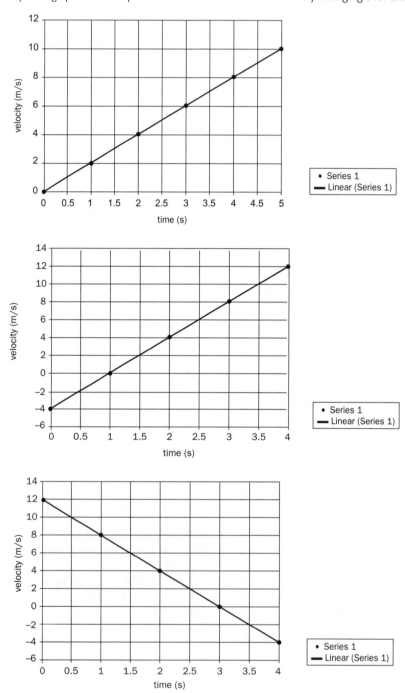

The slope of the velocity-time graph also has a physical meaning. *Since acceleration is defined as* $\frac{\Delta v}{\Delta t}$ *, the slope of the v-t graph is equal to the acceleration of the object.* For example in the first of the three graphs the velocity starts at $v = 0$, and is increasing by 2 m/s each second giving an acceleration equal to 2 m/s² which is equal to the slope of the line. In the second graph the acceleration is also 2 m/s². In this case the velocity starts out moving in the negative direction at 2 m/s, it slows to an instantaneous stop and then increases its speed in the positive direction at a rate of 2 m/s per second. For the entire motion the acceleration is in the positive direction. In the third graph the acceleration is always in the negative direction at a rate of 4 m/s². At $t = 0$ the object is moving in the positive direction but continually slowing by 4 m/s every second. At $t = 3$ seconds the object reverses direction and picks up speed.

Area under the v-t graph

Another useful piece of information about the motion of an object can be obtained by the area underneath a *v-t* graph. Below is an example of a puck sliding along the ice at a constant velocity of 5 m/s.

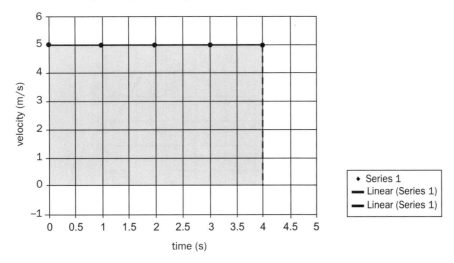

For the 4 seconds of motion shown the puck travelled a distance of 20 m, which is exactly equal to the area in the shaded rectangle shown. The velocity in fact does not need to be constant. *The area underneath any velocity-time graph is equal to the distance travelled during that period of time.* For example the puck described by the graph below starts from rest and constantly increases its speed to 5 m/s during a 4 second time period.

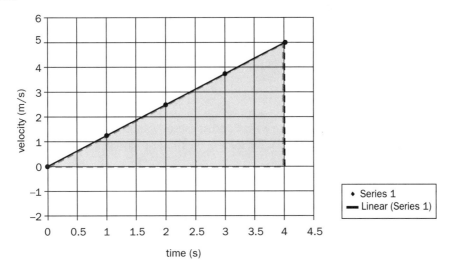

The puck does not cover as much distance as the puck moving for the same time interval at a constant 5 m/s because on average it is moving at a slower rate. In this case the puck has an average velocity of 2.5 m/s resulting in it covering only 10 m which is exactly equal to the area shaded underneath the graph.

Example: For the motion described by the velocity-time graph shown:

a) Describe qualitatively the motion of the object.

b) Determine the acceleration from $t = 0$ to $t = 4$, from $t = 4$ to $t = 8$ and from $t = 8$ to $t = 10$.

c) Determine the distance travelled by the object during the 10 seconds of motion.

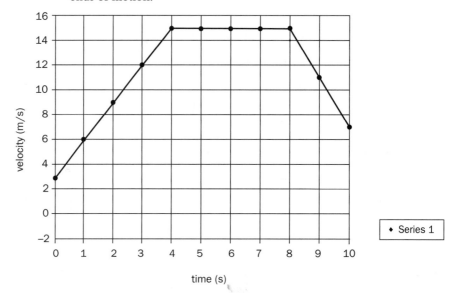

Solution: a) The object starts at an initial velocity of 3 m/s, constantly speeding up to a velocity of 15 m/s in the first 4 seconds. The object then maintains a constant speed of 15 m/s for the next 4 seconds. In the final 2 seconds the object slows to a final speed of 7 m/s. b) Since $a = \dfrac{\Delta v}{\Delta t}$ = the slope of the graph, $a = (15\text{m/s} - 3 \text{ m/s})/4\text{s} = 3 \text{ m/s}^2$ from $t = 0$ to $t = 4$. From $t = 4$ to $t = 8$, $a = 0$, and from $t = 8$ to $t = 10$ $a = (7\text{m/s} - 15 \text{ m/s})/2\text{s} = -4 \text{ m/s}^2$. c) The distance traveled is equal to the total area under the graph $= 140$ m.

NEWTON'S LAWS

In the first section we *described* motion. Here we will discuss causes of motion, or more specifically what causes an object to change its state of motion. The study of the causes of changing motion is called **dynamics**.

Forces

A **force** is a push or a pull acting on an object. The push or pull is due to another object interacting with it, applying that force. Force is a vector quantity having both magnitude and direction. The SI unit of force is the Newton. $1\text{N} = 1 \text{ kg m/s}^2$. An object may have multiple forces acting on it due to its interaction with multiple other bodies. Sometimes these forces all cancel, or balance each other, and we say that there is no net force acting on the object. If the forces do not all cancel out, we say there is an **unbalanced** or **net force**.

Newton's First Law of Motion and Inertia

Newton's First Law of Motion states: an object in motion will stay in motion at a constant velocity (or an object at rest will stay at rest) unless acted on by a net, or unbalanced force. Newton's First Law is also sometimes called the Law of **Inertia**. Inertia is a term that refers to an object's resistance to a change in motion. The mass of an object is a quantitative measure of its inertia. The more inertia an object has, the harder it is to change its motion, and the more force is required to do so. For example it is much harder to accelerate or change the velocity of a bowling ball than it is a tennis ball. The important point of Newton's First Law is that for an object to stay at a constant velocity the absence of force is required, specifically the absence of a net force. It is easy to draw the erroneous conclusion that a constant force is required to maintain constant velocity. Consider a box sliding across the floor. The force one would need to apply to keep it moving is not the only force acting on the box. Friction is acting against its motion, and to keep the object at constant velocity the force we apply is exactly balancing the friction force resulting in a net force of zero. If the applied force is greater than the friction force the object will speed up. If less, or if no push is applied at all, it will slow down until it stops. Once the box stops there is no longer a friction force so the net force is zero, and the box stays at rest.

Newton's Second Law of Motion

According to the First Law, if an object does not experience a net force, it will maintain a constant velocity; however, if it does experience a net force then the object will change its velocity and accelerate. *Newton's Second Law of Motion states that if an object experiences a net force then it will accelerate in the direction of the net force. The acceleration will be directly proportional to magnitude of the net force and inversely proportional to the mass of the object.* Mathematically,

$$F_{net} = ma$$

Example: A 15 kg box is being pulled forward by a rope as shown below. The pulling force = 100 N, and there is a 70 N friction force opposing the motion. What is the acceleration of the box?

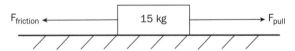

Solution: The net force is 100N − 70N = 30N. Therefore since $a = \dfrac{F}{m}$, $a = \dfrac{30N}{15kg} = 2.0m/s^2$ to the right.

Example: A 2.0 kg mass experiences the forces shown in the diagram below.

a) What is the magnitude and direction of the net force acting on the mass?

b) What is the acceleration of the mass?

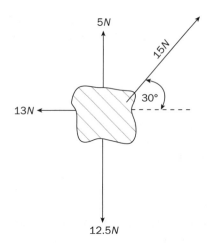

Solution: a) Add up all of the horizontal and vertical forces separately. The 15N force can be broken down into a vertical, and a horizontal component. Using trigonometry the horizontal component $= 15\cos30 = 13$N, and the vertical component $= 15\sin30 = 7.5$N.

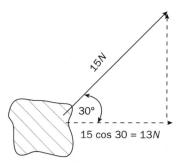

The net horizontal force is then 13N $- 3$N $= 10$N, and the net vertical force is 5N $+ 7.5$N $- 12.5$N $= 0$. Therefore the net force is in the horizontal direction to the right with a magnitude of 10N.

b) $a = \dfrac{F}{m} = \dfrac{10\text{N}}{2.0\text{kg}} = 5.0\text{m/s}^2$ in the same direction as the net force.

Contact versus non-contact forces

Forces can be divided between **contact** and **non-contact** forces. These categories are exactly as they sound. Contact forces require direct contact between the interacting objects. For example pushing a box, or pulling a mass with a string are contact forces. Non-contact forces are also called fundamental forces. These forces act at a distance, across empty space, and include gravity, the electromagnetic force and nuclear forces. In reality all forces are ultimately due to these fundamental forces. Contact forces are actually due to the electromagnetic force at the atomic level. When you push on an object it is electrostatic repulsion between the electrons in your hand and in those in the object that is ultimately responsible for the force that is exerted between you and the object.

The weight force

The force of gravity is a fundamental force which is always attractive, that acts between objects. It is dependent on the mass of each object. The magnitude of the gravitational force between any two masses is given by **Newton's Universal Law of Gravitation**:

$$F = \frac{Gm_1 m_2}{r^2}$$

where F is the force between the two masses m_1 and m_2, r is the distance between the centres of each mass and G is called the Universal Gravitation Constant and is equal to 6.67×10^{-11} Nm^2/kg^2. This force law is very similar in form to Coulomb's Law which describes the electrostatic force between charges. Like Coulomb's Law, the Law of Gravitation is an inverse square law, and diminishes rapidly with distance between the interacting objects. Because the constant G is extremely small, the force of gravity is actually extremely weak compared to the other fundamental forces. It requires at least one of the objects that are being attracted to each other to be very large for the force to be noticeable. Therefore at the Earth's surface, objects experience a noticeable pull towards the Earth. This force of gravity on an object is called the **weight force**. From the Law of Gravitation we can see that the larger the object, the greater the weight force acting on it.

However, it can be shown experimentally that if objects of different mass are dropped, as long as air resistance is not a major factor, they will all experience the same acceleration due to gravity of 9.8 m/s^2. This acceleration is often represented by the constant g (lower case). *It is important to note that the value of g given only pertains at the Earth's surface or close to it. Once an object moves a significant distance from the surface, the value of g can be seen to decrease noticeably*. If an object is dropped just above the surface, and air resistance is negligible, we can show that the value of g is the same for objects of different mass from the Universal Law of Gravitation.

$$F = \frac{Gm_{Earth} m_{object}}{(r_{Earth})^2} = m_{object} a_{object}$$

Therefore $a = \dfrac{Gm_{Earth}}{(r_{Earth})^2}$ which is independent of the mass of the object being accelerated towards the Earth. If the values for G, the mass and radius of the Earth are plugged in the result is:

$$a = 9.8 \text{ m/s}^2 = g$$

and the weight force on an object at or near the Earth's surface reduces to $W = mg$

Example: A 500 kg mass is being lifted by a cable. If the mass is accelerating upward at a rate of 1.0 m/s^2, what is the force that the cable is exerting on the mass?

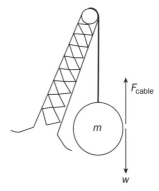

Solution: $F_{net} = ma$. Therefore $F_{net} = 500kg(1.0 \text{ m/s}^2) = 500N$

Since $F_{net} = F_{cable} - W$, $F_{cable} = F_{net} + W = F_{net} + mg = 500N + (500kg)(9.8m/s^2) = 5400N$

Mass versus weight

The concepts of mass and weight are sometimes confused. For example it is common to hear a statement like "the rock *weighs* 3 kg". However, kilograms are a measure of mass not of weight. Mass is a statement of how much *matter* an object contains. Since the amount of matter relates to the object's inertia, its mass can also be thought of as its resistance to a change in motion. An object's mass is independent of where it is. If a rock is floating around in deep space it has no weight, but it still has the same mass as it would have on Earth. Weight is a measure of the **force** that gravity exerts on a mass. In fact as seen above $W = mg$ on the Earth's surface. Weight does not exist in the absence of gravity. It is sometimes misleading to see a scale that measures in kilograms. The scale is actually measuring weight/force but since $m = \dfrac{W}{g}$, and g is a constant at the Earth's surface, the scale is calibrated to convert the weight into the amount of mass that would have that weight on Earth. If you took the scale to the Moon, it would not record the correct mass because g on the Moon is $\dfrac{1}{6}$ that on Earth. However if you had a scale with units of pounds, then this scale would measure your correct weight on the Moon which would be $\dfrac{1}{6}$ your weight on Earth.

Air resistance and terminal velocity

Because Earth has an atmosphere, objects in free fall may experience a significant friction force due to collisions with air molecules, this friction is commonly called **air resistance**. The force of air resistance on an object increases with its velocity (and is also dependent on the shape of the object.) Because this is true an object in free fall will have an acceleration that decreases over time. The figure below shows a skydiver at three different moments. First when he or she has just jumped out of the airplane, then a short while later and finally some time after jumping.

an instant after jumping	a short while after jumping	a long while after jumping (terminal velocity)

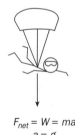

$F_{net} = W = ma$
$a = g$

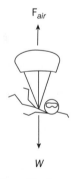

F_{air}

W

$F_{net} = W - F_{air} = ma$
$a < g$

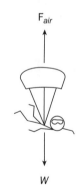

F_{air}

W

$F_{net} = W - F_{air} = 0$
$a = o$

At first the only force acting on the skydiver is the weight force $= mg$, and therefore the diver accelerates at rate g. However, as the skydiver's velocity increases the force of air resistance builds up. Therefore, the net force on the skydiver decreases. Since $F_{net} = ma$ the acceleration will now be less than g. The skydiver will still be speeding up, but at a lesser rate. Eventually as the velocity and air resistance increase, the air resistance force will equal the force of gravity. At that point the net force will equal 0 and acceleration will stop. The velocity at which this occurs is called the **terminal velocity**. Since the weight force on a feather is so small, it takes very little air resistance to balance the weight, and therefore it gains very little speed before it reaches a terminal velocity. Because a skydiver has considerably more weight than a feather, the skydiver's terminal velocity is much greater.

> **Example:** A skydiver achieves terminal velocity when the force of air resistance = 800N. What is the mass of the skydiver?

Solution: Since the skydiver is at terminal velocity, the force of air resistance must equal the skydiver's weight. Therefore $W = 800N = mg$, and $m = \dfrac{W}{g} = \dfrac{800N}{9.8m/s^2} = 82$ kg .

Sliding Friction

Friction is a force that opposes motion or potential motion. Whenever two surfaces are in contact, and one of the surfaces is sliding along the other, there is a force of **kinetic friction** that exists between the surfaces, acting against the motion of each object. Unlike the force of air resistance, the force of kinetic friction is independent of the relative speed of the objects. It does depend on how "sticky" the two surfaces are when in contact with each other, and how hard the surfaces are being pushed together. For example, dry ice sliding along a Formica tabletop experiences much less friction than a brick sliding along a concrete surface. And a book on a table will experience a much greater friction force if it is being pushed down into the table.

Static friction may exist when an object is not in motion relative to the surface on which it rests. For example say a book is at rest on a table and a small force is applied in an attempt to push it along the table, and yet the book does not move. This is because a static friction force is acting against the pushing force, resulting in net force of zero on the book. Static friction opposes potential sliding between two surfaces. Like kinetic friction, it is also dependent on the material properties of each surface, and how hard the surfaces are being pushed together. Static friction will only be as strong as it needs to be to balance the forces that would cause an object to slide. Therefore it will increase as it balances these forces. However, it has a certain maximum value and once the pushing forces exceed that value, the object will start sliding.

> **Example:** A crate is in the back of a flatbed lorry, when the lorry begins to accelerate. If the crate accelerates along with the lorry what force is responsible for its acceleration?

Solution: The force responsible for accelerating the crate is *static* friction. There is no sliding between the bed of the lorry and the crate, although there is potential to slide. If there were no friction at all the lorry would just drive out from underneath the crate. The crate would be sliding relative to the lorry in that case. If there was some friction but not enough to keep the crate accelerating with the lorry then there would be a kinetic friction force acting on the crate. However, in this case the static friction force is able to "grip" the crate and pull it along with the lorry.

Newton's Third Law of Motion

Newton's Third Law is often quoted as "for every action there is an equal and opposite reaction", however to be more specific: if object A exerts a force on object B, then object B exerts a force of equal magnitude back on object A in the opposite direction to the force that A exerts on B. While the statement is simple it is often misunderstood. First of all the Third Law says that all forces occur in pairs, that is all forces are due to the interaction between objects. And the action-reaction force pairs are always equal to each other. It does not matter what the masses of the respective objects are. For example if a train were to collide head on with a fly moving in the opposite direction, during the collision the two objects would exert equal forces on each other. However, the effect of the forces will be different on the train and the fly. Since $a = \dfrac{F}{m}$, for a certain force, a fly will experience a much greater acceleration than a train experiencing the same force. It is important to note that when applying Newton's Second Law to the motion of an object, only the forces acting on that object count. The reaction forces that object exerts back on other objects, only affect the motion of those other objects.

Example: A 60 kg astronaut is in deep space holding a 5 kg rock in his or her hand. He throws the rock, and during the 0.5 second time the rock is in his or her hand, it speeds up to a final velocity of 15m/s upon release. At what speed will the astronaut be moving in the opposite direction after throwing the rock?

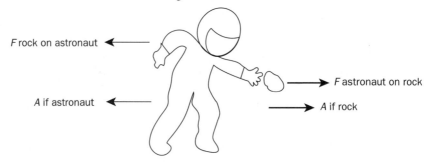

Solution: This problem requires combining several principles. First we can determine the acceleration of the rock.

Since $a = \dfrac{\Delta v}{\Delta t}$, $a_{rock} = \dfrac{(15m/s - 0m/s)}{(0.5s)} = 30m/s^2$. And $F_{net\ on\ rock} = ma = 5kg(30m/s^2) = 150N$. According to Newton's Third Law this force must be equal to the force that the rock exerts back on the astronaut. Therefore

$$a_{astronaut} = \frac{F}{m} = \frac{150N}{60kg} = 2.5m/s^2. \text{ And } \Delta v = \frac{a}{\Delta t} = \frac{(2.5m/s^2)}{(0.5s)} = 5.0m/s.$$

The principle behind rockets is very similar to that illustrated by the above example. In a rocket a force is exerted on the gas that is expelled out of the rocket, and the gas in turn exerts a reaction force back on the rocket causing it to accelerate.

Example: A block sits on a table. a) What forces are acting directly on the block? b) What are the reaction forces to the forces in part a)?

Solution: a) There are two forces acting on the block as shown below: the force of gravity pulling the block towards the Earth, and the force of the table pushing up on the block. The force of the table pushing up must be equal to the weight force down since the block has no acceleration and therefore the net force must be 0.

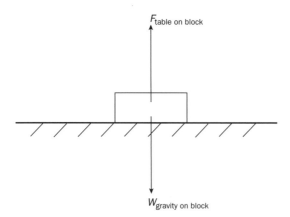

b) The weight force is due to the Earth pulling on the block, and therefore the reaction force to this must be the block pulling back on the Earth. The table pushes up on the block and therefore the reaction to this is the block pushing back down on the table. The weight force and the force of the table on the block are *not* action reaction pairs. Although it is true that the force of the table on the block would not be there if gravity wasn't pulling the block down, these forces act on the same object and cannot be action reaction pairs.

REVIEW QUESTIONS

1. A long distance runner runs 5 miles north in 35 minutes then turns around and runs 5 miles back to where she started in 38 minutes. What is her average speed for the run?

    (A) 5.5 miles/hr
    (B) 0 miles/hr
    (C) 8.2 miles/hr
    (D) 9.6 miles/hr

2. For the runner in question one what is her average velocity?

    (A) 5.5 miles/hr
    (B) 0 miles/hr
    (C) 8.2 miles/hr
    (D) 9.6 miles/hr

3. A train is moving eastward at a velocity = 10 m/s when it puts on the brakes, and slows to 5 m/s over a 60 second time period. During this time what are the magnitude and direction of the acceleration of the train?

    (A) 0.083 m/s eastward
    (B) 0.083 m/s westward
    (C) 0.166 m/s eastward
    (D) The train is not accelerating, it is decelerating.

4. If the train in the example above has a mass = 50,000 kg what is the net force acting on the train as it slows?

    (A) 9300 N eastward

    (B) 4150 N westward

    (C) 9300 N westward

    (D) 4150 N eastward

5. Which of the *v-t* graphs below represent the motion of an object that changes direction?

    (A)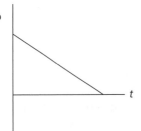

    (B)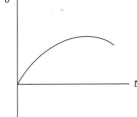

    (C)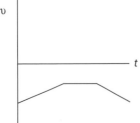

    (D)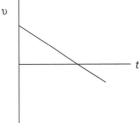

6. Which statement best describes the motion represented by the *x-t* graph below?

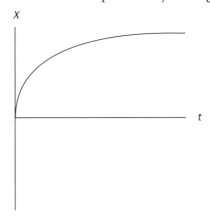

(A) The object starts at a high velocity and gradually slows until it stops.

(B) The object starts with an initial velocity = 0, and speeds up continuously until it reaches some final constant velocity

(C) The object starts at a high velocity and gets faster until achieving some final constant velocity.

(D) The object starts with an initial velocity = 0, speeds up and then slows to a stop.

7. A golf club strikes a golf ball. During the collision,

(A) The club exerts a greater magnitude of force on the ball, than the ball does on the club.

(B) The ball exerts a greater magnitude of force on the club, than the club does on the ball.

(C) They exert equal magnitudes of force on each other.

(D) The club does not accelerate.

8. A person is in a lift. The lift is moving upward but slowing down. Which of the following statements is true during this motion?

(A) The force of the floor on the person is greater than their weight force.

(B) The force of the floor on the person is equal to their weight force.

(C) The force of the floor on the person is less than their weight force.

(D) The person's weight force is less than it would be if the lift were moving at a constant velocity.

Answers and Explanations

1. C

8.2 miles/hr. Since average speed, s = distance/Δt, s = 10 mi/73min = 10 mi/1.22hr = 8.2 mi/hr

2. B

Average velocity, v = Δx/Δt = 0-0/73min = 0 mi/hr. Another way to look at it: on the way there v = 5 mi/35min = +8.6 mi/hr. On the way back v = −5 mi/38 min = −7.9 mi/hr. The weighted average of +8.6 mi/hr for 35 minutes, and −7.9 mi/hr for 38 minutes gives an average velocity = 0.

3. B

a = Δv/Δt = (5 m/s − 10 m/s)/(60 sec) = −0.083 m/s^2 or 0.083 m/s^2 westward.

4. B

F = ma = 50,000 kg(−0.083m/s^2) = −4150 N or 4150 N westward

5. D

The velocity can be read directly off of the graph. Graph d shows an object that starts at a high speed, slows down and stops instantaneously, and then speeds up in the opposite direction to its original motion.

6. A

The steep slope at t = 0 shows an object that is covering a relatively large distance in a short amount of time, as the slope flattens the amount of distance per time decreases and a slope of 0 represents an object that is not moving on an x-t graph.

7. C

According to Newton's Third Law, objects interacting with each other always exert the same magnitude of force on each other.

8. C

In this example the lift is accelerating *downward*, since it is moving upward and slowing down. If it were accelerating upward it would be speeding up. If the acceleration is downward, then the net force must also be downward, according to Newton's Second Law. For the net force to be downward, the upward force of the lift floor on the person must be less than the downward weight force. The weight force cannot change since gravity is constant, but the force that the floor exerts can. The reduced force of the floor on the person when the lift slows is responsible for the feeling of being "lighter" during that motion.

Chapter 18: **Waves**

A wave is a disturbance or an oscillation that travels through a medium in the case of a **mechanical wave**, and through empty space in the case of an **electromagnetic wave**. A wave carries energy as it travels through the medium. Mechanical waves such as water waves, sound waves and earthquake waves require matter to transmit the energy of the wave, while electromagnetic waves consist of oscillating magnetic and electric fields that propagate through empty space. Electromagnetic waves include visible light as well as a continuum of longer and shorter wavelengths such as radio waves, x-rays, gamma rays etc.

MECHANICAL WAVES

There are two basic types of mechanical waves, **transverse waves** and **longitudinal** or **compressional waves**. Each type is defined by the direction of the wave oscillation. In the case of transverse waves, the disturbance oscillates perpendicular to the direction of wave propagation. For example, if a rope is fixed at one end, and the other end is shaken up and down, the vibration would travel through the rope as shown below. Water waves are another example of transverse waves. As the wave travels through the water, the water rises and falls perpendicular to the direction of the wave motion.

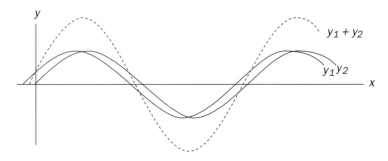

The same type of transverse wave could be generated with a spring rather than a rope; however, if instead of shaking the spring up and down, it was pushed forward and backward along the line of the spring, a compression would be generated that would propagate through the spring oscillating parallel to the spring. This is a longitudinal or compressional wave.

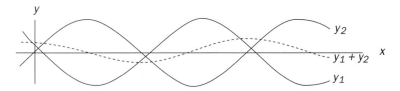

A wave consists of the transfer of energy through the medium not the transfer of matter. Although the medium is disturbed as the wave passes through it, the result is matter oscillating in place while the wave itself continues on through the medium. The wave energy is carried to other points in the medium which then oscillate at that location and so on.

GENERAL PROPERTIES OF A WAVE

The graphs shown below represent two views of a sinusoidal or simple harmonic travelling wave. Both graphs show the displacement of the medium from equilibrium on the *y*-axis. However, the first graph shows this displacement as a function of horizontal position along the medium at a specific time. It is like a photograph of the wave at some instant. The second graph shows the displacement at a specific horizontal point in space along the wave as a function of time. It is in fact a position-time graph showing the motion of the oscillation of the medium at that point.

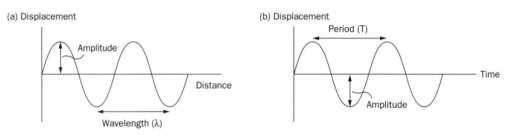

Amplitude

The *y*-axis on both graphs represents the displacement from equilibrium of the medium as it oscillates. We define the **maximum** displacement from equilibrium as the **amplitude** *(A)* of the wave. The amplitude represents the maximum displacement of the oscillations perpendicular to the direction of wave propagation in the case of a transverse wave, and the maximum displacement of the oscillations parallel to the wave direction for a longitudinal wave.

Wavelength, period and frequency

On the *y-x* graph it can be seen that the wave travels through one complete cycle over a specific distance called the **wavelength** (λ). While on the *y-t* graph the time for the wave to travel through one complete cycle is called the **period (T)** of the wave. The reciprocal of the period, called the **frequency (f)** is equal to the number of wave cycles per time. One cycle per second is also known as 1 Hertz (Hz)

Velocity of a traveling wave

The velocity of a wave can be related to the above quantities as follows.

$$v = f\lambda \quad \text{or} \quad v = \frac{\lambda}{T}$$

Example: The wave represented by the graph below has a frequency of 100Hz. Determine a) the wavelength b) the amplitude c) the period d) the velocity of the wave.

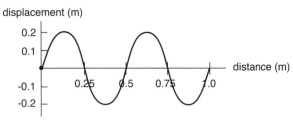

Solution: a) The wavelength can be determined by the distance between successive wave peaks. In this case $\lambda = 0.5$ m. b) The amplitude is the maximum displacement from equilibrium. A = 0.20m. c) $T = \frac{1}{f} = 0.01$s d) $v = f\lambda = (100\text{Hz})(0.50\text{m}) = 50$ m/s.

Reflection, refraction and diffraction of waves

Reflection of a wave can occur when the wave encounters a barrier. The **law of reflection** states that the angle at which the wave is incident upon the barrier will be equal to the angle of reflection, providing that the barrier surface is smooth. By convention, the angle of incidence and reflection are measured relative to a line perpendicular to the barrier called the **normal line**.

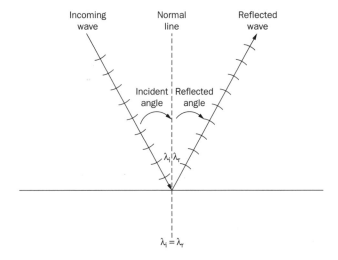

Refraction occurs when the direction of a wave is changed when it travels from one medium to another.

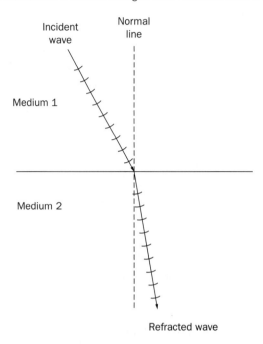

When a wave travels from one medium into another, the wavelength and speed of the wave will both change, although the frequency will remain unchanged. Since $v = f\lambda$ if the velocity of the wave is reduced as it passes into a medium, the wavelength will also decrease and vice versa. As a wave passes from one medium into another usually not all of the energy will be transmitted; some will be reflected back. So, in general, at a boundary some of the wave energy is reflected back, and the rest is transmitted through the boundary as shown.

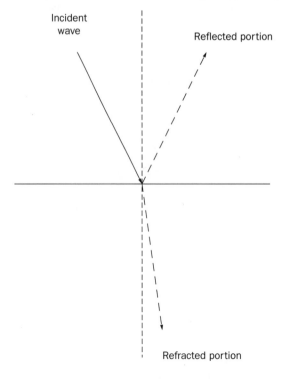

Diffraction is the bending of a wave that occurs as it passes around a barrier. For example water waves passing through a small opening in a barrier will be slower at the edges due to their interaction with the barrier, while the waves are faster in the middle. Therefore the waves will spread out as they pass through the barrier.

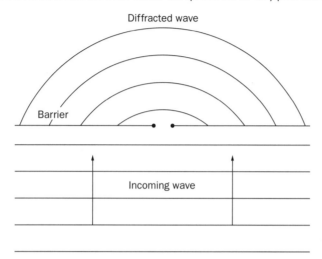

Interference of waves

When two or more waves pass through the same location in space at the same time they will **interfere** with each other. The interference may be **constructive** or **destructive**. Constructive interference occurs when the waves are **in phase** with each other. This means that the displacement of each wave is in the same direction. When the displacements are in phase they will augment each other, resulting in a larger wave than either of the individual waves during the period of time that they overlap. Once the waves move past each other they each return to their original form. For example, two waves traveling toward each other along a rope from opposite directions will interfere as shown below.

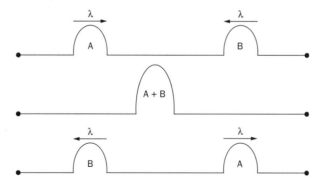

Destructive interference occurs when the waves are **out of phase**. This occurs when the displacements of each wave are in opposite directions. When waves interfere destructively, if they are of equal magnitude they will cancel each other out as they pass through each other as shown below.

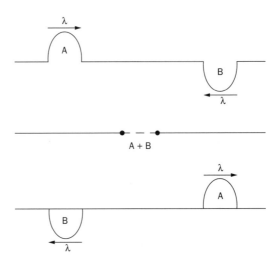

The examples in the figures above show only waves that contain a single pulse with a single phase direction. However, continuous or more complex wave patterns may interfere in such a way that part of the interference is constructive, while part is destructive.

Standing waves

Standing waves are interference phenomena that occur when two waves continuously travelling in opposite directions interfere with each other in such a way that certain areas of the medium experience continuous constructive interference, and other regions experience continuous destructive interference, forming a "standing" pattern. The areas of constructive interference are called **antinodes**, and those with destructive interference are called **nodes**. Standing waves can be demonstrated using a rope and fixing one end rigidly to a wall. If the rope is shaken up and down continuously, a wave will be generated along the rope. The wave will reflect off of the wall and on the way back this reflected wave will then pass through and interfere with the wave that is still travelling towards the wall. If the oscillation is given the right frequency then there will be points along the rope that will constantly be experiencing destructive interference (nodes), and other points constantly experiencing constructive interference (antinodes.) A certain fundamental frequency of oscillation will result in a single antinode in the middle of the wave, while multiples of this frequency will result in multiple antinodes. There will be no standing waves when the frequencies are in between these.

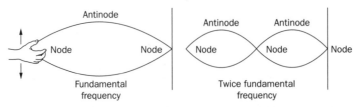

Sound waves

Sound waves are longitudinal or compressional waves. They are mechanical waves and require a medium through which they can travel, such as air or water. Sound cannot propagate through a vacuum, therefore even a supernova explosion in space would make no sound. A sound wave is initiated when a disturbance in a medium creates a region of high pressure. This compression then travels through the medium. The compression is followed by a region of lower pressure, and if the sound source is continuous then the low pressure region is succeeded by another region of high pressure etc. For example a tuning fork oscillates back and forth in the air. The oscillation of the tuning fork is transmitted into the air as regions of higher and lower pressure as shown.

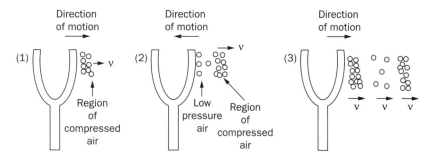

The human ear is able to detect sound between frequencies of 20Hz-20,000Hz.

The speed of sound

The speed of sound in air is around 340 m/s, although it varies slightly with temperature. Sound travels much faster in water or solid materials than it does in air.

> **Example:** A pitch pipe plays the note A which has a frequency of 440 Hz. What is the wavelength of the sound wave?

Solution: Since $v = f\lambda$, $\lambda = \frac{v}{f} = 340$ m/s/440 Hz $= 0.77$m

Volume and pitch

The amplitude of a sound wave is perceived by the ear as volume, or loudness of the sound, while the frequency of the sound is perceived by the ear as pitch. The higher the frequency of sound, the higher the pitch that we hear. Most sounds are combinations of several frequencies mixed together. Usually there is a fundamental frequency, which is the lowest of the frequencies, in conjunction with higher multiples of this frequency called harmonics. The pitch that we hear is the fundamental frequency, but the "colour" of the sound depends on which harmonics are present. For example, a trumpet and a flute can play the same note, and our ear perceives that they are playing the same note, but we hear a difference in the quality or colour of the sound due to each instrument having different harmonics.

> **Example:** Below are shown three different displacement time graphs of three different sound waves. The scales on each graph are the same. Which sound is the loudest? Which sound has the highest pitch?

Solution: Graph (a) represents the loudest sound, because it has the largest amplitude. Graph (c) has the highest pitch, because it has the highest frequency.

Ultrasound

Ultrasound waves have frequencies above 20,000 Hz and therefore cannot be detected by the human ear. A common medical application of ultrasound is in pre-natal screening. The reflection of the sound waves off of the fetus can be used to generate a picture of the fetus. A detector is able to measure the time between the sound wave leaving the source and returning to the detector thus giving a sense of how far away the object is. Since different parts of the fetus are different distances away from the detector, the data can be analysed using computers to create a detailed image. Ultrasound is also used in industrial applications to probe for defects in materials. For example a piece of metal with no defects will allow the sound waves to travel straight through; however, a crack will reflect the waves back to the detector which can then locate the defect.

The Doppler Effect

When a fire engine drives past with the siren on, it is easy to hear that the pitch seems to be higher when it approaches, and lower when it recedes. This is due to an apparent frequency shift that occurs due to the relative motion of an observer with the source of the sound. When either the source and/or the observer are moving towards each other, the frequency is shifted upward, and when moving apart the frequency is shifted downward. For a moving source, because it moves a distance between emitting each successive compression it will shorten or lengthen the distance between peaks thereby changing the frequency that arrives at the observer. For a moving observer although the frequency of the sound is not actually changed relative to the air, because the observer is moving towards or away from the source of sound, they will encounter the compressions more or less frequently than if they were standing still, and thus hear a different frequency.

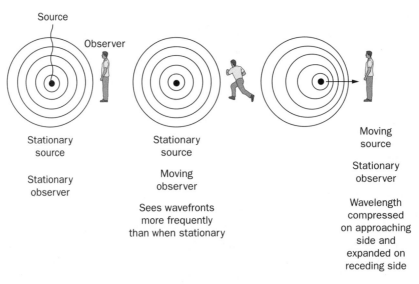

Electromagnetic waves such as light, which we will discuss in more detail below, also exhibit a Doppler shift. Objects that are moving away from us in space are seen to have the frequency of their light shifted towards longer wavelengths, or lower frequencies. These objects are said to display a "red shift" because red is at the lower frequency end of the light spectrum. Objects moving towards us are said to display a "blue shift" because their light is shifted towards shorter wavelengths and higher frequencies. The amount of shift can be used to determine the speed at which these objects are moving relative to the Earth.

> **Example:** Two identical cars drive away from you in the same direction. Each is honking on their horn. If car A is moving faster from which car do you hear the higher-pitched horn?

Solution: You will perceive a lower frequency for both cars compared to if they had been standing still. This is due to the longer wavelengths, and correspondingly lower frequencies of sound arriving at your ear due to the cars moving away. However since car B is not moving as fast as car A, the frequency of the sound arriving from B will be higher than that arriving from car A.

LIGHT AND THE ELECTROMAGNETIC SPECTRUM

An **electromagnetic wave** is an oscillating electric and magnetic field that propagates through space at an extremely high speed. Because the oscillations are perpendicular to the direction of the wave velocity, electromagnetic waves are transverse waves. Light is merely electromagnetic (e-m) radiation within a certain frequency range. The **speed of light**, and all e-m radiation, $c = 3.0 \times 10^8$ m/s in a vacuum. The speed is very nearly the same in air, but will propagate more slowly in more dense materials such as water or glass. The entire spectrum of e-m radiation is shown below.

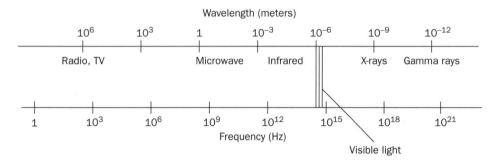

The higher the frequency of e-m radiation the higher the energy the radiation has. Therefore, gamma rays have the highest energy and radio waves the lowest.

Gamma rays and x-rays

Gamma rays are primarily produced as a product of radioactive decay of unstable elements, while x-rays can be produced when electrons collide with atoms. Neither can be seen or felt. Gamma rays usually pass through tissue but some can be absorbed by cells, damaging them. Significant exposure can cause cancer; however, they can also be used as a medical tool to target and kill cancer cells. Gamma rays can also be used to kill bacteria in food and sterilise surgical equipment.

X-rays have less energy than gamma rays. They pass through most tissue but generally not through bone or metal, and are therefore useful as a diagnostic tool in checking for broken bones. Overexposure to x-rays can also cause cells to become cancerous.

Ultraviolet radiation

Just higher than the frequency range of visible light, **ultraviolet** radiation is a component of sunlight. Ultraviolet radiation can cause damage to skin cells. Because darker skin cells absorb more ultraviolet radiation, skin often responds to exposure by turning darker so that less radiation penetrates to deeper skin layers.

The visible spectrum

Between wavelengths of about 400 to 700 nanometers (1 nanometer $= 1 \times 10^{-9}$m), e-m radiation is visible to the human eye. The shortest wavelengths are perceived by the human eye as purple, while the longest wavelengths are perceived as red in colour.

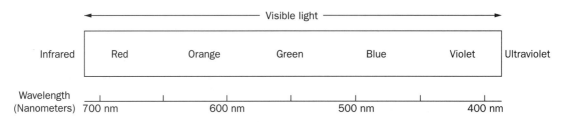

Example: What is the range of *frequencies* at which e-m radiation is visible?

Solution: $v = f\lambda$ and $f = \dfrac{v}{\lambda}$. Since we know that all e-m radiation travels at a speed $c = 3.0 \times 10^8$ m/s in a vacuum, the highest frequencies are in the vicinity of $f_{max} = (3 \times 10^8 \text{ m/s})/(400 \times 10^{-9} \text{ m}) = 7.5 \times 10^{14}$ Hz. The lowest frequencies are around $F_{min} = (3 \times 10^8 \text{ m/s})/(700 \times 10^{-9} \text{ m}) = 4.3 \times 10^{14}$ Hz.

White light, such as that produced by the sun or by an incandescent light bulb, is a mixture of all the frequencies of visible light. When mixed together we perceive the colour to be white. We are able to see objects due to the fact that they reflect light back into our eyes. An object that is white reflects all of the frequencies of light while absorbing none. A black object absorbs all frequencies and reflects none. If an object is a specific colour such as green, it means that the object absorbs all frequencies *except* green which is reflected back off of the object and perceived by the eye.

Infrared radiation

Infrared radiation has wavelengths just longer and frequencies just lower than visible light. When infrared radiation is absorbed by matter it increases the thermal energy of the matter. Therefore, when standing in sunlight or next to a fire, it is the infrared radiation that produces the sensation of heat in our skin. Infrared radiation is used in heaters and toasters, as well is in fibre optics systems.

Microwaves

Microwaves contain wavelengths that are absorbed easily by water molecules. When the water absorbs the microwave radiation it causes the water to heat up, and therefore microwave ovens are used in cooking. Microwaves are also used to transmit signals between mobile phones and to transmit information to satellites in orbit.

Radio waves

The longest wavelength and lowest energy e-m radiation are radio waves. In 1901 Guglielmo Marconi was able to transmit radio waves across the Atlantic Ocean, ushering in the technology of radio and television that dominates the modern world. Radio and television programs are transmitted using e-m radiation in this lowest frequency range. Because radio waves are diffracted as they pass by obstructions such as hills or buildings, televisions and radios do not need to be in a direct line of sight of transmitters to receive signals. Also, radio waves can be transmitted long distances by bouncing them off of the ionosphere, an electrically-charged layer in the upper atmosphere.

Information transmission: Analogue versus digital signals

Analogue signals vary continuously in both amplitude and frequency. FM (frequency modulated) and AM (amplitude modulated) are examples of analogue signals at radio wave frequencies.

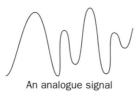

An analogue signal

Digital signals consist of pulses that are generated as square waves. They are either on or off with no amplitudes in between.

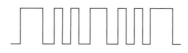

A digital signal

Signals get weaker the longer they travel from their source, and they also may pick up random additional signals as they travel called **noise**. Noise causes static on the radio and may diminish the performance of an internet connection on a computer. Analogue signals are more subject to noise than digital signals are, because as the signal is amplified, so is the amplitude of the noise. However, with digital signals the noise is usually lower in amplitude than the signal, and can be filtered out by the amplifiers. Also, since digital signals are able to carry more information than analogue signals, television and radio broadcasts are gradually changing over to digital.

Refraction and dispersion of light

As discussed earlier, when a wave travels from one medium into another, some of the energy is reflected back, and some is transmitted. If the incident wave approaches at an angle to the interface between the media then it will refract. This can be clearly seen with light. For example, if a narrow beam of light shines on a piece of glass at an angle to the surface we will see some of the light reflected back and some of the light bends as it travels from air into glass.

The amount of bend depends on the difference in velocities of the speed of light in each of the media. The greater the difference in velocity the greater the angle through which the light will bend. If the light travels from a "fast" medium, such as air or a vacuum, into a relatively "slow" medium like glass, the wave will bend towards the normal line. If the light travels from a slow to fast medium it will bend away from the normal line.

Example: Light is traveling through air when it enters the glass prism shown below.

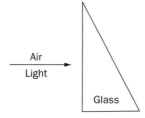

a) What is the path of the light that travels through the prism and out the other side?

Solution: Since the light enters parallel to the normal line, there will be *no* refraction as it enters the prism. It will continue to move in the same direction. However it does strike the other side of the prism at an angle. Since the light is travelling from a slower to a faster medium it will bend away from the normal line and therefore downward as shown.

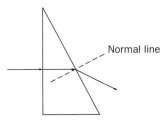

b) In the following case a hollow triangular area of air is cut out of a large piece of glass.

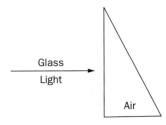

If a beam of light travels through the glass through the hollow area, and back out again, what is the path the light will take?

Solution: Again as the light enters the air, it is parallel to the normal and therefore no refraction will occur. As it exits it will bend towards the normal line because it is moving from a faster to a slower medium, and therefore it bends upward as shown.

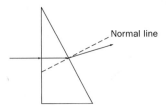

Snell's Law

Snell's Law quantifies the relationship of the incident angle of the wave or beam to the refracted angle.

$$\sin\frac{\theta_{incident}}{V_{in\ incident\ medium}} = \sin\frac{\theta_{refracted}}{V_{in\ refracted\ medium}}$$

Sometimes the velocity of light in the medium is expressed in terms of the **index of refraction (n)** of the medium.

$n = \frac{c}{v}$ where c is the speed of light in a vacuum, and v is the speed of light in the medium in question. For example, the speed of light in most glass is about 2.0×10^8 m/s. Therefore n for glass $= \frac{3.0 \times 10^8}{2.0 \times 10^8} = 1.5$.

N in a vacuum would be 1, and n for air is extremely close to 1 as the velocity of light in air is very nearly that in a vacuum.

Snell's Law can be rewritten in terms of *n* as follows: $n_i \sin\theta_i = n_r \sin\theta_r$.

> **Example:** A beam of light is incident upon a piece of glass ($n = 1.5$) at an angle of 30 degrees to the normal line. What is the angle relative to the normal line as it passes through the glass?

Solution: From Snell's Law: $\sin\theta_r = \dfrac{n_{glass} \sin\theta}{n_{air}} = \dfrac{1.5(\sin 30)}{1} = 0.75$ and inverse sin $(0.75) = \theta = 49$ degrees.

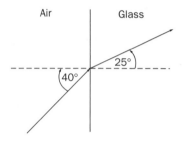

Dispersion

If white light passes through a piece of glass, such as a prism, the various frequencies can be separated out into a spectrum of colours.

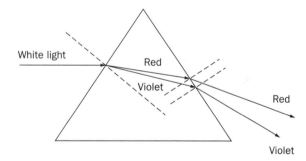

This is because each frequency has a slightly different velocity as it travels through the glass, and will therefore refract at a slightly different angle. As the light passes into the glass, the different frequencies separate out, and as they exit the glass the second refraction separates them even more, so that a rainbow of colour can be seen. The blue end of the spectrum refracts the most, and the red end the least as seen above.

RAINBOWS

Rainbows are caused when sunlight is refracted, dispersed and reflected as is passes through raindrops, which have a higher index of refraction than air. To be able to see a rainbow you must have the Sun behind you, and be looking into a region where there are raindrops in the air. The light from the Sun will enter the raindrops and refract inside them like in a prism. While some of the light will then be transmitted through the raindrop, much of the light will be reflected off of the back wall. This reflected light will then refract again upon exiting the raindrop causing the light to be dispersed into a spectrum of colours.

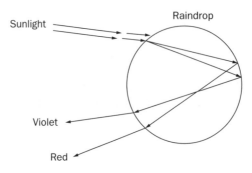

Rainbows always subtend an angle of about 42 degrees giving it its bow-like shape. This occurs because only the dispersed light that reaches your eye will be seen. Light rays coming from different angles in the sky will never reach your eye. They will either pass by above or below you. If there were no ground, the rainbow would be a complete circle, as can sometimes be seen from airplanes as they pass through an area of rain. Sometimes a double rainbow can be seen where a faint rainbow with the colours in the reverse direction sits above the brighter primary rainbow. The secondary rainbow is due to some of the light being reflected a second time within the raindrops.

Total internal reflection

When light travels from a medium where it moves relatively slowly into one where it has a higher velocity, it will bend away from the normal line, and the refracted angle will be greater than the incident angle. Some of the incident light will be transmitted into and refracted by the second medium, and some of the light will be reflected back.

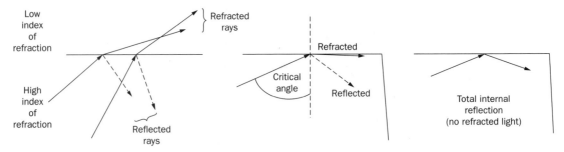

As the incident angle is increased, so is the angle of the refracted light. Eventually, there will be a certain incident angle called the **critical angle** when the resulting refracted angle will be 90 degrees, and move along the interface between the two media. If the incident angle is increased beyond the critical angle, then none of the light will be refracted into the second medium, and all of it will be reflected back. This situation is called **total internal reflection**. For the case of total internal reflection all of the energy of the light is maintained in the first medium, since none can escape.

> **Example:** What is the critical angle for light passing from glass of $n = 1.5$ into air?

Solution: Using Snell's Law: $n_{glass}\sin\theta_{critical} = n_{air}\sin(90)$

Therefore $\sin\theta_{crit} = \dfrac{n_{air}}{n_{glass}} = \dfrac{1}{1.5} = 0.67$ and $\theta_{crit} = 42$ degrees.

FIBRE OPTICS

Fibre optics cables are thin glass rods that use the principle of total internal reflection to transmit information. While electrical signals and radio waves are methods by which information can be transmitted, sending light (visible or infrared) through a fibre optics cable loses less signal and therefore less information than electrical, or radio wave transmission. Light going in at one end of a fibre optics cable undergoes multiple internal reflections, even if the cable is bent and therefore very little of the light signal is lost or attenuated by the time it emerges at the other end.

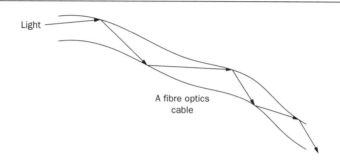

Light

A fibre optics cable

Mirages

The classic example of a mirage is seeing an oasis (water) in the desert where there isn't any. A more common example occurs sometimes when driving on the road on a hot sunny day. It often appears like there are patches of water in the roadway up ahead. In both cases this phenomenon is due to refraction of light. On a hot day the temperature near the ground is much warmer than the air further up. Because light travels slightly faster in warmer air, as light passes through layers of warmer air it will be refracted away from the normal line. Light coming from a source at some elevation above the ground will spread out in every direction. But light rays angled towards the ground will refract away from the normal line, at shallower and shallower angles to the ground. Eventually the light will reach the critical angle to the layer of air below and will undergo total internal reflection. These light rays will then refract back upward.

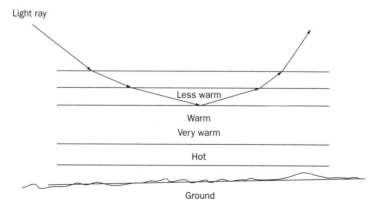

Light ray

Less warm

Warm

Very warm

Hot

Ground

If the light was coming from a treetop in the distance, you would see light rays arriving from a more or less direct path, but you would also see light arriving from the refracted path shown below. Your eye would perceive both where the tree actually is, plus an image of the tree directly back in the direction from which the light rays were coming. Therefore, you would see an image of the tree upside down and beneath where you would also see the actual tree. This would look very much like the reflection of the tree in a pool of water.

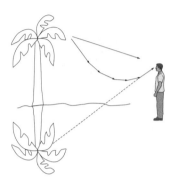

The same effect occurs from light rays coming from the sky itself. Some of these rays are refracted in the manner described above. Your eye perceives sky light, coming up from the ground, which can look very similar to water, and thus the impression of puddles of water in the roadway.

REVIEW QUESTIONS

1. An electric motor causes a ball to oscillate up and down in a tank of water causing waves to propagate outward from the ball. The period of the oscillation is 0.20 seconds.

    Which of the following y-t graphs best represents the wave produced by the oscillating ball?

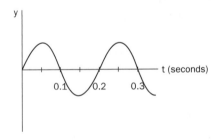

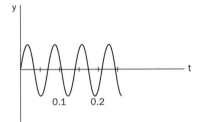

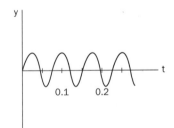

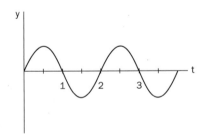

2. The wave described in problem 1) has a velocity of 1.2 m/s. What is the wavelength?

    (A) 0.24 m

    (B) 0.48 m

    (C) 0.12 m

    (D) 1.2 m

3. When a wave is bent as it moves around an obstacle, it is being

   (A) refracted.
   (B) reflected.
   (C) dispersed.
   (D) diffracted.

4. Total internal reflection can occur when light travels in which of the following situations?

   (A) from a medium where it moves faster into a medium where it moves slower.
   (B) from a medium where it moves slower into a medium where it moves faster.
   (C) either (A) or (B)
   (D) only when there is a single medium

5. Ultrasound can be used to map images by

   (A) dispersing high frequency sound off of an object.
   (B) refraction of high frequency sound.
   (C) interference of high frequency sound waves.
   (D) reflecting high frequency sound off of an object.

6. Jelly has an index of refraction of about 1.4. If a beam of light enters a square piece of jelly at a 30 degree angle to the normal line one side of the jelly, in what directions will it travel inside the jelly, and after it has exited back into the air?

   (A) 21 degrees, and 30 degrees to the normal line
   (B) 44 degrees, and 30 degrees to the normal line
   (C) 21 degrees, and 44 degrees to the normal line
   (D) 30 degrees in both cases

7. The following waveforms pass through each other at a certain point in space. At this point when they are completely overlapping, what does the combined waveform look like?

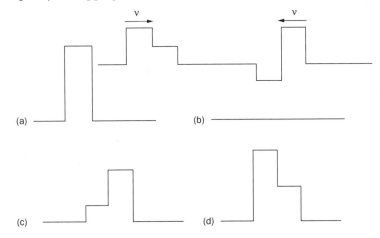

8. Which of the following types of e-m radiation has the highest energy?

    (A) visible light
    (B) ultraviolet radiation
    (C) radio waves
    (D) infrared radiation

Answers and Explanations

1. A

Since we are given a period of 0.2 seconds (which is equivalent to a frequency of 5 Hz) the wave pattern repeats itself every 0.2 seconds, or 5 times a second. Graph A is the only one with the correct period and frequency.

2. A

$v = f\lambda$ or $v = \frac{\lambda}{T}$ therefore $\lambda = \frac{v}{f} = 1.2$ m/s/5 Hz $= 0.24$ m.

3. D

Diffraction is the phenomenon of light bending around obstacles.

4. B

It must move from a slower into a faster medium. If it was the opposite light would bend towards the normal rather than away, and the critical angle would never be reached.

5. D

Ultrasound works by reflecting the waves off of an object and back to a detector. The data is then fed to a computer which interprets the location and form of the object, producing an image.

6. A

Using Snell's Law $n_{air} \sin(30) = n_{jello} \sin\theta_{jello}$, $_{wa} = \sin\theta_{jello}$, and $\theta_{jello} = 21$ degrees. Coming back out of the Jello just gives the above equation in reverse order.

7. C

Due to constructive interference where the waves are in phase, and destructive interference where they are out of phase.

8. B

Of the frequencies listed ultraviolet has the highest frequency and therefore the highest energy. Gamma rays have the highest energy of all e-m radiation.

Chapter 19: **Energy**

Energy is defined as the ability to do work. There are two general categories of energy: **potential energy** and **kinetic energy**. Potential energy consists of energy that is stored in some fashion as in some of the examples in the previous chapter. Kinetic energy is the energy associated with the motion of an object, or objects. When potential energy is released it becomes kinetic energy.

In this chapter we will look at energy and related concepts. Energy is often associated with such things as heat, motion, electricity, the Sun, food etc. In some cases energy is in a stored or **potential** state, such as the electrical energy stored in a battery, or chemical energy stored in a gallon of petrol. In other cases energy is in an active or kinetic state, such as a ball flying through the air. While the practical definition of energy is contained in a simple statement, it is really not a simple task to clearly articulate what energy actually is in a satisfying way. However the concept of energy is intrinsically connected to an idea of an overall balance in nature. This is seen in the principle of Conservation of Energy, one of the most simple, powerful and useful ideas in physics.

WORK

Work has a very specific definition in physics. The work done on an object by a force is the product part of the force that is exerted in the direction of motion of the object times the distance over which the object moves.

$$W = F_x \, \Delta x$$

Therefore if an object does not move, no matter how hard a particular force is pushing on it, that force is doing no work on the object. Also if a force has no part (or component) parallel or anti-parallel to the direction of motion then it does no work. If you were to push on a wall very hard for an hour you may be very tired but you will have done no work on the wall. Work is a scalar quantity.

Example: A block is being pulled along the floor by a rope. The rope is pulled in a horizontal direction with a 100 N force. If the block is moved 10 metres, how much work does the rope force do on the block?

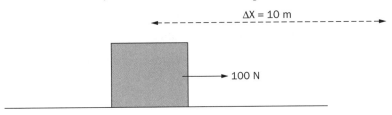

$$\Delta X = 10 \text{ m}$$

100 N

Solution: Since the force is parallel to the direction of motion $F_x = 100N$ and $W = 100N(10m) = 1000 \text{ Nm} = 1000$ Joules (J)

Example: The block above is now pulled by the same rope force over the same 10 m distance along the floor. This time the rope is pulled at an angle of 30 degrees above the horizontal. How much work does the rope force do on the block in this case?

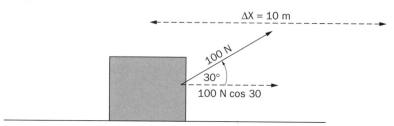

Solution: Here we only take the component of the rope force parallel to the motion. $F_x = F\cos(30) = 100N$ $(.866) = 87N$ and $W = 87N(10m) = 870$ J

Although work is a scalar quantity, if an object is in motion while a force is being applied in the opposite direction to the motion, the force is said to be doing negative work. So for example if a block is sliding along the floor and a force is applied to bring it to a stop over a certain distance then the force has done negative work on the object. Another way of defining work is the energy that is transferred while the force is being applied.

Work may be done by several forces on an object simultaneously.

Example: A block is pulled by a 100 N force acting horizontally. A 40 N friction force acts opposite to the motion. (A) What other forces must be acting on the object? (B) How much work is done by each of the forces after the block has moved a distance of 5 metres?

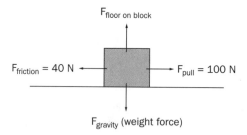

Solution: (A) In addition to the pulling force and the friction force there is a force of gravity (or weight force) acting downward on the block. There is therefore also a force of the floor pushing upward on the block balancing the gravity force.

(B) Since the weight force and the force of the floor are both acting perpendicular to the motion, they each do no work on the block.

$W_{\text{pulling force}} = (100N)(5m) = 500J$, $W = -40N(5m) = -200J$

In the previous example we may also express the **net work** done on the block as the total of the amounts of work done by the individual forces. So in that case the net work done $= 300J$. Alternatively, the net work could be calculated as the work done by the net force. For example the net force above is 60J. Therefore the net work $= (60J)(5m) = 300J$.

POWER

Work can be done slowly or quickly. The amount of work done by a force says nothing about how long it took to do that work. For example 500 J of work may have taken an hour or a minute to accomplish. Therefore **power** is defined as the rate at which work is done, or alternatively the rate at which energy is transferred, or converted from one form to another:

$$P = \frac{W}{t} \quad \text{or} \quad P = \frac{E}{t}$$

The SI units of power are J/s where 1 J/s = 1 Watt.

Example: A 100 kg crate is lifted from the ground by a crane. It takes 10 seconds to raise the crate to a height of 15 m above the ground. If the crate is lifted at a constant velocity, at what power must the crane work to lift the crate to this height?

Solution: $P = \frac{W}{t}$. The work done by the crate $= F_{crane}$ h, and since it is lifting the crate at a constant velocity $F = mg$. Therefore $P = \frac{mgh}{t} = \frac{(100\text{kg})(9.8\text{m/s})(15\text{m})}{10\text{s}} = 1470\,\text{Watts}$.

KINETIC ENERGY

Kinetic energy, the energy associated with an object's motion is defined mathematically as follows: $KE = \frac{1}{2}mv^2$.

If net work is done on an object, then a net force is acting on the object, and therefore the object will change its velocity. It turns out that the net work done on the object is exactly equal to the change in KE of that object. This relationship is referred to as the **Work-Energy Theorem**:

$$W_{net} = \Delta KE$$

Example: The block in the previous example has a mass of 20 kg and starts from rest. During the 5 metres of motion, (A) what is the change in kinetic energy of the block? (B) What is the velocity of the block at the end of the 5 metres of motion?

Solution: (A) $W_{net} = \Delta KE = 300J$

$$\Delta KE = 300\,J = KE_{final} - KE_{initial} = \frac{1}{2}mv_{final}^2 - \frac{1}{2}mv_{initial}^2$$

(B)
$$300\,J = \frac{1}{2}(5\text{kg})v_{final}^2 - \frac{1}{2}(5\text{kg})(0) \quad v_{final} = \left(\frac{600}{5}\right)^{\frac{1}{2}} = 11\text{m/s}$$

POTENTIAL ENERGY

Energy can be stored in a variety of different forms of potential energy. It can be stored in chemical bonds, in electric and magnetic fields, in the form of mass in the case of nuclear energy, in gravitational fields, and in elastic materials among others. We will look at some of these in turn.

Gravitational potential energy

Gravitational potential energy is energy stored by an object due to its position in a gravitational field. For example if a ball is lifted off of the ground it gains gravitational potential energy. This energy can then be converted into kinetic energy by dropping the ball. As the ball falls it continuously gains kinetic energy, and the amount of kinetic energy that it gains is exactly equal to the amount of gravitational potential energy lost.

Since, when work is done on an object, the amount of work done is equal to the amount of energy transferred, we can quantify the gravitational potential energy of an object near the surface of the Earth as follows. Consider a book being lifted from the ground to some height, h, above the ground.

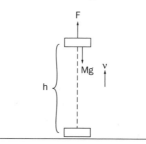

Except for a very short period of time when the book is accelerated to the lifting speed, and another very short time when it is brought to a stop at height h, we will assume that the book is lifted at a constant velocity. Therefore according to Newton's Second Law the amount of the lifting force must be equal to the weight force since the book is not accelerating. The work done by the lifting force is: $W_{lifting\ force}$ = Fh =mgh. This amount of work done is equal to the change in gravitational potential energy of the book in lifting it from the ground to h. So $\Delta PE = mgh$.

> **Example:** A 1.0 kg book is lifted off of the ground to a height of 2.0 m above the ground and placed on a book shelf. The book slips back off of the shelf and then falls back to the ground. (A) How much potential energy does the book gain by being lifted up to the shelf? (B) How much kinetic energy does the book have just before it hits the ground after falling? (C) What is the speed of the book just before hitting the ground? (D) What is the speed of the book when it has fallen a distance of 1.0 m down from the shelf?

Solution: (A) $\Delta PE = mgh = (1.0\ kg)(9.8\ m/s^2)(2.0m) = 19.6\ J$

(B) PE lost = KE gained so since all 19.6 J of PE is lost upon hitting the ground, KE must = 19.6 J.

(C) $KE = \frac{1}{2}\ mv^2$ so $v = (2(KE)/m)^{\frac{1}{2}} = (2(19.6\ J)/1.0kg)^{\frac{1}{2}} = 6.2\ m/s$.

(D) At 1.0 m above the ground the book has lost 9.8 J of PE, and it has 9.8 J left. The 9.8 J lost is equal to the KE gained, so $v = (2(9.8\ J)/1.0kg)^{\frac{1}{2}} = 4.4\ m/s$.

Elastic potential energy

When a rubber band or a spring is stretched or when a bouncy ball is compressed as it hits the ground, energy is stored in the form of **elastic potential energy**. For example when the stretched rubber band is released the stored elastic energy is then converted to kinetic energy. For many springs it is possible to quantify the potential energy stored. The energy stored depends on how far the spring is stretched (or compressed) from its equilibrium or relaxed state (Δx), and the stiffness of the spring measured by the spring constant (k). The larger the value of k for a spring, the more energy that the spring can store, for a given displacement from equilibrium.

$$PE = \frac{1}{2}\ k(\Delta x)^2$$

Example: A 0.50 kg block is placed on a frictionless surface and pushed against a spring that has spring constant k = 200 N/m. The block compresses the spring a distance 0.10 m, and then is released.

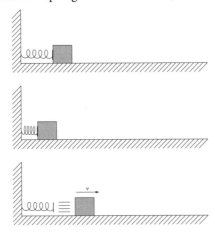

a) What is the maximum amount of energy stored in the spring?

b) What is the velocity of the block the instant after it is released by the spring?

Solution: (A) $PE = \frac{1}{2} k(\Delta x_{max})^2 = \frac{1}{2}(200N/m)(0.10m)^2 = 1.0$ J

c) At the instant of release all of the PE of the spring has been converted to KE of the block. Therefore

$KE = \frac{1}{2} mv^2 = 1.0$ J $v = (2KE/m)^{\frac{1}{2}} = (2(1.0J)/0.5kg)^{\frac{1}{2}} = 2.0$ m/s.

Thermal energy

Thermal energy refers to kinetic energy at the molecular or atomic level. All matter is in constant motion. At the level of thermal energy, the motion may be due to translational (linear) motion, vibrations, or rotations of molecules or atoms. The total thermal energy of a macroscopic object consists of the total kinetic energy of all the particles within that object. **Temperature** is a measure of the average kinetic energy of the particles within the object. The term **heat** technically refers to the transfer of thermal energy from one location to another. For example if two objects at different temperatures are placed in contact with each other, thermal energy from the hotter object will flow spontaneously into the colder object until the two are at the same temperature. The amount of energy transferred is the heat.

Modes of heat transfer

Heat transfer from one location to another can occur via three possible mechanisms: **conduction, convection** and **radiation.**

Conduction occurs more readily in solids than in liquids or gases. Metals are particularly good conductors of heat. In conduction the energy of thermal vibrations is transferred through the material, while matter itself is not transferred. Regions of a material at higher temperature will have particles vibrating more vigourously than cooler regions. Therefore as these higher energy particles oscillate some of their energy will be transferred to neighbouring particles at lower energy when they interact/collide with them. Metals are particularly good

conductors of heat (and electricity) because they contain free electrons that can easily move within the structure of the metal thus transferring energy between metal nuclei. Materials that do not conduct very well are called **insulators**.

Convection occurs when actual matter is transferred from one location to another. This occurs more easily in fluids (liquids and gases.) When a region of a fluid becomes warmer than its surroundings, it expands thus becoming less dense. Because it is less dense it will tend to rise within the fluid due to buoyant forces. As it rises it will displace cooler more dense regions that will descend in the fluid, setting up convection currents of rising and falling matter. Winds are examples of convection currents that occur in the atmosphere.

As discussed in the previous chapter, electromagnetic radiation consists of oscillating electric and magnetic fields propagating through space. These electromagnetic waves carry energy with them. E-m radiation in the **infrared** frequency range is generated by thermal vibrations in matter. This radiation then travels through space and when it interacts with an object it will then increase the thermal energy of that object. Because it is e-m radiation that is transferring energy, this mode of heat transfer is called radiant heat transfer or radiation. Radiant heat transfer can occur across a vacuum unlike conduction or convection. Some surfaces are better at absorbing infrared radiation, while other materials will tend to reflect this type of radiation. For example dark dull objects tend to absorb very well, and reflect very little, while light shiny objects do the opposite. Good absorbers of radiation are also good emitters, so it would be most efficient to have a domestic heating radiator in a house or apartment painted dull black.

> **Example:** To keep a house warm in winter it is desirable that the loss of heat through the walls is minimised. Due to a temperature difference between the inside and outside of the house, heat will conduct through the floors, walls, windows and ceiling to the outside. To minimise these losses what types of materials should be included in the walls and ceiling of a house?

Solution: The rate of conduction through a material depends on the temperature difference on either side of the material, the thickness and surface area, and the conducting properties of the material. The walls and particularly the ceiling, which has a large surface area, should be padded with **insulating** materials such as foam to reduce the rate at which heat is conducted through the walls. Double pane windows which incorporate an insulating air space between two panes of glass also can reduce conduction through the windows.

Heat loss can also occur due to convection currents, which can exist if there are gaps in doors or windows. Energy can be lost due to radiation through the walls, ceiling and windows as well.

Chemical potential energy

When chemical reactions occur energy can either be released or absorbed in the reaction. This is because energy can be stored in the configuration of the chemical bonds between atoms and molecules. In chemical reaction specific chemical bonds are broken and others are formed. If the total energy contained in the bonds of the reactants is greater than the total energy in the bonds of the products of a reaction, then energy will be released as a result of the reaction. For example the combustion of petrol results in the release of heat that can be used to drive an internal combustion engine in an automobile.

Nuclear potential energy

Nuclear energy is the result of energy stored within the mass of subatomic particles. Einstein's famous equation $E = mc^2$ in fact describes the amount of energy contained within a mass. For example if you were to add the total mass of two individual protons, you would find that they would add up to be greater than the total mass of a deuterium nucleus. (Deuterium is an isotope of hydrogen that consists of two protons fused together.) The difference in mass is equal to the energy that will be released in creating a deuterium nucleus by slamming two protons together. This type of reaction is called a nuclear fusion reaction because particles are fused together as a result of the reaction. A fission reaction occurs when a heavy atom such as uranium is split into smaller atoms. The total combined mass of the smaller atoms is less than the mass of the uranium, and therefore energy is released in the reaction. Fission has been able to be harnessed commercially in the production of electrical power, while fusion energy at present cannot be harnessed economically.

Electric and magnetic energy

Electric charges produce electric fields whether the charges are static or in motion. Moving electric charges produce magnetic fields. For example a current flowing through a wire generates a magnetic field surrounding the wire. Energy is stored in these fields in the same way that gravitational energy is stored in gravity fields. It is the energy stored in an electric field of a battery, for example, that is responsible for the forces exerted on electric charges within a wire that cause an electric current to flow.

Sound

Sound is mechanical wave energy released by vibrating objects, which is in a frequency range that the human ear can detect.

Electromagnetic radiation

As discussed above, infrared radiation is one mode by which heat can be transferred. In fact electromagnetic radiation of any frequency transfers energy. Since electric and magnetic fields store energy, and e-m radiation consists of propagating electric and magnetic fields, it must be carrying energy. Clearly this must be the case when we consider that the Sun which ultimately provides the Earth with almost all of its energy (consider that fossil fuels are derived from plant material that originally used radiant energy from the Sun to grow), transfers this energy into space completely by electromagnetic radiation.

CONSERVATION OF ENERGY

Conservation of Energy is one of the fundamental concepts of physics. This principle apparently reflects a balance inherent in the natural universe. All experience and observation to date lead to the following conclusion: *The total amount of energy in the universe is a constant. Energy can change form but it can never be created or destroyed.*

For an isolated system—one that cannot exchange energy with its surroundings—the total energy of that system will remain a constant. If the system is not isolated, that is if work can be done on or by the system, or if energy can be added to or taken away from the system, then while the system may not conserve energy, a larger system that encompasses the objects responsible for the adding or subtracting of energy and the smaller system, must conserve energy.

We did two or three examples above that illustrated the principle without stating it so explicitly. For example, consider the system of a ball sitting a height h above the ground. The ball has gravitational potential energy due to its height above the ground. That gravitational potential energy is the total energy of the system. As the ball falls, we are assuming an isolated system, and therefore however much PE is lost as the ball falls must be exactly equal to the amount of KE that the ball gains. Although the energy transfers from one form to another, the *total* amount of energy is the same, it is simply redistributed. The assumption of an isolated system is reasonable as long there is not significant air resistance. However if there is, then we can deduce that if the amount of total energy of the ball decreases, then that missing energy will have gone into increasing the energy of the atmospheric particles by that amount, mostly by increasing the thermal energy of the air molecules.

Example: A 50 kg rollercoaster car is moving at a velocity of 10 m/s on a frictionless track at point A shown below. (A) What is the total energy of the rollercoaster car? (B) Use conservation of energy to find its velocity at points B, and C.

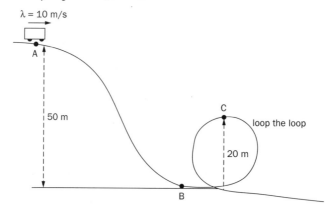

Solution: If there is no friction then the rollercoaster car is an isolated system. Therefore the total energy at point A = the total energy at point B = the total energy at point C. It is simply redistributed between PE and KE.

Total E can be calculated from the kinetic and potential energies at point A.

$$KE_A + PE_A = \frac{1}{2}\, mv_A^2 + mgh_A = \frac{1}{2}(50kg)(10m/s)^2 + 50kg(9.8m/s^2)(50m) = 27{,}000\ J.$$

a) Total $E = KE_A + PE_A = KE_B + PE_B = KE_C + PE_C$

At point B: $27{,}000\ J = \frac{1}{2}\, mv_B^2 + mgh_B = \frac{1}{2}(50kg)v_B^2 + (50kg)(9.8m/s^2)(0)$

$V_B = 33$ m/s.

At point C: $27{,}000J = \frac{1}{2}(50kg)v_C^2 + (50kg)(9.8m/s^2)(20m)$

$V_C = 26$ m/s.

The path of the car is not important as long as the system is isolated. Energy of the system is constant, and a situation that would be very difficult to analyse using Newton's Laws becomes quite simple using Conservation of Energy.

Example: A 65 kg skydiver jumps out of an airplane, and after falling a distance of 1000m is moving at a terminal velocity of 70 m/s. How much of the skydiver's original energy has been converted to thermal energy in the atmosphere at this point?

Solution: The skydiver has fallen a distance of 1000 m and therefore has lost an amount of potential energy, $\Delta PE = mg\Delta h = (65kg)(9.8\ m/s^2)(1000m) = 637{,}000\ J$

The amount of kinetic energy the skydiver has at that point is
$KE = \frac{1}{2}\, mv^2 = \frac{1}{2}(65kg)(70m/s)^2 = 159{,}250\ J.$

Therefore the amount of energy lost into the atmosphere is
637,000 J – 159, 250 = 477,750 J.

> **Example:** You push a box along the floor at a constant velocity. The pushing force applied to the box is 40N. (A) What is the net work done on the box as it is pushed a distance $x = 20$m? (B) How much work do you do on the box during this motion? (C) How much work is done by the friction force during this motion? (D) What happens to the work/energy that you are putting into the box?

Solution: (A) The net work done on the box is 0. Since the velocity of the box is constant, there is no net force on the box, and therefore no net work.

(B) $W_{\text{pushing force}} = F\Delta x = 40\text{N}(20\text{m}) = 800$ J

(C) $W = F\Delta x = (-40\text{N})(20\text{m}) = -800$ J

(D) The energy that you put in goes out of the system due to friction. It is converted to thermal energy in the ground and box.

ENERGY RESOURCES

The principles of conservation of energy and energy transfer are important in assessing the resources that we use to power the modern world. In order to generate electricity, heat and light, energy must be converted from one form to another. In this section we will survey a variety of methods by which energy is converted into a usable form. Some examples of energy transfers are shown in the diagrams below. In one case chemical potential energy stored in the chemical bonds of petrol is converted into thermal energy. This thermal energy is then converted to kinetic energy in the engine and wheels of a car. In the second example kinetic energy is converted by an electromagnetic generator into electrical energy. This electrical energy is then converted to light and heat energy inside of an incandescent light bulb.

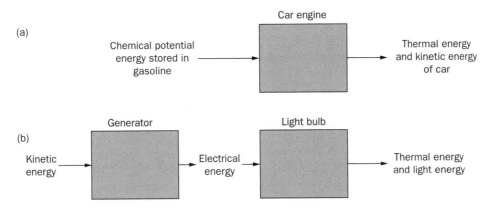

Efficiency

When analysing energy transfer into a useable form, the concept of *efficiency* becomes important.

Efficiency = (useful energy transferred/total energy supplied) × 100

Conservation of Energy says that energy cannot be created or destroyed, it can only be transferred from one form to another. However, some forms of energy are not able to be easily harnessed into a usable form. In fact in any energy transfer process in which we attempt to produce usable energy, for example electrical energy, or kinetic energy as in the examples above, a fraction of the energy converted from the source is "lost" into the surroundings. Most often the lost energy is in the form of heat that spreads out into the surrounding environment. In a car engine, it turns out that only about 15% of the energy released from the chemical bonds of the petrol actually is converted into kinetic energy of the car. Around 85% of the original potential energy is released as waste heat. So for every 100 J of energy supplied by the petrol only 15 J goes into useable kinetic energy. The efficiency of the engine is therefore:

$$e = \left(\frac{15\,J}{100\,J}\right) \times 100 = 15\%$$

The schematic diagram below represents way the energy is distributed.

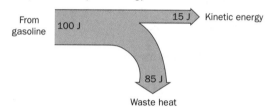

An electric light bulb is also not very efficient—only about 10%. For every 100 J of electrical energy supplied to the light bulb only 10% goes into light, while the other 90% is lost as heat.

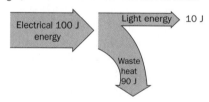

Non-renewable resources

Non-renewable resources are those that have a limited supply. Once the supply of these resources is depleted, they can not be re-stocked or re-made.

Fossil fuels

Fossil fuels are the most commonly used sources of energy. These include oil, coal and natural gas. Fossil fuels are so called because they are derived from the remains of ancient living organisms that were buried and compacted. Fossil fuels release heat when they are burned. The heat is then used to turn water into steam which expands. The kinetic energy of the expanding steam then drives a turbine transferring the energy again into electricity.

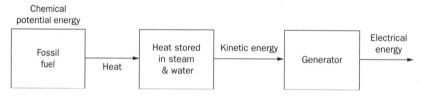

Because it takes natural processes that require millions of years to make fossil fuels, they are non-renewable energy sources, and therefore will eventually run out. Also, among the byproducts of the combustion of fossil fuels are pollutants such as carbon dioxide, and sulphur dioxide. Carbon dioxide contributes to the greenhouse effect and global warming, and sulphur dioxide reduces the pH of rainwater resulting in "acid rain". Sulphur dioxide can also contribute to breathing problems.

Nuclear energy

Because a relatively substantial amount of mass can be converted to energy in nuclear reactions, certain elements can be used to produce nuclear energy. At present nuclear **fission** reactions are the only type that can easily and economically produce energy. A fission reaction is one where the nucleus of a large radioactive atom, usually **uranium** or **plutonium** splits or fissions into smaller atoms. The total mass of the original atom is greater than the total mass of the products, with the difference being given off as energy. The amount of energy is given by $E = mc^2$ where m is the mass difference between the "parent" and total mass of the "daughter" atoms. C is a constant which equals the speed of light, 3.0×10^8 m/s. This does not mean that the atoms are in motion at the speed of light. The constant c is required in the derivation of the above equation. This relation between mass and energy is part of Einstein's Theory of Special Relativity. Heat energy is given off in these reactions, and subsequently electrical energy is produced by the same steps as those used with fossil fuels.

Like fossil fuels, nuclear fuels are non-renewable. An accident at a nuclear plant could release dangerous amounts of radioactive material, and nuclear waste is highly radioactive for thousands of years. Waste disposal is a difficult problem.

Nuclear **fusion** reactions on the other hand are those in which light elements like hydrogen nuclei collide at high speeds. The nuclei fuse together, and energy is given off due to an overall loss of mass. In the case of fusion the fuel is abundant, in that hydrogen is a major constituent of water (although extracting hydrogen from water is not an energy free process.) Also, the byproducts of fusion reactions are generally not radioactive.

Unfortunately the technical difficulties in controlling fusion reactions such that they can be made economically feasible are formidable. Although much research is being done into the potential of nuclear fusion as an energy source, most researchers agree that solutions to the current technical obstacles are decades away.

Renewable resources

Renewable resources are those that for all practical purposes have an unlimited supply. Although these resources are free, the technical difficulties in converting the energy into useable forms in an economical way are not trivial.

Moving water as a source of energy

The kinetic energy of moving water can be used to generate electricity. Perhaps the most commonly used method is in **hydroelectric** power stations. These use the water falling over a dam built across a river to drive electric generators usually built inside the dam. In hydroelectric power, the potential energy of the falling water is converted to kinetic energy. The moving water then spins turbines which convert the kinetic energy into electrical energy.

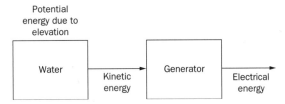

The energy in **waves** and **tides** can also be harnessed to drive electric generators. In both cases the kinetic energy of moving water is converted into electric energy; however, it is difficult to produce large amounts of electricity.

Wind energy

The kinetic energy of wind can be converted to electrical energy in wind farms. Wind farms consist of multiple wind turbines which have large blades mounted on towers. The wind blows spinning the blades which drive an electric generator. The amount of electricity generated depends on the strength of the wind.

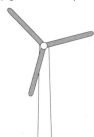

Solar energy

The electromagnetic radiation from the Sun is a constant source of energy, and life on Earth could not exist without it. Converting this energy into electricity can be accomplished using **solar cells**; however, they are expensive and highly inefficient. To produce significant amounts of electricity large arrays of solar cells must be constructed.

Solar panels receive heat energy from the Sun and use it to heat water.

Geothermal energy

Thermal energy is produced in the interior of the Earth due to decay of radioactive substances. This energy tends to rise to the Earth's surface forming volcanoes. In the regions surrounding these volcanoes subsurface water may be heated and converted to steam. The steam can then be used to drive electric generators. In areas where the rock is heated but there is no water, deep wells can be drilled, and cold water pumped down. This water can then heat up and rise to the surface as hot water and steam. There are however a limited number of areas in the world where geothermal energy can be exploited.

REVIEW QUESTIONS

1. A ball is dropped from a bridge. As the ball falls which of the following is NOT true? Assume air resistance is negligible.

   (A) The potential energy of the ball decreases and the kinetic energy increases.
   (B) The gravitational force does work on the ball.
   (C) The total energy of the ball is constant.
   (D) The total energy of the ball decreases.

2. The driver of a car slams on the brakes, and the car slows to a stop. What happens to the kinetic energy of the car?

   (A) It is converted to thermal energy in the lining of the brakes.
   (B) It is converted to potential energy.
   (C) It is converted to electrical energy in the body of the car.
   (D) It decreases the power of the engine.

3. A spring with a spring constant k = 500 N/m is placed on the ground facing upward as shown. A 0.10 kg block is placed on the spring and the spring is compressed a distance of 0.05 m and released. What is the maximum height above the spring that the ball will reach after the spring is released?

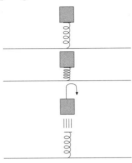

(A) 12.7 m

(B) 0.64 m

(C) 0.25 m

(D) 0.05 m

4. Which of the following energy sources is non-renewable?

(A) Nuclear energy

(B) Geothermal energy

(C) Solar energy

(D) Hydrothermal energy

5. The diagram below shows the energy transfer that occurs at a nuclear power plant. Heat energy is generated from nuclear fission reactions and converted to electricity. Heat is produced at a rate of 1590 MW (million watts). The plant has an output of 540 MW of electrical energy.

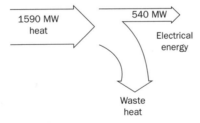

What is the efficiency of the power plant?

(A) 294%

(B) 17%

(C) 34%

(D) 100%

6. For the power plant described above how much total electrical energy does it produce every day?

(A) 1.3×10^{10} J

(B) 5.4×10^{8} J

(C) 1.6×10^{9} J

(D) 4.7×10^{13} J

7. Weather fronts are large masses of air that move through the lower atmosphere (the troposphere). These fronts are ultimately due to the transfer of heat from one location to another. Which of the following processes is the most important in the motion of weather fronts?

   (A) convection
   (B) conduction
   (C) radiation
   (D) magnetic forces

8. Geothermal energy is not a viable replacement for fossil fuels as a major energy source because

   (A) it is too difficult to convert energy from steam into other forms of energy.
   (B) geothermal power plants are too disruptive to the environment.
   (C) there are not enough locations in the world that produce geothermal energy.
   (D) there is not sufficient funding for geothermal research.

Answers and Explanations

1. D

As long as there is not significant air resistance the system will remain isolated and will not lose energy. As the ball falls the total energy is therefore constant. Potential energy decreases as it loses height, with the amount of kinetic energy increasing exactly equal to the amount of potential energy that is lost. Gravity is a force acting on the ball as it falls, and therefore does work on the ball.

2. A

The kinetic energy is lost as the motion of the tyres is slowed by the brakes due to friction acting between the brakes and tyres. The initial kinetic energy is converted into thermal energy in the tyres and brake lining.

3. B

The elastic potential energy stored in the spring will be converted into kinetic energy and then gravitational potential energy. At the top of its flight, all of the original elastic potential energy will now be in the form of gravitational potential energy.

$$\frac{1}{2}kx^2 = mgh \quad h = \frac{1}{2}(k)x^2 / mg = \frac{\frac{1}{2}(500\text{N/m})(0.05\text{m})^2}{(0.1\text{kg})(9.8\text{m/s}^2)} = 0.64\text{m}$$

4. A

Nuclear energy is non-renewable because there exists a limited amount of uranium and plutonium.

5. C

Efficiency = useful energy/total energy supplied × 100 = 540MJ/s/1590MJ/s × 100 = 34%

6. D

The electrical energy is produced at a rate of 540 million joules/second. Therefore the total energy produced in one day = 540 × 10^6 J/s × 60 s/min × 60 min/hr × 24 hr/day = 4.7 x 10^{13} J (47 trillion joules)

7. A

Weather fronts are in motion in the atmosphere due to winds which are convection currents.

8. C

There are not that many locations where geothermal is a viable energy source.

| PART VII |

Mathematics Review

Chapter 20: **Arithmetic**

Arithmetic means nothing without numbers and the number system. Here is a review of those topics.

SETS OF NUMBERS

The **real numbers**, all of the numbers that are encountered each day, are classified into various sets and subsets. All real numbers are either **rational** numbers or **irrational** numbers.

Rational Numbers

The **rational numbers** are the numbers that can be expressed as a fraction in the form $\frac{a}{b}$, where a and b are integers and $b \neq 0$.

The **rational numbers** can be classified into subsets:

> The **natural numbers**, also known as the counting numbers: { 1, 2, 3, 4, 5, 6, 7… }.
>
> The **whole numbers** are the natural numbers, plus 0: { 0, 1, 2, 3, 4, 5, 6, 7… }.
>
> The **integers** are the whole numbers and their opposites: { …−3, −2, −1, 0, 1, 2, 3… }.

A rational number can take various forms: 5 can also be written as $\frac{5}{1}$; 1.2 can be written as $\frac{12}{10}$ or $\frac{6}{5}$; −7 can be written as $-\frac{7}{1}$; and $0.\overline{3}$ can be written as $\frac{1}{3}$. When written as a decimal, a rational number is either *terminating* or *repeating*.

More information about integers follows.

Integers

Integers are the set of whole numbers and their opposites. As a set, the integers are written as {…, −3, −2, −1, 0, 1, 2, 3, …}.

Each integer has a location on a real **number line**, where the sign of the number determines to which side of 0 the number is located. For example, positive 5, which can also be written as +5 or simply 5, is located 5 units to the right of 0, as shown in the number line here.

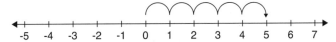

It is important to remember that the number 0 is neither positive nor negative.

Here is more information about **integers**:

- All numbers greater than 0 are positive numbers.
- All numbers less than 0 are negative numbers.
- Zero is neither positive nor negative.
- The **even** integers are divisible by 2, and include the number 0.
- The **odd** integers are not divisible by 2.

ORDERING INTEGERS

The value of an integer is determined by its location on the real number line, where negative numbers appear to the left of 0 and positive numbers are located to the right of 0. A number farther to the right will be larger in value than a number farther to the left. For example, when comparing –8 and –9, –9 is farther to the left on a number line–therefore, –9 is less than –8. This concept can also be written using the symbol for less than, and would appear as –9 < –8.

Irrational Numbers

The **irrational numbers** cannot be expressed as fractions. Some examples are $\sqrt{2}$, $\sqrt{3}$, $\sqrt{5}$, and π. When irrational numbers are expressed as decimals, they are *non-terminating* and *non-repeating*. Some examples of irrational decimals are:

3.1415926535897932384…, or 7.030030003…, or 8.81811811181111…

NUMBER PROPERTIES

There are common properties of numbers that are frequently used to make adding and multiplying easier. These properties give "licence" to change the order of operations in certain situations. In addition to making addition and multiplication of number terms easier to calculate, these properties are frequently used in solving algebraic equations, as explained later in the chapter.

The **commutative property of addition** states that changing the order of the addends in a sum does not change the sum.

$a + b = b + a$, where a and b are any real numbers

The **commutative property of multiplication** states that changing the order of the factors in a product does not change the product.

$a \times b = b \times a$, where a and b are any real numbers

The **associative property of addition** or **multiplication** states that changing the grouping (parentheses or brackets) of addends in a sum or the grouping of factors in a product does not change the resulting sum or product.

$a + (b + c) = (a + b) + c$, where a, b and c are any real numbers

$a \times (b \times c) = (a \times b) \times c$, where a, b and c are any real numbers

Remember, the **commutative and associative properties** can be combined. For example, to simplify the expression 2.1 + 8.07 + 7.9 + 24.93, scan the addends and recognize that (2.1 + 7.9) and (8.07 + 24.93) will produce whole numbers. Use the commutative property to get 2.1 + 7.9 + 8.07 + 24.93. Then use the associative property to get (2.1 + 7.9) + (8.07 + 24.93). Now the addition is easy to finish: 10 + 33 = 43.

The **distributive property of multiplication over addition** or **subtraction** states that multiplication distributes over addition and subtraction.

$a \times (b + c) = (a \times b) + (a \times c)$, where a, b and c are real numbers

$a \times (b - c) = (a \times b) - (a \times c)$, where a, b and c are real numbers

The **distributive property** can also be used in reverse. For example, if you were instructed to simplify $(12 \times 6.4) + (12 \times 3.6)$, order of operations would have you evaluate parentheses first, which involves decimal multiplication. If you notice that both terms are multiplied by 12, use the distributive property to "factor out" the 12: $(12 \times 6.4) + (12 \times 3.6) = 12 \times (6.4 + 3.6) = 12 \times 10 = 120$.

INTEGER OPERATIONS

First is a brief review of absolute value and then come the topics of adding and subtracting integers, multiplying and dividing integers, and finally the order of operations. Please be sure to review these topics carefully as they are the foundation for other maths concepts in this chapter.

Absolute Value

Absolute value is the number of units a number is away from 0 on a number line. Since absolute value is a measure of distance, it is always a positive value. The symbol for absolute value is two bars on either side of a numerical value or expression. For example, the absolute value of 4 is written as $|4|$, and since it is 4 units away from 0 on a number line, $|4| = 4$. The absolute value of -7 is written as $|-7|$, and since -7 is 7 units away from 0 on a number line, $|-7| = 7$.

WORKING WITH OPERATIONS AND ABSOLUTE VALUE

When working with absolute value, expressions are simplified in much the same way as expressions that contain parentheses. Any operations contained within the absolute value bars are evaluated first. Take the expression $|-16 + 7|$. First combine -16 and 7, which equals -9. Remember, the -9 is still inside the absolute value bars. Now, evaluate the absolute value of -9: $|-9| = 9$. In a contrasting example such as $|-16| + |7|$, only single values are contained within the absolute value bars. Evaluate the absolute values first. Since $|-16| = 16$ and $|7| = 7$, the problem then becomes $16 + 7 = 23$. The key for both of these examples is to simplify any absolute value problem down to a single value within the absolute value bars first.

Adding Integers

When adding integers, the sign of the numbers involved is very important. In order to visualise adding integers, think of any positive integer as a group of that many positives, and any negative integer as a group of that many negatives. Thus, +5 would be represented as 5 positives. In the same way, −7 would be represented as 7 negatives.

Now, keep in mind that any time one positive and one negative are grouped together, they cancel each other out, making a neutral. Consider this as $+1 + -1 = 0$. When adding integers that have the same sign, just add the absolute values of the numbers and keep the sign.

For example, $+6 + +7 = +13$ and $-4 + -8 = -12$.

When adding integers that have different signs, recall that each negative sign can pair with a positive sign to form a neutral. Each member of the pair cancels the other out. Therefore, the solution to an addition problem with integers of different signs will be the remaining positives or negatives that did not form a pair. For example, in the problem $-3 + 5$, 3 negatives pair with 3 of the 5 positives to form 3 neutral pairs.

There are now 2 positives left over that did not form a pair. Therefore, the solution to the problem $-3 + 5$ is 2.

A general rule for adding integers with different signs is to subtract their absolute values and keep the sign of the number with the larger absolute value as the answer. In the example $18 + -25$, subtract the absolute values to get $25 - 18 = 7$. Since -25 has a larger absolute value, take the negative sign for the answer, -7.

Subtracting Integers

The subtraction of any two integers can also be expressed as adding the opposite of the number being subtracted. This way, the concept can be simplified into an addition problem, and there are only two rules to commit to memory.

Remember, when **adding integers**:

1. If the signs are the same: add, and keep the sign.
2. If the signs are different: subtract, and take the sign of the number with the larger absolute value.

Multiplying and Dividing Integers

Multiplication and division of integers is slightly more straightforward than adding and subtracting. Regardless of the numbers' signs, multiply or divide the absolute values of the numbers. The only question is whether the solution is positive or negative. Since multiplication is repeated addition, use the principles of addition to make sense of the rules. In the example $6 \times (-2)$, this is the same as adding 6 groups of -2. Therefore, the answer would be -12.

For the problem $(-5) \times (-3)$, this is the same as the opposite of adding 5 groups of -3. This would have a result of 15. There are two negatives in the problem, so they cancel each other out.

Since division follows the same principle, a problem such as $-12 \div 4$ would result in an answer of -3. There is only one negative in the problem, so the answer will also be negative. The negative has nothing to cancel out with.

In the example $-4 \times -9 \times -2$, the result will be the opposite of the product of 4, 9, and 2, which is -72. The solution here is negative because there are two negatives that pair up to cancel out and one negative sign left over.

Remember, when multiplying and dividing integers, if there is an *even* number of negatives in the problem, the solution will be **positive**. If there is an *odd* number of negatives, the solution will be **negative**.

The Order of Operations

A predetermined **order of operations** is used to evaluate mathematical expressions. There is a mnemonic for remembering the order of operations: PEMDAS. It is often remembered by the expression "Please Excuse My Dear Aunt Sally". The order of operations is:

P Parentheses (grouping symbols)

E Exponents

MD Multiply and divide from left to right

AS Add and subtract from left to right

The "P" in PEMDAS stands for parentheses, or grouping symbols. Grouping symbols include parentheses, brackets, the absolute value symbol, and a fraction bar. So to simplify:

$$\frac{18 + 10^2 - 4 \times 2}{20 - 27 \div 3}$$

Treat the fraction bar as a grouping symbol and first evaluate the top (the numerator) then the bottom (the denominator). Then divide for the final step.

To simplify the numerator, first simplify the exponent: $10^2 = 100$. Second, multiply 4 times 2 to get 8. The top is now $18 + 100 - 8$. Evaluate from left to right: $118 - 8 = 110$. To simplify the denominator, first divide 27 by 3 to get 9. Then subtract: $20 - 9 = 11$. Finally, divide 110 by 11 to get 10.

In the order of operations, a radical sign is evaluated on the same level of priority as an exponent. To simplify $550 - \sqrt{9 \times 4} \times 3$, evaluate the radical first. Under the radical sign, multiply 9 times 4 to get 36. The square root of 36 is 6. Now the problem reads $550 - 6 \times 3$. Multiply 6 by 3 next to get $550 - 18$, for a final value of 532.

FRACTIONS

A **fraction** is a rational number in the form $\frac{a}{b}$. The variable a is called the **numerator**, and the variable b is called the **denominator**. There is one restriction on b: The denominator cannot have the value of 0.

The fractional form of any rational number is the most precise way to represent the number, unless the number is an integer. Some fractions, or ratios, show a comparison of two numbers. Fractions can also represent a part-whole relationship. Fractions are usually used to display probabilities, as well. In the upcoming review of fraction operations, you will be asked to find factors of a whole number. It is helpful to be familiar with divisibility rules for whole numbers and other terminology for factors prior to reviewing fractions in greater detail.

Divisibility Rules

Here are the most common divisibility rules:

Divisibility by 2: A number is divisible by 2 if the number is an even number.

Examples: The numbers 24, 50 and 66 are all divisible by 2 because they are all even numbers.

Divisibility by 3: A number is divisible by 3 if the sum of the individual digits in the number is divisible by 3.

Examples: The number 312 is divisible by 3 because 3 + 1 + 2 = 6, which is divisible by 3. The number 9,021 is divisible by 3 because 9 + 0 + 2 + 1 = 12, which is divisible by 3.

Divisibility by 4: A number is divisible by 4 if the last two digits, taken as a two-digit number, are divisible by 4.

Examples: The number 736 is divisible by 4 because 36 is divisible by 4. The number 12,716 is divisible by 4 because 16 is divisible by 4.

Divisibility by 5: A number is divisible by 5 if the last digit of the number is a 5 or a 0.

Examples: The numbers 10, 25, 30, and 75 are all divisible by 5 because the last digit of each is a 5 or a 0.

Divisibility by 8: A number is divisible by 8 if the last three digits, taken as a three-digit number, are divisible by 8.

Examples: The number 3,024 is divisible by 8 because 024, or just 24, is divisible by 8. The number 79,128 is divisible by 8 because 128 is divisible by 8; 128 ÷ 8 = 16.

Divisibility by 9: A number is divisible by 9 if the sum of the individual digits in the number is divisible by 9.

Examples: The number 9,135 is divisible by 9 because 9 + 1 + 3 + 5 = 18, which is divisible by 9. The number 414,972 is divisible by 9 because 4 + 1 + 4 + 9 + 7 + 2 = 27, which is divisible by 9.

Prime Factors of a Number

In order to understand how to perform operations with fractions, first review the concepts of factors and multiples.

A **factor** of a number x is a whole number that divides into x evenly without remainder. All the factors of a number can be reduced down into only prime numbers. Every number has a unique set of prime factors. For example, the number 28 has 2, 2, and 7 as its prime factors.

The Greatest Common Factor

The **greatest common factor (GCF)** is the largest common factor of two or more numbers. The GCF is often used to simplify a fraction. Prime factorisation is a convenient way to find the GCF of two or more numbers. For example, if you find the prime factors of 28 (2, 2, 7) and the prime factors of 80 (2, 2, 2, 2, 5) you can see that each set of factors has two 2's in common. Therefore the GCF of 28 and 80 is the product of these two numbers: 4.

The Least Common Multiple

The **least common multiple (LCM)** is the smallest number that two or more numbers will divide into evenly. The LCM of two or more numbers is used when adding or subtracting fractions. Again, the prime factorisation of numbers is a convenient way to find the LCM. After finding the prime factors two numbers have in common, just multiply *all* of the factors appearing in the diagram and that is the LCM of the two numbers.

Using the same numbers 28 and 80, the LCM is (2 × 2) × 2 × 2 × 5 × 7 = 560; the factors in parentheses are the common pairs.

Equivalent Fractions

Knowing that a fraction is a rational number in the form $\frac{a}{b}$ helps when comparing fractions. A single number can have several equivalent fractional forms. To find an equivalent fraction, just multiply or divide the fraction by the number one, in the special form of $\frac{a}{a}$.

For example, $\frac{5}{35}$ is equivalent to $\frac{1}{7}$ because $\frac{5}{35} \div \frac{5}{5} = \frac{1}{7}$. To find an equivalent fraction to $\frac{3}{4}$, multiply by some fractional form of one: $\frac{3}{4} \times \frac{6}{6} = \frac{18}{24}$. Often, when performing operations on fractions, you will be instructed to simplify a fraction. To simplify a fraction, divide by the greatest common factor of the numerator and the denominator. To simplify $\frac{28}{80}$, divide by $\frac{4}{4}$ because 4 is the GCF; $\frac{28}{80} \div \frac{4}{4} = \frac{7}{20}$.

Fraction Operations

There are special rules for solving operations with fractions. What follows is a review of addition, subtraction, multiplication and division of fractions.

Addition and Subtraction

To add or subtract fractions, first change the fractions so they have common denominators. The best common denominator to use is the least common multiple of the denominators involved. This is called the **least common denominator**.

For example, to add $\frac{13}{15}$ and $\frac{3}{5}$, find the LCM of the denominators. This is 15. Rewrite the problem with denominators of 15:

$$\frac{13}{15} + \frac{9}{15} = \frac{13+9}{15} = \frac{22}{15}$$

Remember, to add or subtract fractions:

    1) Convert the fractions so they have an equivalent **least common denominator**.

    2) Add or subtract the numerators and keep the denominator.

    3) Simplify the resultant fraction if necessary.

Multiplication

To multiply fractions, simply multiply the numerators and then multiply the denominators. An example is $\frac{7}{9} \times \frac{3}{16}$. Cancel out any common factors found in any of the numerators and denominators to make the multiplication easier:

$$\frac{7}{\underset{3}{\cancel{9}}} \times \frac{\overset{1}{\cancel{3}}}{16} = \frac{7 \times 1}{3 \times 16} = \frac{7}{48}$$

Division

To divide fractions, recall that division is the inverse operation of multiplication. The multiplicative inverse of a fraction is the **reciprocal**, or "flip" of the fraction. The easiest and most common way to divide fractions is to take the first fraction and multiply it by the reciprocal of the second fraction. For example, $\frac{5}{8} \div \frac{3}{2}$ is equivalent to $\frac{5}{8} \times \frac{2}{3} = \frac{10}{24}$.

Mixed Numbers

Mixed numbers are numbers in the form $A \frac{b}{c}$. When performing operations using mixed numbers, it is helpful to first change the mixed number into an improper fraction and then use the correct procedure for fractions as previously described. Change $A \frac{b}{c}$ to an improper fraction by multiplying $c \times A$ and adding it to b. Then put this number over c:

$$\frac{(A \times c) + b}{c}$$

Complex Fractions

Complex fractions are fractions whose numerator or denominator is also a fraction. To simplify these fractions, remember that the fraction bar means to divide. Rewrite the fraction as a division problem, and follow the procedure for dividing fractions.

To simplify $\frac{\frac{8}{15}}{4}$, rewrite it as division:

$$\frac{8}{15} \div 4 = \frac{8}{15} \times \frac{1}{4} = \frac{8}{60} = \frac{2}{15}$$

DECIMALS

Decimal form is a convenient way to express a number, because it is based on the powers of 10. This makes comparisons like addition, subtraction, multiplication and division easier to perform.

Look at the decimal form *"abc.def"* to understand place value. The letter a is the digit in the hundreds place, the letter b is in the tens place, c is in the ones place; d is in the tenths $\left(\frac{1}{10}\right)$ place, e is in the hundredths place $\left(\frac{1}{100}\right)$ and f is in the thousandths place $\left(\frac{1}{1,000}\right)$.

As an example, 5.092 is equivalent to 5 and 92 thousandths because the rightmost digit is three places after the decimal point.

Equivalent Decimals

The number 3.5 is equivalent to any other decimal form of that number with trailing zeroes; 3.5, 3.500 and 3.50000 are all equivalent decimal numbers. Each represents 3 and five-tenths. When adding, subtracting or comparing decimals it is often convenient to add trailing zeroes, as demonstrated later.

Conversions

To change a mixed number to a decimal, separate and keep the whole number part; this is the number to the left of the decimal point. Then divide the fractional part. The mixed number $12\frac{3}{4}$ is 12.75 because 3 divided by 4 is 0.75.

Ordering

To order or compare fractions, first convert the fractions to decimals by dividing, and then order the decimal equivalents.

The decimal form of a number makes comparisons easy. Just rewrite each decimal to have the same number of places to the right of the decimal point and then compare the numbers. For example, to order the decimals {1.2, 1.07, 1.019} from least to greatest, rewrite the numbers as 1.200, 1.070, and 1.019. Since the whole number parts are the same, just order the decimal portion. With the trailing zeroes it is evident that 200 > 70 > 19, so the correct order from least to greatest is 1.019, 1.07, 1.2.

Decimal Operations

It is crucial to understand operations with decimals as they will frequently appear on maths exams. Addition, subtraction, multiplication and division are covered here.

Addition and Subtraction

To add or subtract decimal numbers, remember that it is imperative to LINE UP the decimal points! This is the FIRST step before performing addition or subtraction. Add trailing zeroes if necessary to avoid careless mistakes.

For example, to add 2.509 to 234.6, first line up the decimal points as shown here. Two trailing zeroes are added to the end of 234.6 and then addition is performed as shown.

$$
\begin{array}{r}
234.600 \\
+\quad 2.509 \\
\hline
237.109
\end{array}
$$

Multiplication

To multiply decimal numbers, follow these steps:

1. Multiply the numbers without regard to the decimal point and obtain a whole number product.
2. Count the number of digits that are to the right of the decimal point in BOTH factors.
3. Alter the whole number product to have the same number of digits to the right of the decimal point, as counted in step 2.

For example, to multiply 12.9 times 0.07, step 1 instructs you to multiply 129 times 7, which equals 903. In step 2, count the number of digits to the right of both decimal points; there is one digit in 12.9 and there are two digits in 0.07: 1 + 2 = 3. In step 3, take the whole number product, 903, and alter it so that it has three digits to the right of the decimal point, making the answer 0.903.

Division

To divide decimal numbers, follow these steps:

1. Set up the long division problem.
2. Count how many digits are to the right of the decimal point in the divisor (the number you are dividing with).
3. Move the decimal point in the dividend (the number you are dividing into) the amount from step 2.
4. Raise the newly-placed decimal point up to the quotient.
5. Divide as usual as if there were no decimal points.

For example, to divide 0.39 by 2.6, look at the divisor. 2.6 has one digit to the right of the decimal point. Therefore, move the decimal point one place to the right in the dividend. Move this new point position up to the quotient. The answer is 0.15.

$$
\begin{array}{r}
.15 \\
2.6\ )\overline{0.390} \\
\underline{26} \\
130 \\
\underline{130} \\
0
\end{array}
\qquad 0.39 \div 2.6 = 0.15
$$

PERCENTAGES

A **percent** is a special fraction that compares a numerical quantity to 100. They are used so frequently in everyday life that you should review this subject carefully if you are unfamiliar with any of its topics.

Converting between Decimals and Percents

To change a percent to a decimal, remove the percent symbol and divide by 100. To change a decimal to a percent, just multiply by 100. Because of the place value number system, to divide by 100 just move the decimal point two places to the left and remove the percent symbol. For example: 56% is 0.56, 230% is 2.30, and 4% is 0.04. To multiply any number by 100, simply move the decimal point two places to the right and add the percent symbol. For example: 0.76 is 76%, 1.34 is 134%, and 0.06 is 6%.

Converting between Fractions and Percents

Remember that a percent is a fraction that compares a numerical quantity to 100. To convert from a fraction $\frac{a}{b}$ to a percent, use a variable to represent the unknown percent and set up a proportion. To change a fraction to a percent use the proportion $\frac{x}{100} = \frac{a}{b}$ and cross multiply to solve for the variable x.

To convert from a percent into a fraction, just put the given percent over 100, remove the percent symbol and simplify if needed.

The Percent of a Number

Think of a percent as a part-whole relationship. When asked to find the percent of a number, try to find the part of the whole number that is represented by the given percent. The equation "part is percent times number" can be used to solve problems of this type. For example, to find 18% of 250, change 18% to a decimal and then multiply by 250: $0.18 \times 250 = 45$.

When asked to find a missing percent, such as *252 is what percent of 600?* set up a simple equation, substituting an equal sign for "is" and a multiplication sign for "of": $252 = 600x$. Divide both sides by 600 to get 0.42, or 42%. Note that when using the equation method the percent is expressed as a decimal number.

Remember, the key word "of" in mathematics usually means multiply and the key word "is" in mathematics means equals.

Percent Increase or Decrease

Percent increase or decrease is calculated as $\dfrac{\text{change}}{\text{original amount}} = \dfrac{\text{percent}}{100}$. It is important to realise that the part is the change that occurs, and the whole is the starting amount. The new amount does not enter into the formula to calculate the percent. The new amount is only used to calculate the change from the original.

Simple Interest Rates

Simple interest is calculated with the formula $I = prt$, where I is the interest charged or paid out, p is the principal amount that is saved or borrowed, r is the percentage rate written as a decimal and t is the time in years.

This formula is based on the concept that the percent of the whole equals the *part*, that is, percent of the principal amount is the amount of interest. Then multiply this amount by the number of years involved. For example, to find the simple interest earned on £1,700 at 8% interest for 3 years, set up the formula $I = prt$. $I = (1,700)(0.08)(3)$, or interest = £408.00. Note that when using the simple interest formula, change the percent to a decimal equivalent.

RATIOS

A **ratio** is a comparison of two or more different quantities. A comparison of two different values represented by a and b can be written as $\dfrac{a}{b}$, $a : b$ or a to b. A ratio is in its most simplified form if there are no common factors between the values and the values in the ratio are integers. Take the ratio 25 to 75. Since each number has a common factor of 25, the ratio can be reduced to 1 to 3 by dividing each number by 25. Therefore, this ratio can be written as 1 to 3, 1:3, or $\dfrac{1}{3}$.

Rates

A rate is a comparison of two types of units. Some common examples of rates are *kilometres per hour, feet per second* and *kilometres per gallon*. Notice that the key word "per" is often used with rates. A rate with a denominator of 1 is called a **unit rate**.

For example, if you travelled 100 kilometres in 2 hours, this would reduce to a unit rate of 50 kilometres in 1 hour, or 50 kilometres per hour. When dealing with rates of speed, it is often useful to use the equation *distance* = *rate* × *time* to help you. For instance, if you wanted to find the amount of time it would take to travel 660 kilometres while going at a rate of 60 kilometres per hour, you would fill in 660 for your distance and 60 for your rate. 660 = 60*t*. Divide both sides by 60 to get a time of 11. In other words, it would take 11 hours to travel 660 kilometres going 60 kilometres per hour.

Proportion

A **proportion** is a comparison of two ratios. In other words, a proportion is two ratios set equal to each other. To solve a proportion, multiply the numerator from the first ratio by the denominator from the second ratio, and then the denominator from the first ratio by the numerator of the second ratio and set the values equal to each other. After this step, divide each side of this new equation by the number with the variable to get your solution.

An important concept to note is that many problems that involve ratios and proportions can be categorised as either *part to part* or *part to whole* comparisons. These problems involve different parts of a whole set, and the correct way to set up the proportion to solve the question depends on the question asked.

Scale

Scale is using a smaller unit to represent a much larger unit. The blueprints of a building or home, model cars and model airplanes are just a few examples of the use of scale. When working with scale models, the scale is often given as the ratio *model measurement: actual measurement*.

Similarity

When figures have corresponding sides that are in proportion with one another and corresponding angles with the same measure, the figures are **similar**. Proportions can be used to determine that figures are similar, and can also be used to calculate the missing part or parts of known similar figures.

Remember that the ratio of the sides of two similar figures will be the same as the ratio of the perimeters of the same two similar figures. Angles and perimeter will be covered later in the chapter.

Now that you have reviewed the essentials of arithmetic, test your knowledge by completing these practice questions.

REVIEW QUESTIONS

1. Which number below is not in the set of rational numbers?

   (A) $\dfrac{5}{4}$

   (B) $\dfrac{2}{3}$

   (C) π

   (D) $7.\overline{8}$

   (E) 4.125

2. What is the greatest common factor of 24 and 90?

   (A)   6

   (B)   2

   (C)   3

   (D) 180

   (E) 360

3. Hannah deposits £1,250 in a savings account that pays 5% simple interest. How much interest will be earned after 2 years?

   (A)   £62.50

   (B)   £625.00

   (C)   £12.50

   (D) £1,250.00

   (E)   £125.00

4. What is the percent decrease from 90 to 85?

5. The sum of two numbers is 48. If the numbers are in the ratio 3 : 5, what is the smaller number?

Answers and Explanations

1. C

Pi is a constant number that is irrational. An irrational number cannot be exactly expressed as a fraction because in decimal form it neither terminates nor repeats. Rational numbers are numbers that can be written in the form $\frac{a}{b}$, where a and b are integers and $b \neq 0$. Therefore, choices (A) and (B) are by definition rational numbers. In choice (D), $7.\overline{8} = 7\frac{8}{9} = \frac{71}{9}$ a rational number. In choice (E), $4\frac{125}{1,000} = 4\frac{1}{8}$, also a rational number.

2. A

The prime factors of 24 are $2^3 \times 3$. The prime factors of 90 are $2 \times 3^2 \times 5$. The common factors are $2 \times 3 = 6$, the greatest common factor. Choice (B) is a factor of both numbers, but is not the greatest common factor. Choice (C) is also a factor of both numbers, but again, is not the greatest. Choice (D) is a multiple of 90. Choice (E) is the least common multiple of 24 and 90.

3. E

This problem assesses your knowledge of the simple interest. Use the simple interest formula: $I = prt$, where I is the interest earned, p is the principal amount invested, r is the percentage rate, written as a decimal, and t is the time in years. $I = 1,250 \times 0.05 \times 2 = £125.00$.

4. 5.6%

The change is 5 (90 − 85), and the original number is 90. By substitution, $\frac{5}{90} = \frac{x}{100}$. Cross multiply to get $500 = 90x$. Divide both sides by 90 to get 5.6%, rounded to the nearest tenth.

5. 18

Set up the part to whole proportion using the given smaller number: $\frac{3}{8} = \frac{x}{48}$. Then, cross multiply and divide to get $x = 18$. Or, set up the equation $5x + 3x = 48$; $8x = 48$. $x = 6$. Multiply 6×3 (the smaller number) to get the same answer of 18.

Chapter 21: **Algebra**

Algebra builds upon the foundations of arithmetic. Begin by reviewing exponents, which were first mentioned in the discussion of the order of operations.

POWERS AND ROOTS

Exponents (sometimes referred to as **powers**) are a way to write very small and very large numbers in a shortened fashion, which can save both time and space. Some of the topics covered under this subject include exponents as powers, the laws of exponents, negative exponents, fractional exponents (otherwise known as radicals and roots) and scientific notation.

Exponents as Powers

Using exponents is a way to write repeated multiplication more efficiently. The **exponent** or **power** is the total number of times a base is used as a factor.

The number or expression that appears below the exponent is called the **base number** or **base expression**. In the numerical expression 6^4, 6 would be considered the *base number* and 4 the *exponent*. Remember, the exponent in the expression tells how many times to use the base number as a factor. For example, in the expression 6^4, 6 should be used as a factor 4 times:

$$6^4 = 6 \times 6 \times 6 \times 6 = 1,296$$

When an expression is written out showing all of its factors, as done here, this is called the **expanded form** of the expression.

Sometimes a number or expression will have no exponent. If there is not an exponent written with a base number or variable, the exponent is equal to 1. For example, the numerical expression 6 actually means 6^1. In another special case, any base expression to the 0 power is equal to 1. For example, the expressions 5^0, 101^0, and $12,045^0$ all equal 1.

Multiplying Like Bases

When working with exponents there are shortcuts to simplifying expressions. It is important to understand expanded form and apply different laws of exponents. One of the patterns occurs when the base numbers are the same (they are like bases) when multiplying exponents. In the example $2^3 \times 2^5$, 2 is the common base number, or the like base. To multiply with like bases, add the exponents: $a^m \times a^n = a^{m+n}$. The simplified expression is then equal to 28, or 256.

Dividing Like Bases

A pattern also occurs when dividing exponents where the base expressions are the same. To **divide** with like bases, subtract the exponents: $\frac{a^m}{a^n} = a^{m-n}$. So, in the expression $\frac{5^6}{5^4}$, 5 is the common base for each expression. The simplified expression is then equal to 5^2, or 25.

Operations with Powers

Raising a Power to a Power

Occasionally, an exponent, or power, is raised to another power. An example of this is the expression $(2^3)^4$. In this type of problem, use expanded form to help visualize the operation. Since the exponent of 4 is outside of the parentheses, it implies that $(2^3)^4 = (2^3) \times (2^3) \times (2^3) \times (2^3)$. In other words, the base of 2^3 is being used as a factor 4 times. By adding the exponents of the like bases, the result is 2^{12}. Since raising the exponents of 3 to the 4th power gave a resulting exponent of 12, it is clear that the original exponents were multiplied together in order to simplify the expression.

Raising a Product or Quotient to a Power

When a base expression contains more than just one variable or constant and is then raised to another power, this is called raising a product to a power. An example is $(3x^4)^3$, where the entire expression $3x^4$ is raised to the third power. Here, it is essential to multiply each base number or variable's exponent by 3. $(3x^4)^3$ becomes $3^3 x^{4 \times 3}$, which simplifies to $127x^{12}$ using the power to a power multiplication rule.

The product to a power rule also works if an expression contains a fraction. For example, in the expression $\left(\frac{3^2}{2}\right)^3$, the exponent of 3 needs to be applied to the base in the numerator of 3^2 and the base in the denominator of 2. The simplified expression would be $\left(\frac{3^2}{2}\right)^3 = \frac{(3^2)^3}{(2)^3} = \frac{3^6}{2^3} = \frac{729}{8}$.

Negative Exponents

Working with negative exponents can be a challenge. A common misconception is that the negative sign on the exponent makes the base number negative. In fact, a base expression raised to a negative exponent is equal to the *reciprocal* of the base raised to a positive exponent.

Remember, when simplifying an expression with negative exponents: $a^{-m} = \frac{1}{a^m}$.

Scientific Notation

A common application of exponents is **scientific notation**. Scientific notation is often used to write very large or very small numbers more efficiently. To convert a number to scientific notation, first use the non-zero digits to make a number between 1 and 10. Then, multiply by a factor of 10 to a power, where the power is the number of places the decimal moved. If the number is less than 1, the exponent is negative; if the number is greater than one, the exponent is positive.

For example, to change the number 6,400,000 to scientific notation, write the non-zero digits as a number between 1 and 10 and drop the zeros. The number becomes 6.4. Then multiply this number by 10 raised to an exponent; the exponent is the number of places the decimal had to move to get between the 6 and the 4. By counting from the ones place of 6,400,000 to the space between 6 and 4, the decimal moved 6 places to the left.

$$6,\underset{\underset{\text{6 places}}{\frown\frown\frown\frown\frown\frown}}{400,000}$$

Therefore, 6,400,000 written in scientific notation is equal to 6.4×10^6.

Perfect Squares

Another topic that falls under powers and roots is perfect squares. **Perfect squares** are numbers that are the result of multiplying two of the same integers together. Some examples are:

$1 \times 1 = 1$ $2 \times 2 = 4$ $3 \times 3 = 9$ $4 \times 4 = 16$ $5 \times 5 = 25$

Therefore, the perfect squares listed are 1, 4, 9, 16 and 25.

Finding the square root of a number, or a radicand, is the opposite of finding the square of a number. To find the **square root** of a number, find the integer that you would multiply by itself to equal the number. The number under the **radical sign** is called the **radicand**.

For example, since $4^2 = 4 \times 4 = 16$, then $\sqrt{16} = 4$. Four is the square root of 16.

The root of a number can also be written as an exponent. However, when the root of a base number is involved, the exponent will be in fraction form. The numerator of the fraction is the power of the base number, and the denominator is the root of the base number. Because of this fact, fractional exponents can be written as $a^{x/y} = \sqrt[y]{a^x}$.

For any square root, the fractional exponent will always be $\dfrac{1}{2}$, where the root (or index) is 2 and the power is 1.

Square Roots That Are Not Perfect Squares

Not all square roots are perfect squares. If the number in the radicand is not the product of a number and itself, then the number is irrational. But just like fractions, most radicals can be expressed in a reduced, or simplified form, even if they are not perfect squares. To simplify radicals, look for the perfect square factors of the number in the radical. In other words, find the largest perfect square that divides evenly into the radicand without a remainder.

For example, the square root of 8, or $\sqrt{8}$. Since 8 is the product of 4 and 2, then $\sqrt{8} = \sqrt{4} \times \sqrt{2}$. Because the square root of 4 is equal to 2, this expression can be simplified to $2 \times \sqrt{2}$ or $2\sqrt{2}$. Four is the largest perfect square factor of 8, and simplifying this factor reduces the radical to simplest radical form.

An additional twist to simplifying radicals happens when there is a coefficient, or a number in front of the radical. In this situation, simplify the radicand as previously explained, and then multiply the coefficient by any number taken out of the radical. For example, take the expression $5\sqrt{44}$. Since the largest perfect square factor of 44 is 4, the expression becomes $5 \times \sqrt{4} \times \sqrt{11}$. The square root of 4 is 2 so the expression is $5 \times 2 \times \sqrt{11}$, which simplifies to $10\sqrt{11}$.

Always keep in mind that a radical is in simplest form if there are no perfect square factors contained in the radicand.

Operations with Radicals

Addition and Subtraction

Adding and subtracting radicals is very much like adding and subtracting with fractions—there must be like terms. In the case of radicals, there must be the same radicand in order to add and subtract, instead of a common denominator. If the terms being combined do not have the same radicand to begin with, simplify each term to see if a common radicand is possible and then only add the terms with this common radicand (i.e. $\sqrt{2} + \sqrt{5}$ cannot be combined).

Multiplication and Division

When multiplying and dividing radicals, no common radicand is necessary. Multiply (or divide) coefficients with coefficients, and radicals with radicals. For example, $2\sqrt{5} \times 3\sqrt{3} = 6\sqrt{15}$.

Note that any radical in simplest form *cannot* be written with a radical in the denominator of a fraction. To take care of this, the denominator must be rationalised. Take $\dfrac{3}{\sqrt{2}}$. To rationalise the denominator, multiply both the denominator and numerator by $\sqrt{2}$. When doing this, you are really just multiplying the fraction by 1. But performing this simple operation will take the radical out of the denominator by creating a perfect square within the radical sign.

$$\frac{3}{\sqrt{2}} \times \frac{\sqrt{2}}{\sqrt{2}} = \frac{3\sqrt{2}}{\sqrt{4}} = \frac{3\sqrt{2}}{2}$$

Since there are no common coefficients between the denominators of 3 and 2 and the denominator is rational, the expression is simplified. Similarly, any radicand that is a fraction needs to be rationalised. In the radical $\sqrt{\dfrac{4}{3}}$, divide the fraction into numerator and denominator by placing each number under its own radical sign and simplify.

$$\sqrt{\frac{4}{3}} = \frac{\sqrt{4}}{\sqrt{3}} = \frac{2}{\sqrt{3}}$$

Notice that since 4 is a perfect square, the square root is an integer. Now, rationalise the denominator by multiplying by $\dfrac{\sqrt{3}}{\sqrt{3}}$.

$$\frac{2}{\sqrt{3}} \times \frac{\sqrt{3}}{\sqrt{3}} = \frac{2\sqrt{3}}{3}$$. This fraction is simplified.

A radical is in simplified form if:
- There are no perfect square factors of the radicand other than 1.
- There are no fractions under the radical sign.
- There are no radicals in the denominator of a fraction.

ALGEBRAIC EXPRESSIONS

Algebra is a mathematical language that uses numbers and symbols to create statements and solve problems. The **variables**, or unknown quantities, are commonly represented by letters such as x or n. Before starting the study of algebraic concepts, it is important to be able to translate word sentences and word problems into algebraic expressions and equations. When translating word phrases into symbols, look for key words that represent certain operations and symbols.

Add (+)	Subtract (−)	Multiply (×)	Divide (÷)	Equal (=)
Sum, increased by, more than, plus, exceeds	difference, decreased by, less than, minus, reduced	product, multiplied by, of, times	quotient, divided by, into	is, result, total, equal to

It is important to understand the difference between an algebraic expression and an equation. An **algebraic expression** contains numbers, variables, and operations to state a relationship. An **equation** is two algebraic expressions set equal to each other. Therefore, an equation contains an equal sign, where an expression does not.

To convert a statement into an expression or equation, identify the key words for the operations mentioned and translate the statement. For example, to translate the statement *"6 times a number n, added to 4"*, you would look for the key word *times* which represents multiplication and the phrase *added to* which indicates addition. Note that n represents the unknown number in the statement. Using the numbers in the statement, translate in order from left to right. Therefore, the expression would read $6 \times n + 4$, or $6n + 4$.

Monomials and Polynomials

Algebraic expressions containing terms created by the product of constants and variables are called **polynomials**, in which the prefix *poly-* means *many*. A single term is called a **monomial**, in which the prefix of *mono* means *one*. Some examples of monomials are 3, $4x$, $-6ab$, and $24x^2y$. Expressions such as $a + b$ or $3x - 4yz$ are called **binomials** because they contain two terms that do not have exactly the same variables and exponents. Binomials are polynomials with two terms; the prefix *bi-* means *two*. A **trinomial** is a polynomial with three distinct terms, such as $x^2 + 3x - 4$. The prefix *tri-* means *three*.

Adding and Subtracting Polynomials

There are special rules for performing the basic operations with polynomials. The first, which involves adding and subtracting polynomials, is called combining like terms. The phrase like terms refers to polynomial terms that contain exactly the same variable(s) and exponent(s). Some examples of like terms are $3x$ and $4x$, $5ab$ and $-10ab$, and $8r2t$ and $-9r2t$. Notice that in like terms, the variables and exponents must be the same, but the coefficients do not have to be the same. When adding and subtracting polynomials, only like terms can be combined.

Multiplying Polynomials

When multiplying polynomials, coefficients are multiplied separately from variables. It is important to note the rules for multiplying the exponents of like bases.

Here are four situations that occur when multiplying polynomials.

1) When multiplying a *monomial by a monomial*, multiply the coefficients and then follow the rules for multiplying the exponents of like bases. In the example $3x^2 \times 4x^3$, multiply the coefficients and add the exponents of the like bases. Thus, the result is $3x^2 \times 4x^3 = 12x^5$.

2) To multiply a *monomial by a polynomial*, use the distributive property. For the expression $6y^3(2y + 3)$, multiply the factor of $6y^3$ by both terms inside the parentheses. The expression then becomes $6y^3 \times 2y + 6y^3 \times 3$. Now, simplify each term by multiplying the coefficients and adding the exponents of the like bases. The result is $12y^4 + 18y^3$.

3) To multiply a *binomial by a binomial*, use a special form of the distributive property known by the acronym FOIL.

FOIL

The acronym **FOIL** can be used when multiplying two binomials together. In the expression $(x + a)(x + b)$:

First: Multiply the first term in each binomial $x \times x = x^2$

Outer: Multiply the outer terms in each binomial $b \times x = bx$

Inner: Multiply the inner terms in each binomial $a \times x = ax$

Last: Multiply the last term in each binomial $a \times b = ab$

Final result is $x^2 + bx + ax + ab = x^2 + (a + b)x + ab$

Factoring

In order to simplify algebraic expressions, it is necessary to know how to factor them. The factors of a number or expression are the pieces of the number or expression that multiply together to form the expression. Finding the factors of a number or expression is the opposite of finding its product.

For example, to find factors of the number 6, think of all of the numbers that can be a part of the product of 6. In other words, think of any number that would divide evenly into 6 without a remainder. The factors of 6 are 1, 2, 3, and 6.

To find the factors of an algebraic expression such as $2x^2y$, break down the expression into smaller pieces. $2x^2y$ can be expressed as the product of $2 \times x \times x \times y$. These are all factors of $2x^2y$.

Using a Greatest Common Factor

When an expression contains more than one term, it is often helpful to find the GCF between the terms in order to simplify. To find the GCF of any polynomial, look for common factors in the coefficients, and common variables between each term. For example, in the trinomial $3x^3 - 6x^2 + 9x$, each term has a coefficient factor of 3 and variable factor of x. Factor out $3x$ from each term: $3x^3 - 6x^2 + 9x = 3x(x^2 - 2x + 3)$

The Difference Between Two Squares

There are some special cases of factoring polynomials. One of these cases is finding the difference between two perfect squares, like $x^2 - 25$, $y^2 - 49$, or $4c^2 - 9$. In order to factor the difference between two perfect squares, take the square root of each term. For example, in the binomial $x^2 - a^2$, x is the square root of x^2 and a is the square root of a^2. Then, write the factors in the form $(x - a)(x + a)$. Following this model—$x^2 - a^2 = (x - a)(x + a)$—the factors of the expressions mentioned are as follows:

$$x^2 - 25 = (x - 5)(x + 5)$$

$$y^2 - 49 = (y - 7)(y + 7)$$

$$4c^2 - 9 = (2c - 3)(2c + 3)$$

$ax^2 + bx + c$

When factoring certain trinomials, the result will often be two binomials. To factor a trinomial in the form $ax^2 + bx + c$, where a, b and c represent real numbers, take a look at the values of a, b and c. If the value of a is 1, then the second terms in each binomial factor must have a sum of b and a product of c.

For example, take the expression $x^2 + 5x + 6$. The value of $a = 1$, $b = 5$ and $c = 6$. Find the factors of this expression:

First, list factors of 6 (c): 1 and 6, −1 and −6, 2 and 3, and −2 and −3. The only pair of factors that has a sum of 5 (b) is 2 and 3. So now, use the 2 and 3 as the second terms in the binomial factors. This makes the factors of the expression equal to $(x + 2)(x + 3)$.

To check to see if these binomials are the correct factors, use FOIL to multiply them together:

$$(x + 2)(x + 3) = x^2 + 3x + 2x + 6 = x^2 + 5x + 6, \text{ which was the original trinomial.}$$

When factoring any factorable polynomial in the form $ax^2 + bx + c$ where $a = 1$, the constant terms of the factors have a sum of b and a product of c. If the value of $a \neq 1$, use the factors of c with trial and error to find the factors.

One thing to keep in mind is that not all trinomials are factorable. An example of a non-factorable trinomial is $x^2 + 3x - 1$. There are no factors of −1 that will also have a sum of 3.

Perfect Square Trinomials

A perfect square trinomial is another special case that is the product of two equal binomials. These trinomials are factored in the same way as previously mentioned, looking for the sum of b and the product of c. An example of a perfect square trinomial is $x^2 + 10x + 25$. Factors of 25 that will have a sum of 10 are 5 and 5. The factors then become $(x + 5)(x + 5)$, or $(x + 5)^2$. Another example of a perfect square trinomial is $n^2 - 6n + 9$. Since the factors of 9 that will have a sum of −6 are −3 and −3, the factors of the trinomial are $(n - 3)(n - 3)$, or $(n - 3)^2$.

A perfect square trinomial has two equal binomial factors. They have two forms and are factored as follows:

$$x^2 + 2ax + a^2 = (x + a)^2 \text{ and } x^2 - 2ax + a^2 = (x - a)^2.$$

Factoring Completely

In order for polynomials to be factored completely, the expression must be broken down into its smallest possible factors. Take the expression $2x^2 - 128$. First, look for any common factors between the terms, or the GCF. Each term contains a factor of 2, so the expression becomes $2(x^2 - 64)$. Since the binomial within the parentheses is the difference between two squares, break it down even more. The factors now become $2(x - 8)(x + 8)$. The expression is now factored completely.

Use the following steps to make sure that the expression is factored completely:

1. Factor out the GCF, if it exists.
2. Factor the difference between two squares.
3. Factor the trinomial into two binomials (FOIL).

Rational Expressions

Simplifying

A rational expression is an expression that may involve constants and/or variables in the form $\frac{a}{b}$, where b cannot equal 0. When a fraction contains any common factors between the numerator and denominator, it can be reduced or simplified. Take the rational expression $\frac{3x}{6x^2}$. When examining the numerator and denominator, each has a factor of 3x. Divide each by this common factor (3x) to simplify the expression: $\frac{1}{2x}$.

When simplifying rational expressions, it is important to factor first and be sure to only cancel factors.

Adding and Subtracting

When adding and subtracting rational expressions, it is necessary to find a common denominator. To find the **least common denominator** (LCD), find the smallest expression that each denominator will divide into without a remainder. When this denominator is found, multiply both the numerator and denominator of the rational expressions by the missing factor needed to make the LCD. Then combine the expressions and keep the common denominator.

For example, in order to add the expressions $\frac{2}{x^2} + \frac{5}{x}$ find the least common denominator of the terms. The LCD of x^2 and x is x^2. Now, multiply each term by the necessary factor to make each denominator equal to x^2. Since the first fraction already has this denominator, keep it as is. In the second fraction, the denominator of x needs to be multiplied by another factor of x to make it x^2. Therefore, both the numerator and denominator of the second term need to be multiplied by x. $\frac{2}{x^2} + \frac{5}{x} = \frac{2}{x^2} + \frac{5 \times x}{x \times x} = \frac{2}{x^2} + \frac{5x}{x^2}$

Now that there is a common denominator, add the numerators and keep the common denominator to get $\frac{2+5x}{x^2}$. Since there are no common factors between the numerator and denominator, the fraction is simplified.

Multiplying and Dividing

When performing multiplication and division with rational expressions, a common denominator is not necessary. For these problems, first factor each fraction in the numerator and denominator when possible, and cancel out any common factors between the numerators and denominators. Then multiply across any remaining factors. The difference between dividing and multiplying rational expressions boils down to one step: dividing by a fraction is the same as multiplying by its reciprocal. Therefore, when the operation is division, simply take the reciprocal of the fraction being *divided by*, and then multiply as previously explained.

Take the example $\dfrac{xy^2}{ab} \times \dfrac{b^2}{xy}$. Each part of the expression is the product of factors, so no factoring is necessary.

Now, cancel the common factors of xy and b from both fractions and multiply across the remaining factors. The expression becomes $\dfrac{\cancel{x}y^{\cancel{2}}}{a\cancel{b}} \times \dfrac{b^{\cancel{2}}}{\cancel{xy}} = \dfrac{yb}{a}$.

Another example is $\dfrac{x^2 - 25}{2x - 10} \times \dfrac{2x^2 + 4x}{x + 5}$. First, factor each part of the fractions to get

$\dfrac{(x-5)(x+5)}{2(x-5)} \times \dfrac{2x(x+2)}{x+5}$. Cancel the common factors. $\dfrac{\cancel{(x-5)}\,\cancel{(x+5)}}{\cancel{2}\,\cancel{(x-5)}} \times \dfrac{\cancel{2}x(x+2)}{\cancel{x+5}}$. The expression

simplifies to $x(x + 2)$ or $x^2 + 2x$.

Now take the quotient $\dfrac{36 - x^2}{4ab} \div \dfrac{x - 6}{2a}$. First take the reciprocal of the second fraction and change the operation to multiplication, so the expression becomes $\dfrac{36 - x^2}{4ab} \times \dfrac{2a}{x - 6}$. Now, factor to get

$\dfrac{(6 - x)(6 + x)}{4ab} \times \dfrac{2a}{x - 6}$. Cancel any common factors. Since two of the factors are $x - 6$ and $6 - x$, a little more work needs to be done before cancelling. First change $6 - x$ to $-x + 6$, and factor out a -1. This expression now becomes $-1(x - 6)$. Therefore, when you cancel $x - 6$ and $6 - x$ the result is -1, not $+1$. In addition, when the 2 from the numerator of the second fraction is cancelled with the 4 from the denominator of the first fraction, a 2 will remain where the 4 once was, since $4 \div 2 = 2$. $\dfrac{(\overset{-1}{\cancel{6 - x}})(6 + x)}{\underset{2}{\cancel{4}}\,ab} \times \dfrac{2\cancel{a}}{\cancel{x - 6}}$. The product

becomes $\dfrac{-1(6 + x)}{2b} = \dfrac{-6 - x}{2b}$.

Simplifying Complex Fractions

A complex fraction is a fraction that contains other fraction(s) in the numerator and/or denominator. One way to simplify complex fractions is to find the least common denominator of each fraction within the complex fraction, and multiply each term by this LCD.

In the example $\dfrac{\frac{1}{x}}{\frac{6}{x^2}}$, the LCD is x^2. By multplying each term by x^2, the result is $\dfrac{\frac{1}{\cancel{x}} \times x^{\cancel{2}^1}}{\frac{6}{\cancel{x^2}} \times \cancel{x^2}} = \dfrac{x}{6}$ after the common factors are cancelled out.

For another example, look at the complex fraction $\dfrac{\frac{x}{y} + x}{\frac{1}{y^2} + \frac{1}{y}}$. The LCD is y^2, so multiply each of the four terms by y^2: $\dfrac{\dfrac{x}{y} \times y^2 + x \times y^2}{\dfrac{1}{y^2} \times y^2 + \dfrac{1}{y} \times y^2}$. Simplify by cancelling common factors to get $\dfrac{xy + xy^2}{1+y}$. Factor the numerator to

get $\dfrac{xy(1+y)}{1+y}$, which reduces to just xy.

EQUATIONS

An **equation** is a mathematical sentence that states that two expressions are equal. An equation contains at least one variable and an equal sign. When solving an equation, first the expressions are simplified, and then other operations are performed until the variable is alone on one side of the equation. This is called **isolating the variable**.

When performing a mathematical operation on an equation, whatever is done to one side must be done to the other side so the equation stays in balance. Every action or operation performed on an equation will change the equation into a simpler form, until the variable is isolated.

One-Step Equations

The simplest type of equation to solve is one that requires only one step in order to isolate the variable, like $x + 5 = 12$, $\dfrac{1}{3x} = 21$ or $\dfrac{x}{15} = 3$. In these examples, only one mathematical operation is present on the side of the equation that contains the variable. In order to isolate the variable, perform the inverse operation to both sides of the equation.

For example, in the first equation, you should subtract 5 from both sides, since subtraction is the inverse of addition. The equation then becomes $x + 5 - 5 = 12 - 5$, which simplifies to $x = 7$.

After solving an equation, check your answer. Just substitute in the answer value for the variable in the original equation and verify that the statement is true.

Two-Step Equations

Two-step equations are equations in which two operations are present and therefore two steps are required to isolate the variable. When performing the inverse operations, always undo the addition or subtraction operation first, and then undo the multiplication or division.

For example, in the equation $5x + 12 = -13$, there are two operations present, multiplication and addition. First, subtract 12 from both sides: $5x + 12 - 12 = -13 - 12$. This simplifies to $5x = -25$. Now, divide both sides by 5, to isolate the variable: $\dfrac{5x}{5x} = \dfrac{-25}{5x}$, or $x = -5$.

SOLVING EQUATIONS

Advanced equations require some steps prior to performing the inverse operations previously explained. Generally speaking, these additional steps are: applying the distributive property, combining like terms and moving the variable to one side of the equation.

Applying the Distributive Property

When an equation has parentheses on either side, the first step is to simplify the expression containing the parentheses. Usually, the distributive property is needed to simplify this type of expression. After applying the distributive property, solve as described for a two-step equation.

For example, to solve $-4(x + 5) = -64$, first apply the distributive property to get rid of the parentheses: $(-4 \times x) + (-4 \times 5) = -64$, or $-4x - 20 = -64$. Now, add 20 to both sides to get $-4x - 20 + 20 = -64 + 20$, or $-4x = -44$. Finally, divide both sides of the equation by -4: $\frac{-4x}{4x} = \frac{44}{-4x}$, or $x = 11$.

Check the result by substituting in the value of 11 for x: $-4(11 + 5) = -64$, which simplifies to $-4 \times 16 = -64$, and $-64 = -64$.

Combining Like Terms

If an equation has any like terms on either side, combine these like terms before performing any inverse operations. If an equation has both parentheses and the need to combine like terms, the best approach is to first apply the distributive property, then combine like terms, and finally, solve the resulting one or two step equation.

For example, in the equation $6x - 25 - 3x = 26$, first combine the like terms. Applying the commutative property, and then combining the variable terms, simplifies the equation to a two-step equation.

$6x - 3x - 25 = 26$, or $3x - 25 = 26$. Now, add 25 to both sides to get $3x - 25 + 25 = 26 + 25$, or $3x = 51$. Finally, divide both sides by 3 to isolate the variable: $\frac{3x}{3x} = \frac{51}{3x}$, and thus $x = 17$.

Verify your work with a check on the original equation: $(6 \times 17) - 25 - (3 \times 17) = 26$. Use the order of operations to simplify: $102 - 25 - 51 = 26$, or $77 - 51 = 26$, or $26 = 26$.

Solving Equations with Variables On Both Sides

After simplifying each side of an equation separately by removing parentheses and combining like terms, the next step is to get the variable on one side of the equation. Identify the smaller variable term and add the opposite of this term to both sides of the equation.

For example, in the equation $9x + 70 = 3x - 2$ there are no parentheses present and no like terms to combine on the separate sides. There is, however, a variable term on both sides. $3x$ is the smaller of the variable terms, so add the opposite of $3x$ $(-3x)$, to both sides of the equation: $9x + -3x + 70 = 3x + -3x - 2$, which simplifies to $6x + 70 = -2$. This is now a two-step equation. Subtract 70 from both sides:

$6x + 70 - 70 = -2 - 70$, or $6x = -72$. Finally, divide both sides by 6: $\frac{6x}{6} = \frac{-72}{6}$, or $x = -12$.

Check this result: $(9 \times -12) + 70 = (3 \times -12) - 2$. This simplifies to $-108 + 70 = -36 - 2$, or $-38 = -38$.

Remember, when solving an equation, follow these steps:

1) Simplify each side of the equation separately:
   - Apply the distributive property when needed.
   - Combine like terms when needed.
2) Move the variable to one side of the equation.
3) Perform the inverse operations of either addition or subtraction.
4) Perform the inverse operations of multiplication or division.
5) Check the answer, by substituting the value of the variable into the original equation.

SYSTEMS OF EQUATIONS

A system of equations is a set of equations containing two variables, typically x and y. To solve a system of equations, find the values of x and y that will make every equation in the system true. There are two algebraic methods of solving a system: the substitution method and the elimination method.

The Substitution Method

The **substitution method** of solving a system of equations is to solve one of the equations for one of the variables, say y, and then to substitute in the resultant expression in the second equation for y. The second equation then becomes an equation with one variable, in this case x. For example, to solve the following system of equations:

$$3x + y = -2$$
$$7x - 3y = -26$$

Solve the first equation for y. First, isolate the variable y by subtracting $3x$ from both sides of the equation to get $y = -3x - 2$. Take $-3x - 2$ and substitute it into the second equation in place of y to get $7x - 3(-3x - 2) = -26$. The second equation now contains only one variable, so you can find a solution. Apply the distributive property: $7x + 9x + 6 = -26$. Combine like terms, and subtract 6 from both sides: $16x + 6 - 6 = -26 - 6$. This simplifies to $16x = -32$. Divide both sides by 16 to get $x = -2$. This is the value for x in the system of equations.

Now, use one of the equations and substitute in -2 for x to then solve for y: $3x + y = -2$ becomes $3 \times -2 + y = -2$, or $-6 + y = -2$. Add 6 to both sides to get $y = 4$. The solution to the system is the ordered pair $(-2, 4)$. This means that in both equations the solutions are $x = -2$ and $y = 4$.

Keep in mind that there are an infinite number of solutions to each of these equations separately; there is usually one unique solution for the system of two or more equations. Just as for all equations, you can check this solution. It is important to check the solution in both given equations in the system. To check the equation $3x + y = -2$, substitute: $(3 \times -2) + 4 = -2$, or $-6 + 4 = -2$ which is the true statement $-2 = -2$. To check the second equation, use the same procedure: $7x - 3y = -26$ becomes $(7 \times -2) + (-3 \times 4) = -26$. This simplifies to $-14 + -12 = -26$, and then to $-26 = -26$.

The Elimination Method

The **elimination method** of solving a system of equations involves multiplying each term of one of the equations by some factor, so that when the two equations are combined together, one of the variables will be eliminated. Here is the previous system now being solved with the elimination method:

$3x + y = -2$
$7x - 3y = -26$

Look at the variable terms. Since the y term in the first equation has a coefficient of 1, and the y term in the second equation has a coefficient of −3, multiply each of the terms in the first equation by positive 3:

$9x + 3y = -6$
$7x - 3y = -26$

Now, combine the like terms of the two equations, and notice that the y terms will be eliminated: $(9x + 7x) + (3y + -3y) = -6 + -26$. This simplifies to $16x = -32$, and again, as in the other method, $x = -2$. From this point, follow the procedures outlined in the substitution method to arrive at the value of 4 for y, and perform the check on both equations.

To solve the next system, look at the equations and find the most convenient variable to eliminate:

$-4x + 2y = -6$
$-2x + 3y = 11$

It is easy to find a common factor for the coefficients of −4 and −2. To turn the coefficient of x in the bottom equation to a +4, multiply each term of the second equation by −2, so that the x variable terms will be eliminated when the equations are combined:

$-4x + 2y = -6$
$4x + -6y = -22$

Combine the like terms in the two equations: $(-4x + 4x) + (2y + -6y) = -6 + -22$. This simplifies to $-4y = -28$. Divide both sides by −4, to get $y = 7$. Now, use this value of 7 for y in the first equation to solve for x: $-4x + (2 \times 7) = -6$, or the simplified version $-4x + 14 = -6$. Subtract 14 from both sides, $-4x = -20$, and then divide both sides by −4 to get $x = 5$. The solution to the system is $(5, 7)$, that is $x = 5$ and $y = 7$. You can check this system in the same manner that you performed the check on the other system of equations.

QUADRATIC EQUATIONS

A **quadratic equation** is an equation that has the form $ax^2 + bx + c = 0$, where a is non-zero.

Factoring

To solve a quadratic equation, get all terms of the equation to one side of the equation; the other side should equal zero. Then, try to factor the quadratic into two binomials.

For example, to solve the quadratic equation $x^2 + 12 = 7x$, first add $-7x$ to both sides of the equation to get all terms on the left side. The equation is now $x^2 - 7x + 12 = 0$. Try to factor this trinomial. The factors are $(x - 3)(x - 4)$. Now write the equation using these factors: $(x - 3)(x - 4) = 0$. This equation says the product of two factors is equal to 0. This means that if either the first factor $(x - 3)$ or the second factor $(x - 4)$ is zero, the equation will be true. Solve each of these simple one-step equations to find the two solutions to the quadratic equation. When $x - 3 = 0$, $x = 3$; and when $x - 4 = 0$, $x = 4$. The two solutions to the quadratic are $x = \{3, 4\}$.

Check by substituting in the values for x to ensure that the simplified statement is true. Use the original equation of $x^2 + 12 = 7x$. Check 3 as the value of x: $3^2 + 12 = 7 \times 3$, or $9 + 12 = 21$, and $21 = 21$. Check 4 as the value of x: $4^2 + 12 = 7 \times 4$, or $16 + 12 = 28$, and $28 = 28$.

Sometimes a quadratic equation will have two identical solutions. Consider the equation $x^2 + 16x = -64$. Again, the first step is to get all of the terms on one side. Add 64 to both sides to get $x^2 + 16x + 64 = 0$. Factor the trinomial. This trinomial is a perfect square, or $(x + 8)(x + 8) = 0$. If either of these factors is 0, the equation will be true. In both cases, the one-step equation is $x + 8 = 0$. When you subtract 8 from both sides, the value of $x = -8$. Now, check this solution in the original equation: $x^2 + 16x = -64$. $(-8)^2 + (16 \times -8) = -64$. This simplifies to $64 + -128 = -64$, which results in the true statement $-64 = -64$.

Sometimes, when solving quadratics with real world problems, you may have to reject one of your two solutions. This usually occurs when you are solving for a length and one of the solutions is negative. You cannot have a negative length.

The Quadratic Formula

If you cannot factor the resultant trinomial after transforming a quadratic to be equal to 0, then either the quadratic has no real solution or the solutions are not rational numbers. The formula used to solve a quadratic equation is called the quadratic formula. This formula will find solutions to any quadratic equation, whether or not the trinomial could have been factored.

The **quadratic formula** is a formula used to solve a quadratic equation in the form $ax^2 + bx + c = 0$. The solutions to the equation are found by substituting in the values of the coefficients a, b and c into the formula:

$$\frac{-b \pm \sqrt{b^2 - 4ac}}{2a}$$

Notice the plus-minus symbol in the formula. This will yield the two solutions to the quadratic equation. Take as an example the equation $2x^2 + 8x + 3 = 0$. You cannot factor the trinomial, so you must use the quadratic formula, where $a = 2$, $b = 8$ and $c = 3$. Substitute these values into the formula to get:

$x = \dfrac{-8 \pm \sqrt{8^2 - 4 \times 2 \times 3}}{2 \times 2}$, or $x = \dfrac{-8 \pm \sqrt{40}}{4}$. Simplify the radical to get $x = \dfrac{-8 \pm 2\sqrt{10}}{4}$. Divide out a common factor of 2 and the solutions are thus $x = -2 \pm \dfrac{\sqrt{10}}{2}$, or $x = -2 + \dfrac{\sqrt{10}}{2}$, and $x = -2 - \dfrac{\sqrt{10}}{2}$.

Sometimes, a quadratic equation has no solutions in the set of real numbers. Consider the following equation: $4x^2 + 2x + 9 = 0$. This trinomial cannot be factored, so use the quadratic formula, where $a = 4$, $b = 2$ and $c = 9$. $x = \dfrac{-2 \pm \sqrt{2^2 - 4 \times 4 \times 9}}{2 \times 4}$, or $x = \dfrac{-2 \pm \sqrt{4 - 144}}{8}$, which simplifies to $x = \dfrac{-2 \pm \sqrt{-140}}{8}$. In the set of real numbers, the square root of a negative number does not exist. There is no real solution to this quadratic equation.

Transforming Graphs

Transformations in the coordinate plane can occur with graphs of algebraic equations. For example, take the equation $y = x^2$. The graph of this function is a parabola, or u-shape, as shown here.

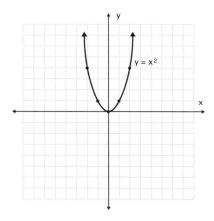

The graph of the equation $y = x^2 + 2$ is the same as $y = x^2$, but moved up, or translated, 2 units. Notice that the +2 at the end of the equation changes the y-intercept from 0 to 2, but the rest of the figure remains the same shape. The translation is shown here.

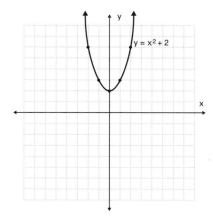

See "Geometry" for additional information about transformations.

Now that you have reviewed the essentials of algebra, test your knowledge by completing these practice questions.

REVIEW QUESTIONS

1. $(2x - 1)(3x^2 - 5x + 2) =$ _____

2. $\dfrac{r^2 - 81}{2t} \times \dfrac{6t^2}{r + 9}$

3. What is the solution to $10x - 2(x - 12) = 59$?

4. Solve the system of equations:

$y = 6x + 10$

$2x + 3y = 110$

(A) (5,40)
(B) (7,52)
(C) (4,34)
(D) (34,4)
(E) (40,5)

5. Solve for x: $x^2 - 14x = -49$

(A) {−7}
(B) {7}
(C) {−7,7}
(D) {40,9}
(E) {−40,9}

Answers and Explanations

1. $6x3 - 13x2 + 9x - 2$

Multiply using the distributive property. $(2x - 1)(3x^2 - 5x + 2) = 6x^3 - 10x^2 + 4x - 3x^2 + 5x - 2$. Combine like terms to get $6x^3 - 13x^2 + 9x - 2$.

2. $3t(r - 9)$

First factor, and then cancel any common factors between the numerators and denominators.

$\dfrac{r^2 - 81}{2t} \times \dfrac{6t^2}{r+9} = \dfrac{(r-9)(r+9)}{2t} \times \dfrac{\cancel{3}6t^{\cancel{2}}}{r+9}$. Multiply the remaining factors to get $\dfrac{3t(r-9)}{1}$, or $3t(r - 9)$.

3. 4.375

Apply the distributive property and then combine like terms: $10x - 2x + 24 = 59$, $8x + 24 = 59$. Subtract 24 from both sides to get $8x = 35$. Divide both sides by 8 to isolate x.

4. C

The first equation is already solved for the variable y, so use the substitution method and substitute in the expression $6x + 10$ for the value of y in the second equation: $2x + 3(6x + 10) = 110$. Apply the distributive property: $2x + 18x + 30 = 110$. Next, combine like terms: $20x + 30 = 110$. Subtract 30 from both sides of the equation to get $20x = 80$. Divide both sides by 20 and $x = 4$. Using the value of 4 for x, use the first equation to find y: $6(4) + 10$, or $y = 34$. The solution is the ordered pair (4, 34).

5. B

First, add 49 to both sides to get the equation in the correct form: $x2 - 14x + 49 = 0$. The left-hand side is a perfect square trinomial when factored: $(x - 7)(x - 7) = 0$. When either of these factors are 0 the equation is true, so the solution is $x = 7$.

Chapter 22: **Geometry**

To start, here are some basic terms and definitions.

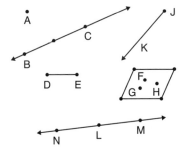

Point—a position in space. A point has no length or width. An example is point A.

Line—The shortest distance between two points determines a line. A line has no width, and an infinite length. An example is line $\overleftrightarrow{BC}$.

Line segment—a piece of a line. A segment includes two points, called endpoints, and all the points in between. An example is $\overline{DE}$.

Plane—Any three non-collinear points determine a plane. A plane has an infinite width and length. An example is plane *FGH*.

Ray—one-half of a line. A ray includes an endpoint and all the collinear points on one side of this endpoint. An example is $\overrightarrow{JK}$, or $\overrightarrow{LM}$ (one half of line $\overleftrightarrow{NM}$).

When naming lines, line segments or planes, the order of the points does not matter. In the given definitions, segment $\overline{DE}$ could also be named $\overline{ED}$; line $\overleftrightarrow{BC}$ could also be named $\overleftrightarrow{CB}$ and plane *FGH* could also be named *GFH*, or other variations. But when naming a ray, the endpoint must be named first. In the previous figure, there is a ray $\overrightarrow{LM}$ and a different ray $\overrightarrow{LN}$. Both have the same starting point of L, but they contain all other points that are different on the opposing sides of the line $\overleftrightarrow{NM}$. As a rule, line segments, lines, planes and rays all have an infinite number of points.

Two geometric figures are **congruent** if each has the same measure. This relationship can apply to several geometric figures. The symbol for congruence is ≅ .

A segment **bisector** is a line or line segment that divides the segment into two congruent segments.

The **midpoint** of a segment is where the bisector intersects the segment.

SPECIAL LINES

There are three kinds of special lines:

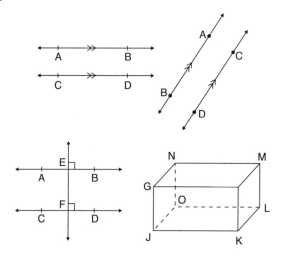

Parallel lines—lines in the same plane that do not intersect. In the previous figure, lines $\overrightarrow{AB}$ and $\overrightarrow{CD}$ are parallel as shown by $AB \parallel CD$. Line segments, rays and planes can also be parallel.

Perpendicular lines—lines in the same plane that intersect at one point and form four 90° angles. In the previous figure, line $\overleftrightarrow{EF}$ is perpendicular to both of the lines $\overleftrightarrow{AB}$ and $\overleftrightarrow{CD}$. This is shown by the symbols $EF \perp AB$ and $EF \perp CD$.

Skew lines—lines in different planes that do not intersect. Skew lines exist in three dimensions. In the rectangular solid in the previous figure, segments *NM* and *KL* are skew.

ANGLES

An **angle** is defined by two distinct rays that have the same endpoint. The common endpoint the rays share is called the *vertex* of the angle. When naming an angle, use the symbol for angle (∠) and name the vertex of the angle in the middle of the three letters. In the following figure, there are several angles, which are numbered for clarity.

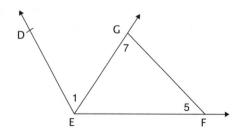

∠1 can be named ∠*DEG* or ∠*GED*. ∠5 can be named ∠*EFG* or ∠*GFE*. ∠7 can be named ∠*FGE* or ∠*EGF*. Note that ∠5 and ∠7 use the same three points, but name different angles, based on the vertex point.

An **angle bisector** is a ray in the interior of the angle that divides the angle into congruent angles with the same measure.

In the following figure, ray $\overrightarrow{BD}$ is an angle bisector: ∠*ABD* ≅ ∠*DBC*. Note how congruent angles are indicated on the figure.

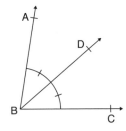

Angle Classification

Angles are classified according to their degree measure.

An **acute** angle is an angle whose measure is between 0° and 90°.

A **right** angle measures exactly 90°. Right angles are designated by a small box in the interior at the vertex.

An **obtuse** angle is an angle whose measure is between 90° and 180°.

A **straight** angle measures exactly 180°.

Special Angle Pair Relationships

Complementary angles are any two angles whose combined measures equal 90°.

Supplementary angles are any two angles whose combined measures equal 180°.

A **linear pair** is two supplementary angles that share a common side and no common interior points. They will form a straight angle, or a line.

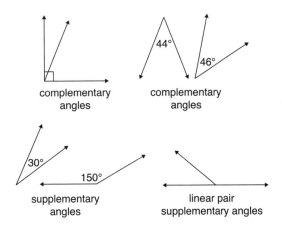

When a line, called a *transversal*, cuts through two parallel lines, eight angles are formed. These angles are numbered 1 through 8 in the following figure for clarity:

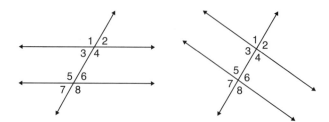

From this condition, several types of conguent angles are defined:

Vertical angles are formed when two lines intersect. They are two angles that share a common vertex but share no common sides. In the previous figure, ∠1 and ∠4, ∠2 and ∠3, ∠5 and ∠8, and ∠6 and ∠7 are all examples of vertical angle pairs.

Corresponding angles are two angles on the same side of the transversal, but one is in the interior of the parallel lines and one is in the exterior of the parallel lines. In the previous figure, ∠1 and ∠5, ∠2 and ∠6, ∠3 and ∠7, and ∠4 and ∠8 are all examples of corresponding angle pairs.

Alternate interior angles are two angles on different sides of the transversal, both in the interior of the parallel lines. In the previous figure, ∠3 and ∠6, and ∠4 and ∠5 are the alternate interior angle pairs in the previous figure.

Alternate exterior angles are two angles on different sides of the transversal, both in the exterior of the parallel lines. In the previous figure, ∠1 and ∠8, and ∠2 and ∠7 are the alternate exterior angle pairs in the previous figure.

Note that in the parallel line figure there are also several examples of linear pairs: ∠1 and ∠2, ∠2 and ∠4, ∠7 and ∠8, and ∠5 and ∠7. In fact, if you study the figure, you will realise that there are actually only two angle measures in the figure. With the exception of a transversal that is perpendicular to the parallel lines, four acute angles and four obtuse angles are formed. All of the acute angles are congruent and all of the obtuse angles are congruent. In addition, any one of the acute angles paired with any one of the obtuse angles forms a supplementary pair.

TRIANGLES

The triangle is the most common geometric figure used in mathematics. A triangle is a closed geometric figure that has three sides and three angles. Triangles are classified according to their angles and their side lengths.

Triangles are classified according to their angles as follows:

An **acute** triangle has three acute angles.

An **obtuse** triangle has exactly one obtuse angle and two acute angles.

A **right** triangle has exactly one right angle, and two acute angles.

Triangles are classified according to their sides as follows:

A **scalene** triangle has three sides of different length.

An **isosceles** triangle has two sides of the same length. This triangle also has two angles with the same measure—the angles opposite to the sides of the same length.

An **equilateral** triangle has all three sides of the same length. This triangle also has three congruent angles, each with measure of 60°.

The figure here gives some examples of triangles and their classifications.

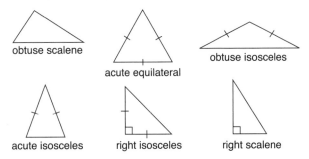

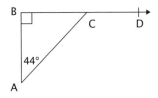

The Angles of a Triangle

There are some important facts about triangles that are important to understand when performing operations with angles.

The sum of the measures of the angles in a triangle is 180°.

The measure of an exterior angle to a triangle is equal to the sum of the two remote interior angles of the triangle.

In a right triangle, the two acute angles are complementary, that is, the sum of the measures of these angles is equal to 90°.

For example, in the following figure, △ABC is a right triangle. Therefore, ∠BAC and ∠ACB are complementary. The measure of ∠ACB = 90 − 44 = 46°. In addition, the measure of ∠ACD, which is an exterior angle to triangle △ABC, is equal to the sum of ∠CAB and ∠ABC, the two remote interior angles. The measure of ∠ACD = 90 + 44 = 134°. You may also notice that ∠ACD and ∠BCA form a linear pair, and therefore their angle measures sum to 180°.

The Sides of a Triangle

The sum of the lengths of any two sides of a triangle must be larger than the length of the third side. For example, to determine if 4, 7, and 12 can be the sides of a triangle, check each sum pair: $4 + 7 = 11$, which is not greater than 12. This set cannot be the sides of a triangle. However, 4, 4, and 7 can be the sides of a triangle. Test the sides: $4 + 4 = 8$, which is bigger than 7; the other two tests would be $7 + 4 = 11$, which is bigger than 4.

The Pythagorean Theorem

One of the most widely used theorems in mathematics is the Pythagorean theorem, which is based upon right triangles. The Pythagorean theorem states that in every right triangle, the sum of the squares of the legs is equal to the square of the hypotenuse. This is commonly shown as $a^2 + b^2 = c^2$, where a and b are the lengths of the legs of the right triangle and c is the length of the hypotenuse.

The converse of the Pythagorean theorem is also true: if a triangle has sides whose lengths follow the relationship that $a^2 + b^2 = c^2$, then the triangle is a right triangle. The Pythagorean theorem is used to find the missing length of a side of a triangle when any two of the lengths are known. For example, given that a right triangle has legs with length of 12 mm and 5 mm, the length of the hypotenuse, c, is found with the theorem $a^2 + b^2 = c^2$. Substitute in 12 and 5 for a and b to get $12^2 + 5^2 = c^2$. Simplify: $144 + 25 = c^2$. or $169 = c^2$. The length of the hypotenuse is the square root of 169, or 13 mm.

QUADRILATERALS

Quadrilaterals are four-sided polygons. There are two major classifications of common quadrilaterals:

A **trapezoid** is a quadrilateral with one pair of parallel sides. Examples here are trapezoid *ABCD* and trapezoid *EFGH*.

A **parallelogram** is a quadrilateral with two pairs of parallel sides. An example here is parallelogram *JKLM*.

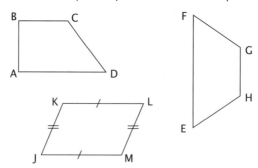

For every quadrilateral, the sum of the measure of the angles is 360°. In a parallelogram, both pairs of opposite sides are parallel and congruent. Opposite angles are also congruent. Trapezoids and parallelograms can be further classified into subcategories.

A **rectangle** is a parallelogram with four right angles, as shown in rectangle *LMNO* and *STUV*. Like all parallelograms, the rectangle has opposite sides and opposite angles that are congruent. In addition, the diagonals are congruent.

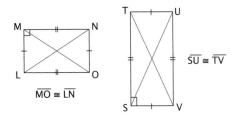

$$\overline{MO} \cong \overline{LN}$$

$$\overline{SU} \cong \overline{TV}$$

A **rhombus** is a parallelogram with four congruent sides, as shown in rhombus *ABCD* and *WXYZ* below. Like all parallelograms, the rhombus has opposite sides and opposite angles that are congruent. In addition, the diagonals are perpendicular.

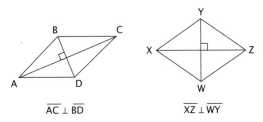

$$\overline{AC} \perp \overline{BD}$$

$$\overline{XZ} \perp \overline{WY}$$

A square is both a rhombus and a rectangle. Therefore it is a parallelogram with four 90° angles, and all sides are congruent. In addition, the diagonals of a square are both congruent and perpendicular. A square is shown below, *JKLM*.

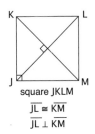

square JKLM

$$\overline{JL} \cong \overline{KM}$$

$$\overline{JL} \perp \overline{KM}$$

The tree below summarises the relationship between the different classifications of special quadrilaterals. The characteristics are listed under each heading. All polygons lower in the tree share the characteristics of the polygons above them in the tree.

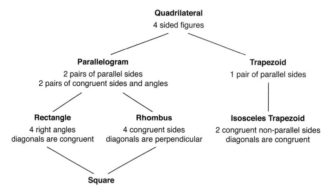

CIRCLES

The radius, *r*, of a circle is the segment whose endpoints are the centre of the circle and any point on the circle. The diameter, *d*, of a circle is a segment that passes through the centre of the circle and whose endpoints are both on the circle. The diameter's length is twice the length of the radius.

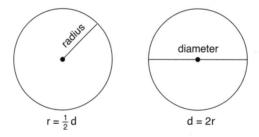

For example, to find the circumference of a circle with diameter of 34 centimetres, use the formula $C = \pi d = 3.14 \times 34 = 106.76$ centimetres. To find the area, first calculate the radius, which is one-half of the diameter, or 17 centimetres. Then use the formula $A = \pi r^2$, or $A = 3.14 \times 17 \times 17 = 907.46 \text{ cm}^2$.

COORDINATE GEOMETRY

Coordinate geometry is a way to use a rectangular grid to locate particular places and determine measurements such as area or distance.

The Coordinate Plane

The coordinate plane is formed by the intersection of two perpendicular number lines. The horizontal number line is known as the *x*-axis and the vertical number line is known as the *y*-axis. When the lines intersect, four regions, called quadrants, are formed. They are numbered I, II, III, IV, in anti-clockwise fashion, starting from the upper right-hand quadrant. The point where the two number lines intersect is called the origin, and has the coordinates (0, 0). The number lines are labelled with positive numbers to the right of the origin on the *x*-axis and above the origin on the *y*-axis, and with negative numbers to the left of the origin on the *x*-axis and below the origin on the *y*-axis.

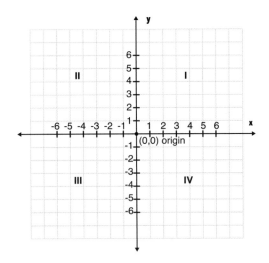

Each point in the coordinate system has a location determined by the number of spaces the point lies to the right or left of the origin, and above or below the origin. Therefore, each point in the system is named with two numbers: an *x*-coordinate and a *y*-coordinate. These coordinates are always written in *x, y* order and placed in parentheses. Take, for example, the point named by the coordinates (4, 5). The first number in the pair is 4, so this point is 4 spaces to the right of the origin on the *x*-axis. The second number is 5, so the point is also 5 spaces above the origin on the *y*-axis. Therefore, to find the location of this point, start at the origin, move 4 spaces to the right and 5 spaces up from there. Note the location in quadrant I of the point (4, 5) in the following figure.

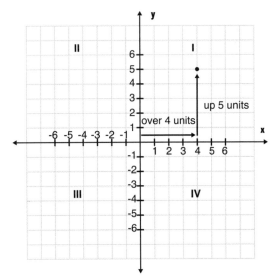

Notice the following pattern when graphing points in the four quadrants:

In quadrant I, both the *x* and *y* coordinates are positive.

In quadrant II, all *x*-values are negative while the *y*-values are positive.

In quadrant III, both the *x* and *y* coordinates are negative.

In quadrant IV, all *x*-values are positive, while the *y*-values are negative.

Formulas

The Midpoint Formula

It is oftentimes helpful to know the halfway point, or midpoint, between two endpoints of a line segment. You can find this location by using the formula $\left(\dfrac{x_1 + x_2}{2}, \dfrac{y_1 + y_2}{2}\right)$ where (x_1, y_1) and (x_2, y_2) represent the two endpoints. To find the midpoint between the points (2, 5) and (4, −3), for example, first, plug in the values of x and y from each point and then evaluate the formula: $\left(\dfrac{x_1 + x_2}{2}, \dfrac{y_1 + y_2}{2}\right) = \left(\dfrac{2+4}{2}, \dfrac{5+-3}{2}\right) = \left(\dfrac{6}{2}, \dfrac{2}{2}\right) = (3, 1)$. The midpoint between the points (2, 5) and (4, −3) is (3, 1). To help you remember the midpoint formula, notice that you are actually finding the sum of the two x-values and dividing it by 2, and then you are doing the same for the y-values.

You can also use this formula to find an endpoint when given the value of the other endpoint and the midpoint. Take the segment $\overline{AB}$ with point A at (4, −7) and the midpoint of $\overline{AB}$ at (−1, −3). To find the location of point B, substitute the known values into the formula and set it equal to the midpoint: $\left(\dfrac{x_1 + x_2}{2}, \dfrac{y_1 + y_2}{2}\right) = \left(\dfrac{4 + x_2}{2}, \dfrac{-7 + y_2}{2}\right) = (-1, -3)$. Now, set each expression in the formula equal to its coordinate at the midpoint: $\dfrac{4 + x_2}{2} = -1$ and $\dfrac{-7 + y_2}{2} = -3$. Cross-multiply in the first equation: $4 + x_2 = -2$, so $x_2 = -6$. Cross-multiply in the second equation: $-7 + y_2 = -6$, so $y_2 = 1$. Therefore, the coordinates of point B are (−6, 1).

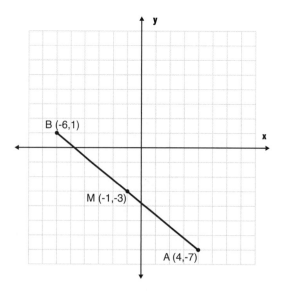

The Distance Formula

Another formula frequently used in the coordinate plane is the distance formula. This formula will help you calculate the distance between any two points in the coordinate plane. To find the distance between any two points (x_1, y_1) and (x_2, y_2), use the formula $d = \sqrt{(x_1 - x_2)^2 + (y_1 - y_2)^2}$, which is based on the Pythagorean theorem. For example, to find the distance between the points $(0, -2)$ and $(5, -2)$, substitute the values for x and y from each point into the formula:

$$\sqrt{(x_1 - x_2)^2 + (y_1 - y_2)^2} = \sqrt{(0 - 5)^2 + (-2 - (-2))^2} = \sqrt{(-5)^2 + (0)^2} = \sqrt{25 + 0} = \sqrt{25} = 5.$$

The distance between the points $(0, -2)$ and $(5, -2)$ is 5 units.

The distance between two points may also be an irrational number. Take the points $(4, 2)$ and $(-3, 6)$. To find the distance between them, substitute into the distance formula:

$$\sqrt{(x_1 - x_2)^2 + (y_1 - y_2)^2} = \sqrt{(4 - (-3))^2 + (2 - 6)^2} = \sqrt{(7)^2 + (-4)^2} = \sqrt{49 + 16} = \sqrt{65}.$$

Notice in this case the final distance is not a perfect square. Since the square root of 65 is approximately equal to 8, the distance can be rounded to 8 units using a calculator, but the exact answer is $\sqrt{65}$ units.

Slope and Its Applications

Slope helps you draw conclusions about the pattern of a graph, and tells you the **rate of change** of a situation. The slope (m) of the line between two points (x_1, y_1) and (x_2, y_2) can be found by using the formula $m = \dfrac{\text{change in } y}{\text{change in } x} = \dfrac{(y_1 - y_2)}{(x_1 - x_2)}$

Slope is commonly known as the *rise over the run*. In other words, the number in the numerator of the fraction tells how many units to move up or down and the number in the denominator tells how many units to move to the right or left. If the slope is written as a whole number, write that value over the number 1. A slope of 3 is written as $\dfrac{3}{1}$ because the rise is 3 and the run is 1.

Special Cases of Slope

There are four major categories that the slope of a line can fall under: positive slope, negative slope, slope of 0 or no slope. **Positive slopes** are lines that go up to the right as you move from left to right. When using the slope, count up and over to the right when plotting the graph.

These lines appear to be "uphill", as shown in the following figure.

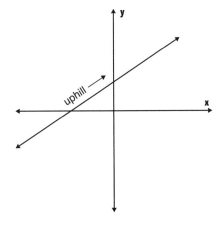

Negative slopes are lines that go up to the left, and appear to be at a downhill slant. With negative slope, count up and over to the left when plotting the graph. The figure here shows a line with negative slope.

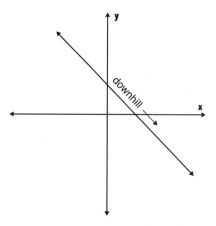

Two additional special cases of slope are horizontal and vertical lines. When the rate of change in the y-values is equal to 0, the line formed will be a horizontal line. In this case, the slope would have a rise of 0 and a run of any real number. This would cause the graph to travel horizontally across, but to not have any steepness. Each horizontal line is in the form $y = k$, where k represents a constant value. A few examples are shown in the following figure.

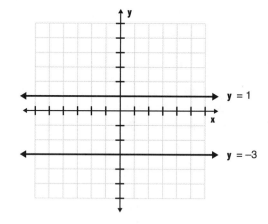

When the rate of change of the x-values is 0, then the line formed is a vertical line. Because the 0 will then be at the bottom of the fraction, no real number slope can exist. Each vertical line is in the form $x = k$, where k represents a constant value. A few examples of vertical lines and their equations are shown in the figure here.

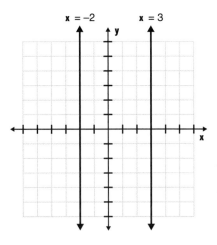

Intercepts

There are two intercepts that are commonly used when graphing lines in the coordinate plane. The first is the **x-intercept**, the location at which a line intersects, or crosses, the x-axis. This point is written in the form $(x, 0)$. Notice that the y-value at the x-intercept will always be 0.

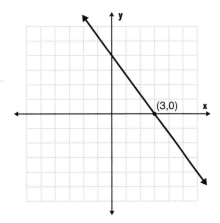

The **y-intercept** is the location at which a line intersects the y-axis. This point is written in the form (0, y). Also notice in this case the x-value at the y-intercept will always be 0.

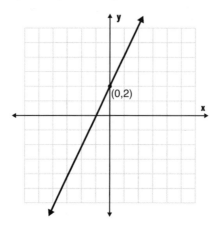

Graphing in Slope-Intercept Form

The **slope-intercept form** of a linear equation is $y = mx + b$, where m is the slope of the line and b is the y-intercept.

In order to graph a line written in slope-intercept form, follow these four steps.

    1) Make sure the equation is in the form $y = mx + b$.

    2) Use b from the equation (the y-intercept) to graph the point $(0, b)$ on the y-axis.

    3) Using the numerator and denominator of m, or the slope of the equation, start at the y-intercept and count up (the amount of the rise) and over (the amount of the run) to find another point. Repeat the process of counting up and over to find additional points on the line.

    4) Connect the points to create your line.

Practise this procedure with the linear equation $y = 3x + 1$.

    1) Since the equation is in the form $y = mx + b$, first identify that $m = 3$ and $b = 1$.

    2) Place a point at the y-intercept of $(0, 1)$.

    3) Since the slope is 3 or $\frac{3}{1}$, count up 3 units and over 1 unit to find another point on the line. This is the point $(1, 4)$. Note that since the slope is positive, count up and over to the right. Repeat the process of counting up 3 and over 1 to the right to find additional points.

    4) Connect the points to form the graph of the line. This equation is graphed in the following figure.

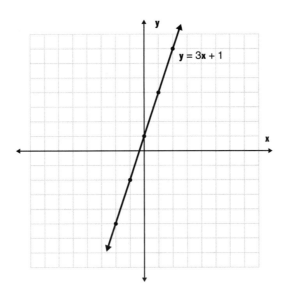

Try another practice example using the equation $2y + x = 4$.

1) Since the equation is not in the form $y = mx + b$, first subtract x from both sides of the equation and then divide each term by 2 to get $y = -x + 2$. Now, identify that $m = -$ and $b = 2$.

2) Place a point at the y-intercept of $(0, 2)$.

3) Since the slope is $-$, count up 1 unit and over 2 units to the left to find another point on the line. This is the point $(-2, 3)$. Note that since the slope is negative, you are counting up and over to the left. Repeat the process of counting up 1 and over 2 to the left to find additional points.

4) Connect the points to form the graph of the line. This equation is graphed in the figure here.

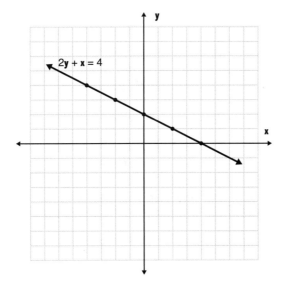

Linear Inequalities

Inequalities use the symbols $<$ (less than), $>$ (greater than), $\leq$ (less than or equal to) and $\geq$ (greater than or equal to) instead of equal signs. Linear inequalities work just like linear equations, except for two differences:

1. The line should be *dashed*, not solid, if the inequality symbol is $<$ or $>$ because the points that lie on the line are not in the solution set.

2. One side of the line, or half-plane, is shaded to show all the points in the solution set.

Here are examples of linear inequalities. Each one is graphed using the slope-intercept method as previously explained.

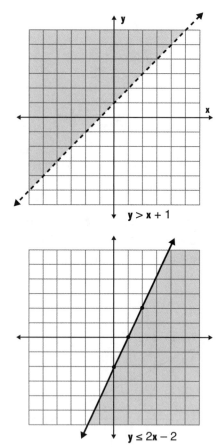

$y > x + 1$

$y \leq 2x - 2$

Note that in the previous figure, the line for the inequality $y > x + 1$ is dashed because the symbol is *greater than* and not *greater than or equal to*. The *greater than* symbol indicates that the graph should be shaded above the line.

In the other figure given, the line for the inequality is solid because the symbol is *less than or equal to*. This symbol also causes the shading to fall below the line.

Solving Systems of Equations

When more than one equation is graphed on the same set of axes, a system of equations is created. To solve a system of equations, look for the intersection of the lines. These point(s) of intersection, if they exist, are the solution(s) to the system.

Here is an example of how to solve a system of equations. Take the system:

$$y = -2x + 3$$
$$y = x - 3$$

First, graph each equation on the same set of axes. In the first equation, the slope is equal to -2 and the y-intercept is 3. In the second equation, the slope is 1 and the y-intercept is -3. The following figure shows these two equations graphed on the same set of axes.

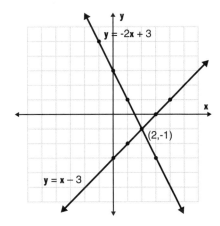

Since the two lines intersect at the point $(2, -1)$, this point is the solution to the system of equations. To check this solution, substitute the coordinates $x = 2$ and $y = -1$ into each of the original equations and check to make sure they are equal.

$$y = -2x + 3 \qquad y = x - 3$$
$$-1 = -2(2) + 3 \qquad -1 = 2 - 3$$
$$-1 = -4 + 3 \qquad -1 = -1$$
$$-1 = -1$$

Special Systems of Equations

There are three different cases of solutions to systems of equations when working with linear equations: **one solution**, **infinite solutions** or **no solution**. The first case happens when two lines intersect at a single point. The second case is when the lines appear to have different equations, but end up being the same line after the equations are transformed to $y = mx + b$ form. These lines are called **coincident lines** and actually share all the same points. Therefore, there are infinite solutions to a system of coincident lines.

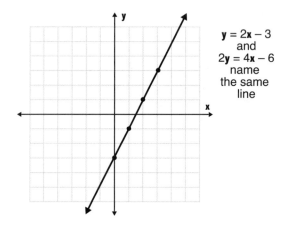

The third case is when the lines do not intersect at all. The only way this can happen in a plane is if the lines are parallel. Parallel lines in the same plane slant at the same rate, running next to each other but never touching. Therefore, parallel lines have the same slope. If two lines on the same set of axes have the same slope, then there is no solution to this system. In the following figure, each line has a slope of -1; therefore the lines are parallel and will not intersect.

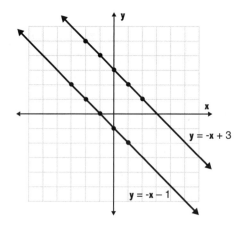

Transformations in the Coordinate Plane

There are four basic types of transformations in the coordinate plane: reflections, translations, rotations and dilations.

When dealing with reflections, think of a mirror image. A **reflection** is also known as a "flip", as the object being reflected appears to flip over a line of reflection. Take the example that follows. Triangle ABC is reflected, or flipped, over the y-axis and triangle A'B'C' is the image of reflection.

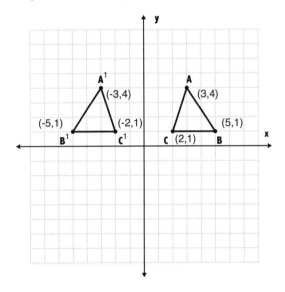

This reflection is written as $\triangle ABC \xrightarrow{Ry-axis} \triangle A'B'C'$, and the line of reflection is the y-axis. Notice that the y-coordinates remain the same, while the x-coordinates become their opposites. In the same manner, if reflecting over the x-axis, the x-coordinates would remain the same while the y-coordinates would become their opposites.

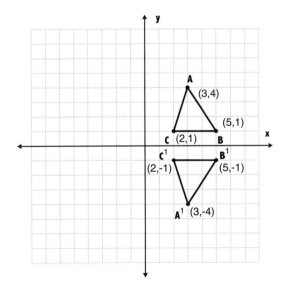

Another common line of reflection is the line $y = x$. In this linear equation, the slope of the line is 1 (the coefficient of x is 1) and the y-intercept is 0 (there is no b in this equation). This line contains all of the points where x is equal to y, such as $(-1, -1)$, $(0, 0)$, $(2, 2)$ etc. When reflecting over this line, all of the coordinates of the points in the object are reversed; in other words, (x, y) is changed to (y, x). An example of this is shown in the following figure.

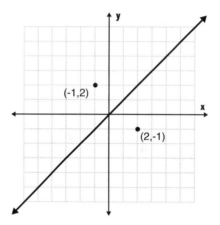

With a **translation**, an object is moved a certain number of units either left or right and then either up or down. A translation is written using the notation $T_{a, b}$ where a is the number of horizontal units (change in the x-coordinates) the point or object will move and b is the number of vertical units (change in the y-coordinates) the point or object will move. If the value of a or b is positive, that number is added to the corresponding coordinates; if the value of either is negative, it is subtracted from the corresponding coordinates. Note the example that follows.

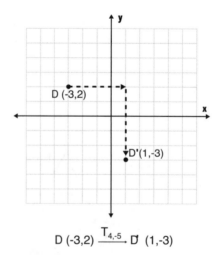

$$D\ (\text{-}3,2) \xrightarrow{\ T_{4,\text{-}5}\ } D'\ (1,\text{-}3)$$

Notice in the translation of point D, 4 was added to each x-coordinate and -5 was added to each y-coordinate to find the image.

A **rotation** is also known as a "turn", as the object is turned much like a wheel would spin about a centre point. The notation *Rot*, or sometimes just *r*, is used to indicate a rotation. The following figure shows a few of the most common types of rotations, each one with the centre at the origin.

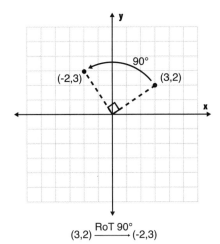

$$(3,2) \xrightarrow{\text{RoT } 90°} (-2,3)$$

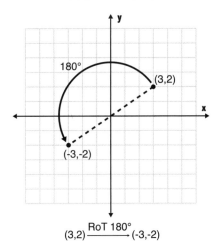

$$(3,2) \xrightarrow{\text{RoT } 180°} (-3,-2)$$

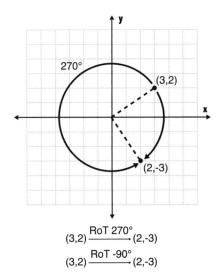

$$(3,2) \xrightarrow{\text{RoT } 270°} (2,-3)$$

$$(3,2) \xrightarrow{\text{RoT } -90°} (2,-3)$$

Note that any positive rotation is in an anti-clockwise fashion, and any negative rotation occurs in a clockwise direction. As shown in the previous figure, a rotation of 270° is the same as a rotation of −90°.

The **dilation** is the only type of transformation that does not preserve the size of the object. In most dilations, the image of the object is smaller or larger than the original object, but always remains in proportion to the original object. Each dilation has a centre (which is usually at the origin in a coordinate plane) and a scale factor. The scale factor indicates how many times larger or smaller the image is of the original figure. In other words, the scale factor is multiplied by the coordinates of the original image to find the coordinates of the new image. The following graph shows a dilation of scale factor 2. Notice how each coordinate is multiplied by 2 to find the coordinates of the image.

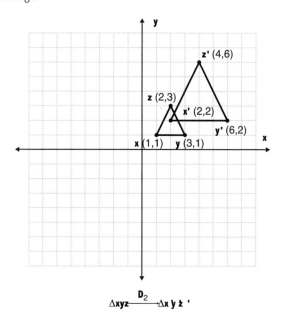

MEASUREMENT

Measurement explores the concepts of perimeter, area, surface area and volume.

Perimeter

The perimeter is the distance around a polygon. To find the perimeter of a polygon, add together the lengths of all its sides. For example, the perimeter of the following trapezoid is $21 + 8 + 5 + 12 = 46$ cm.

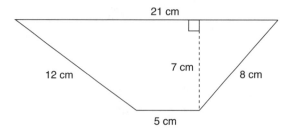

Notice that the height of the trapezoid (7 cm) is indicated on the figure. However, this fact is not needed to calculate the perimeter.

Area

The **area** of a polygon is the amount of square units needed to cover the polygon. Area is calculated by multiplying two entities, so the units are always in square units. To use the formulas to calculate area, you need to know how to recognise and find the height of a polygon.

The **height** of a polygon is the length of the segment that is perpendicular to a side of the polygon (called the base). Study the following figure to recognise the height of different polygons.

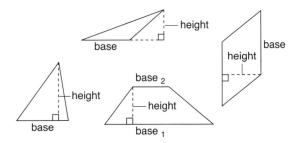

To distinguish the height from a side of the polygon, it is usually shown as a dotted line. Sometimes, as in rectangles and squares, the height is also one of the sides. The formulas used to find the area of common polygons are as shown here:

Area of Common Polygons

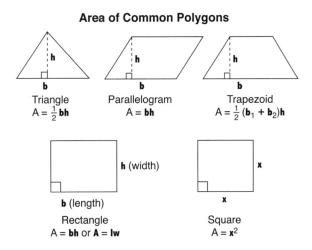

To find the area of a polygon, substitute the given lengths into the formula and simplify. The units for area are always square units.

Surface Area

The measure of surface area applies to three-dimensional solids. A **prism** is a three-dimensional solid with two congruent bases, and any number of other faces that are all rectangles. A **cylinder** has two congruent circular bases, with one rectangular face wrapped around the bases.

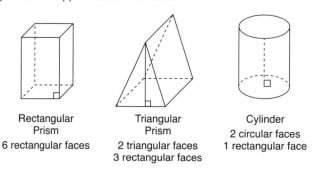

Rectangular
Prism
6 rectangular faces

Triangular
Prism
2 triangular faces
3 rectangular faces

Cylinder
2 circular faces
1 rectangular face

These solids have faces that are made up of common polygons.

To find the surface area of any solid, calculate the area of each of the faces, and then add them all together. The units for surface area are square units.

Volume

The volume of a three-dimensional solid is the amount of cubic units needed to fill the solid. The volume of a prism or a cylinder is the area of one of the bases, B, multiplied by the height, h. For a prism, the formula for volume is the area of the base, B, multiplied by the height. So for a triangular prism, the volume is the area of the triangular base $\frac{1}{2}bh$, multiplied by the height of the prism.

The two most common solids to find the volume of are the rectangular prism and the cylinder. The volume of a rectangular solid is $V = Bh$, or $V = lwh$, where B is the area of the base, that is, $l \times w$, and h is the height. The volume of a cylinder is $V = Bh$, or $V = \pi r^2h$, where B is the area of the base, that is $\pi \times r^2$, and h is the height.

Volume of a Pyramid and a Cone

The pyramid and the cone are special three-dimensional solids that are related to the prism and the cylinder. The pyramid is a rectangular solid in which instead of two congruent faces, there is a point opposite to the base of the solid. The cone is similarly related to the cylinder. Some examples are shown here.

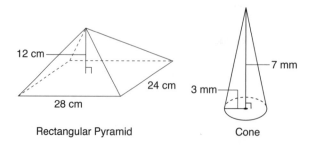

12 cm

28 cm

24 cm

Rectangular Pyramid

7 mm

3 mm

Cone

The volume of a pyramid or a cylinder is $V = \frac{1}{3}Bh$.

The volume of a pyramid is $V = \frac{1}{3}wh$.

The volume of a cone is $V = \frac{1}{3}\pi r^2 h$.

Now that you have reviewed the essentials of geometry, test your knowledge by completing these practice questions.

REVIEW QUESTIONS

1. In the figure below, $AB \parallel CD$. What type of angles are angles $\angle 1$ and $\angle 5$?

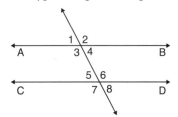

   (A) complementary
   (B) corresponding
   (C) vertical
   (D) alternate interior
   (E) alternate exterior

2. What is the slope of the line between the points $(6, 2)$ and $(3, -2)$?

   (A) 4
   (B) $\frac{4}{3}$
   (C) $\frac{3}{4}$
   (D) 0
   (E) 3

3. Write the equation for the graph below.

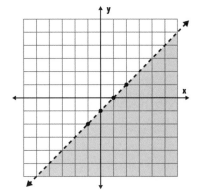

4. Find the surface area of this solid.

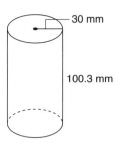

30 mm

100.3 mm

5. How much water will a rectangular reservoir with dimensions of 60m × 24m × 6m hold?

(A) 8,640 m^3

(B) 90 m^3

(C) 1,440 m^3

(D) 540 m^3

(E) 2,880 m^3

Answers and Explanations

1. B

This pair of angles is on the same side of the transversal line, one is in the interior and one is in the exterior of the parallel lines. The name for this special pair is corresponding angles.

2. B

To find the slope, use the formula $m = \dfrac{\text{change in } y}{\text{change in } x} = \dfrac{(y^1 - y^2)}{(x_1 - x_2)}$ and substitute the values of each point.

$m = \dfrac{2-(-2)}{6-3} = \dfrac{2+2}{3} = \dfrac{4}{3}$

3. $y < x - 1$

In this figure, the dashed line and shading below the line indicate a *less than* inequality. In addition, the line has slope of 1 and a y-intercept of -1.

4. 24,548.52 mm^2

This is a cylinder, so the surface area is $(2 \times \pi \times r^2) + (2 \times \pi \times r \times h)$.

SA $= (2 \times 3.14 \times 30^2) + (2 \times 3.14 \times 30 \times 100.3)$

SA $= 5,652 + 18,896.52$

SA $= 24,548.52$ mm^2

5. A

The volume of a rectangular solid is found by multiplying length × width × height. Therefore the volume is $60 \times 24 \times 6 = 8,640$ m^3.

Chapter 23: **Data and Statistics**

Data and statistics encompasses the topics of measures of central tendency such as mean, median, mode, and range, and different types and uses of statistical graphs. In addition, probability and the counting principle are discussed.

MEASURES OF CENTRAL TENDENCY

Measures of central tendency are values that are examined from a set of data in order to make predictions and draw conclusions about that set of data as a whole. Four of the most common measures that we use are mean, median, mode, and range.

Mean

The **mean** of a set of numbers is the sum of the numbers in the set divided by the total number of values in the set. For example, in order to find the mean of the set {8, 9, 22, 14, 12}, first find the sum by adding the numbers: 8 + 9 + 22 + 14 + 12 = 65. Since there are 5 numbers in the set, the mean can be found by dividing the sum of 65 by 5. The mean is 65 ÷ 5 = 13.

Median

The **median** of a set of data is the middle number when the values are listed in order from smallest to largest. In lists containing an odd number of values, one number will be located directly in the middle of the list. If there is an even amount of numbers in the list, two numbers will share the middle. In this case, find the average of those two values to find the median of the entire list.

For example, find the median of the following set of numbers {20, 65, 34, 21, 55, 89, 38, 41, 76}

First, list the numbers in order from smallest to greatest. 20, 21, 34, 38, 41, 55, 65, 76, 89

Since there are nine numbers in the list, the fifth number, 41, is in the middle. The number 41 is the median of the data set.

Mode

The **mode** of a set of data is the number that occurs the most in a data set. For example, find the mode in the data set {8, 9, 10, 4, 5, 8, 8}; the mode is 8. When there is not a number that occurs more than any other in the list, there is *no mode*. Sometimes there is more than one value that occurs as much as another number. If two numbers occur the same number of times and they occur more than any other number in the list, the set is considered to be *bimodal*, meaning there are two modes. It is also possible to have more than two modes in a set of data.

Range

The **range** of a set of numbers is the difference between the largest value in the list and the smallest value in the list. Take the following data set: 34, 54, 22, 84, 90, 55, 60, and 23. The range of this set would be 90 − 22 = 68, since 90 is the largest value in the set and 22 is the smallest.

STATISTICAL GRAPHS

Some of the most common statistical graphs are the bar graph, the line graph, the circle graph, the scatter plot, and the histogram.

Bar graphs are used to compare data. They can be drawn using horizontal bars or vertical bars. The following graph compares the price of a popular video game from four different stores.

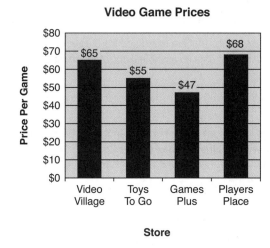

Video Game Prices

A line graph is used to show a trend that occurs over time. Take, for example, the following graph that shows stock prices for a certain company over one month.

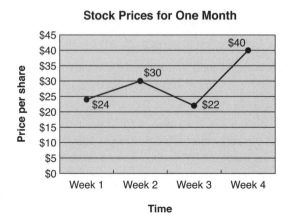

Stock Prices for One Month

A circle graph is used to show parts of whole. Percents are often used within a circle graph; always make sure that any percents used in a circle graph always add to 100%. The following graph shows the breakdown of the participation in extracurricular activities at a secondary school. Each student can be a member of only one club.

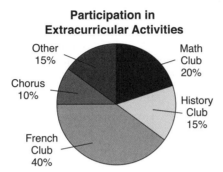

**Participation in
Extracurricular Activities**

Remember:

A **bar graph** is used to compare data.

A **line graph** is used to show trends over time.

A **circle graph** is used to show parts of a whole; the percents in a circle graph must add to 100%.

SCATTER PLOTS

Much like a line graph, a scatter plot is also used to show trends in data. In this type of graph, however, the data points are not connected. Instead, the general trend of the data points is examined. The more the data in the graph appears to form a straight line, the stronger the relationship is among the data in the graph. The following is an example of a scatter plot that shows the relationship between the number of assignments completed and the class average from a certain academic class.

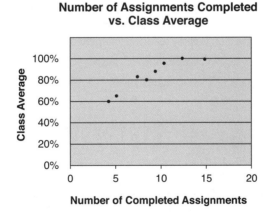

**Number of Assignments Completed
vs. Class Average**

Specific information about the data can be determined from the graph. For example, the greatest number of assignments completed is 15, and the person who completed 15 assignments has approximately a 98% class average.

In a scatter plot, there is usually one of three conclusions that can be made based on the graph. The first is a **positive trend**, or positive correlation: when the *x*-values increase there is also an increase in the *y*-values.

As shown in the given graph, the relationship between the number of assignments completed and the class average in this class is positive.

The second type of trend is a **negative trend**, or negative correlation: when there is a decrease in the *y*-values as the *x*-values increase. An example of a negative correlation might be the cost of a ticket for a show and the number of tickets sold. As the price increases, the number of tickets purchased may decrease.

A third possibility is that there is **no correlation**, or relationship, in the data graphed. The following figure shows what each type of correlation looks like on a graph.

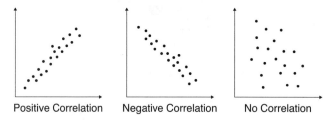

| Positive Correlation | Negative Correlation | No Correlation |

STEM AND LEAF PLOTS

Before constructing certain types of graphs, it is very useful to organize the data in a chart or table for easy reference. One way to organize a list of numbers is a stem and leaf plot. In the stem and leaf plot, there are typically two columns. The first column, known as the stem, often represents the first digit(s) in the number and the second column, known as the leaf, represents the last digit of the number. For example, if placing the number 29 in a stem and leaf plot, the 2 would appear in the stem and the 9 would appear in the leaf.

stem	leaf
2	9

When dealing with more than two digits, such as three-digit numbers, the first two digits would form the stem and the number in the ones place would be the leaf. In a stem and leaf plot, each of the stems is listed in ascending order so that the information is easily read and interpreted. The figure below shows a stem and leaf plot containing 10 data values.

stem	leaf
2	8, 9
3	4
4	1, 2, 9
5	0, 1, 1, 4

The numbers in the plot are 28, 29, 34, 41, 42, 49, 50, 51, 51, and 54. Notice a few things:

a. You can tell the total number of values in the list by counting the leaves. Here there are a total of 10 leaves.

b. You can tell if a number repeats because there will be a leaf with a number or numbers that repeat. The stem of 5 has a leaf of 1 that repeats, so the number 51 is in the data set twice.

c. You can also figure out measures such as mode, median, and range quickly since the numbers are in order. The mode is 51, the median is 45.5 and the range is $54 - 28 = 26$.

HISTOGRAMS

One type of graph where stem and leaf plots are particularly helpful is the histogram. Histograms appear to be much like bar graphs except for two major differences: the bars in the histogram represent number values or intervals of values, and the bars are touching each other.

Assume that the data in the given stem and leaf plot represented the attendance at various performances of a play. The following is an example of a histogram made from the data in this stem and leaf plot. Notice that since the data is already set up in intervals of 10, constructing the histogram is quick and easy.

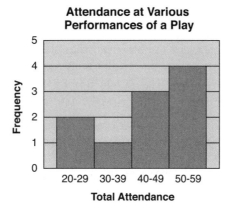

**Attendance at Various
Performances of a Play**

PROBABILITY

Simple Probability

Theoretical probability is the principle used when calculating the chance that these and other events could happen. The **probability** of an event (E) is defined as $P(E) = \dfrac{\text{the number of ways event E can occur}}{\text{the total number of possible outcomes}}$

The **outcome set**, also known as the **sample space**, is the list of all possible outcomes. For example, the outcome set when flipping a coin is {Heads, Tails} because these are the only possible outcomes. To calculate the probability that tails will be shown when flipping a coin, $P(\text{tails}) = \dfrac{1}{2}$ since there is 1 way to get tails out of 2 possible outcomes.

The probability of an event that can't happen, or an impossible event, is 0. The probability of an event that is certain to happen is 1. All other simple probabilities will be between 0 and 1.

Compound Probability

Compound probability occurs when a problem asks for the chance of more than one outcome to occur. The key word used in most compound probability questions is "or".

The formula for compound probability is **P(A or B) = P(A) + P(B) − P(A and B)**. **Mutually exclusive** events are situations that cannot occur at the same instance, so P(A and B) from the preceding formula will be 0.

Two examples of compound probability are finding the probability of getting a 3 or a 6 when rolling a die. In this example, the probability of rolling a 3 is $\dfrac{1}{6}$, the probability of rolling 6 is $\dfrac{1}{6}$, and the probability of rolling both a 3 *and* a 6 is $\frac{0}{6}$. Thus, the probability is P(3 or 6) = $\frac{1}{6} + \frac{1}{6} - \frac{0}{6} = \frac{2}{6} = \frac{1}{3}$.

Note that since the two events were mutually exclusive, the probability that *both* would happen was $\frac{0}{6}$ or 0.

Independent and Dependent Events

More complex situations occur in probability problems when more than one event is taking place at the same time, or when one is taking place right after another. In these circumstances, the probabilities of each event are multiplied together to get the final likelihood of occurrence.

Independent Events

Independent events are two or more events that will occur without the outcome of one affecting the outcome of any other. The probability of the second event will be the same regardless of the outcome of the first event. An example of two independent events is rolling a die and flipping a coin. No matter what was rolled on the die, the probability of getting heads or tails on the coin will always be the same.

Another example would be selecting a card from a deck, replacing the card, and then selecting the next card. In this case, the key word *replace* or the phrase *with replacement* would indicate that the events were independent. Since the first card would be replaced, there will always be 52 cards to choose from when selecting a card. The probabilities would be the same each time.

Dependent Events

Dependent events are situations where the outcome of the first event *does* affect the probability of the second event. These are often events presented much like the ones mentioned above, but there is *no replacement*.

THE COUNTING PRINCIPLE

Sometimes when there are many choices to select from, the number of possible choices can seem unlimited. However, when the number of choices in a situation is known, the actual number of possibilities can be calculated. For example, when ordering a sandwich at a deli you may have 3 different choices of condiments, 4 choices of bread, and 5 choices of meat, or main ingredient, for the sandwich. To find the total number of possible sandwich combinations, multiply the number of choices in each category together: 3 × 4 × 5 = 60 different sandwiches. Multiplying the number of choices together is a concept called the **counting principle**. This strategy is also used when solving the next two types of situations presented: permutations and combinations.

Permutations

A **permutation** of objects is the number of possible arrangements for that set of objects. With permutations, it is all about order. Every time the order changes, a new permutation of the objects is formed. If 6 different books are placed on a shelf, there are 6 choices for the first spot on the shelf, 5 choices for the second, 4 for the third, 3 for the fourth, 2 for the fifth, and only 1 book left for the sixth. Thus, the total number of arrangements for those 6 books can be represented by an operation that looks like this: 6! = 6 × 5 × 4 × 3 × 2 × 1 = 720. This is known as 6 *factorial*.

The **factorial** of a whole number is the product of that whole number and each of the natural numbers less than the number. It is written as $n! = n \times (n-1) \times (n-2) \times \ldots \times 1$. In other words, the number of permutations of *n* objects taken *n* at a time is $_nP_n = n!$.

However, sometimes not all of the objects are considered for each different arrangement. In this case, n represents the total number of objects available to choose from and r is the number of objects actually selected to be arranged. The formula for the permutation of n objects taken r at a time is $_nP_r = \dfrac{n!}{(n-r)!}$.

Combinations

With combinations, the order is not important. The grouping of objects changes the number of combinations that exist. A **combination** is the total number of groupings of a set of objects. The formula for the number of combinations of n objects taken r at a time is $_nC_r = \dfrac{n!}{r!(n-r)!}$

Note that $_nC_n$ will always be equal to 1. There is only one way to select *all* the members of a group or committee.

Now that you have reviewed the essentials of data and statistics, test your knowledge by completing these practice questions.

REVIEW QUESTIONS

1. Given the following set of data, which of the following statements is NOT true?

   $\{2, 5, 6, 8, 10, 12, 20\}$

   (A) The mode is 8.
   (B) The range is greater than the median.
   (C) The median is 8.
   (D) The mean is 9.
   (E) The mean is less than range.

2. The following graph shows the weekly pizza sales at a pizzeria for four different kinds of pizza. If a total of 200 pizzas were sold, how many more pepperoni pizzas were sold than mushroom pizzas?

Weekly Pizza Sales

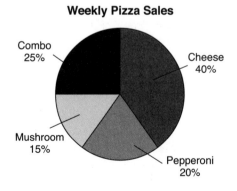

   (A) 100
   (B) 70
   (C) 40
   (D) 30
   (E) 10

3. According to the histogram below, what interval is the mode of the set of grades? _____

Frequency of Grades on a Science Test

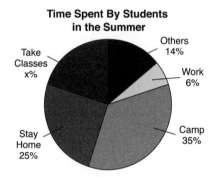

Intervals of Grades

4. The following circle graph shows the breakdown of summer activities of certain students.

Time Spent By Students in the Summer

Others 14%
Take Classes x%
Work 6%
Camp 35%
Stay Home 25%

According to the graph, what percent of students attended classes during the summer?

(A) 1%

(B) 10%

(C) 15%

(D) 20%

(E) 25%

5. When selecting a card from a standard deck, what is the probability of selecting a king or a red card?

(A) $\frac{26}{52}$

(B) $\frac{28}{52}$

(C) $\frac{30}{52}$

(D) $\frac{32}{52}$

(E) $\frac{34}{52}$

6. A bag contains 6 red, 4 blue, 10 orange, and 3 yellow candies. What is P(red or yellow)?

    (A) $\dfrac{3}{23}$

    (B) $\dfrac{23}{23}$

    (C) $\dfrac{10}{23}$

    (D) $\dfrac{9}{23}$

    (E) $\dfrac{9}{46}$

7. Find $_4P_4$.

8. At an ice cream shop, Kerensa can choose from 8 different flavours of ice cream, 3 different toppings, and 2 types of cones. If she selects 1 flavour of ice cream, one topping, and one type of cone, how many different combinations can she make?

    (A) 12

    (B) 13

    (C) 24

    (D) 36

    (E) 48

Answers and Explanations

1. A

To solve this question, it may be helpful to find a few of the measures mentioned in the answer choices. Starting with choice (A): The mode is the number that appears most often, and in this list there is no mode, making (A) false and the correct answer. Since the numbers are already listed in ascending order, the median is 8, making choice (C) true. The range is the smallest value subtracted from the largest value: $20 - 2 = 18$. Since 18 is greater than 8, the range is greater than the median and answer choice (B) is true. The sum of the list of numbers is 63; $63 \div 7 = 9$, so the mean is 9, making answer choice (D) true. Since 9 is less than 18, then answer choice (E) is also true because the mean is less than the range.

2. E

To find the number of pepperoni pizzas, find 20% of 200. Set up the proportion $\dfrac{20}{100} = \dfrac{x}{200}$. Cross-multiply to get $4,000 = 100x$; divide each side of this equation by 100 to get 40. To find the number of mushroom pizzas, find 15% of 200 using the same procedure. Set up the proportion $\dfrac{15}{100} = \dfrac{x}{200}$, cross-multiply to get $3,000 = 100x$, then divide to get $x = 30$. Since $40 - 30 = 10$, there were 10 more pepperoni pizzas sold than mushroom pizzas. Another approach to this question is to subtract the percents first; $20 - 15 = 5\%$. Then find 5% of 200. This number will be the difference in the number of pizzas. Set up the proportion

$\dfrac{5}{100} = \dfrac{x}{200}$, cross-multiply to get $1{,}000 = 100x$, and divide to get $x = 10$.

3. 91 – 100

Because the tallest bar is the interval 91 – 100, then the most grades occur in that interval.

4. D

Since the percents in a circle graph need to add to 100%, add the known percents and subtract that sum from 100: $14\% + 6\% + 35\% + 25\% = 80\%$; $100\% - 80\% = 20\%$.

5. B

The probability of a compound event is $P(A \text{ or } B) = P(A) + P(B) - P(A \text{ and } B)$. The probability of selecting a king from a standard deck of 52 cards is $P(\text{king}) = \dfrac{4}{52}$. The probability of selecting a red card is $P(\text{red card}) = \dfrac{26}{52}$. Since there are 2 kings that are also red, the $P(\text{king and a red card}) = \dfrac{2}{52}$. The equation becomes $P(\text{king or red card}) = \dfrac{4}{52} + \dfrac{26}{52} - \dfrac{2}{52} = \dfrac{28}{52}$.

6 D

There are a total of 23 candies in the bag. Because there are 6 red and 3 yellow, the probability of $P(\text{red or yellow})$ is $\dfrac{6}{23} + \dfrac{3}{23} = \dfrac{9}{23}$.

7. 24

$_4P_4 = 4 \times 3 \times 2 \times 1 = 24$.

8. E

Use the counting principle to multiply the total number of choices together: $8 \times 3 \times 2 = 48$ different combinations.

PART VIII

How to Approach the Writing Task

The BMAT Writing Task

The final section of the BMAT is the Writing Task. You'll be presented with three prompts and have 30 minutes to write a coherent essay in response to **one** of those prompts.

Writing under time pressure is probably not one of your favourite things and the Writing Task may well be the part of the BMAT you're least looking forward to. But fear not! We have a chapter full of tips and strategies that will prepare you for the Writing Task and help you write your best on test day.

THE WRITING PROMPTS

On essay exams, some students like being told what to write about; others want the freedom to choose their topic. The BMAT offers a fair compromise—you have three possible topics to choose from. All three prompts will consist of two parts: a **proposition** and **questions** about that proposition.

Proposition: This will be a brief statement, most likely a quotation, most likely controversial, definitely debatable. The topic will be of general, medical, or scientific interest. In other words, it will be a proposition anyone should be able to respond to—you won't need any specialised knowledge to write an intelligent response.

Questions: The proposition will be followed by a series of questions to guide your response. The questions will ask you to:

- explain the proposition
- offer an alternative to the proposition
- suggest a way to synthesise or reconcile the differing positions or points of view

Here's a sample prompt:

Art is I; science is we.
(Claude Bernard)
Explain what you believe the author means by this statement. Are there any ways in which art can be a communal act and science an individual act? How might we reconcile this apparent difference between these two disciplines?

HOW YOUR ESSAY IS SCORED

Your essay will be marked by two readers, each of whom will give your response a score between 0–15 on a 3-point scale (0, 3, 6, 9, 12, 15). Scores are based on a holistic reading that takes into consideration the *overall effectiveness* of your response. That means a few minor errors aren't likely to relegate an otherwise powerful essay to a single-digit score. Style, substance and correctness all count.

If your two readers give your essay the same mark, that's the score you'll receive. If the two marks are different but adjacent on the scale (e.g., 9 and 12), those two marks are averaged for your score (10.5). On the rare occasion that there is a larger discrepancy in the two marks, a third reader will mark the essay and the final score will be checked by the Writing Task Assessment Manager.

Scoring Scale

0: Trivial, irrelevant, or absent response.

3: Answer has some relevance to the prompt but does not respond appropriately or fully to the questions asked. Essay lacks organisation and focus and/or has serious errors that render much of it incoherent or confusing.

6: Essay fulfills most of the task but may misinterpret an important aspect of the proposition, fail to consider one or more of its main implications, and/or fail to present a strong alternative position. Organisation is reasonably logical but may have some weaknesses, and there may be many errors in grammar or mechanics.

9: Essay addresses all aspects of the prompt, presenting both a reasonable argument and counter-argument. Argument is rational, though it may lack sophistication and scope. There may be some weaknesses in style, grammar or mechanics, but the writing is reasonably clear and effective.

12: A good essay with few of the weaknesses of a score 9 response. All aspects of the prompt are addressed, organisation is strong, and writer shows a strong sense of reader awareness. A few minor grammar or mechanical errors may be present.

15: An excellent response with virtually no weaknesses. The writing is superior—clear and compelling with effective organisation and an argument that is sophisticated and firmly grounded in unassailable logic. Style is sophisticated and engaging throughout.

Remember that the BMAT is designed to be difficult, and an essay scoring a 15 is a rarity. Most essays fall in the middle score ranges (6–9); the mode (most common) score on the 2004 BMAT was 7.5. That doesn't mean that you shouldn't aim for a 15; it simply means that the standards are very high, and a 9 is still a strong score.

What Readers Are Looking For

How exactly do readers arrive at these scores? Here are the six things readers will be looking for as they read your essay.

1. Response to the assignment. A strong essay completely fulfills the assignment, addressing each task in the prompt. It should include:

   - a thoughtful analysis of the proposition—its meaning and implications
   - consideration of counter-arguments—how and why one might disagree with the proposition or offer an alternative view
   - suggested means of assessing the merits of each point of view or resolving the conflicting positions

2. Support. A strong essay provides specific examples and evidence and uses general knowledge and opinions effectively and appropriately.

3. Organisation. A strong essay divides ideas into coherent paragraphs and arranges paragraphs in a logical and effective order.

4. Style. A strong essay has a compelling style with variety and sophistication in vocabulary and sentence structure.

5. Clarity. A strong essay expresses ideas in a clear and straightforward manner.

6. Correctness. A strong essay follows the conventions of written English for grammar, spelling and punctuation.

FIVE STEPS TO A STRONG BMAT ESSAY

1. Identify the task
2. Brainstorm
3. Create an Outline
4. Write
5. Review

Step 1: Identify the Task

As soon as you are allowed to turn to the prompt page, read each prompt and quickly decide which one you'll use. Go with your gut instinct—which prompt immediately intrigues you? (Do *not* spend too much time choosing the prompt! You must get started and keep moving.)

Once you've picked your prompt, pick it apart. Read it carefully to identify each of the specific tasks you need to complete in your essay.

Step 2: Brainstorm

Draft a short response to each of the tasks in the prompt. Generally this is as simple as answering the questions or responding to each statement in the prompt. But don't rely on simple answers; the propositions are chosen because they present complex issues requiring complex thought, not just a simple yes/no response.

Brainstorm *on paper* so you can see your ideas in front of you and work out the best way of expressing them. For each main idea, think of at least two supporting ideas. Remember that you are *brainstorming*—coming up with ideas—so write down every thought that comes to mind. You can always cross it out in the next step if it doesn't really belong or offer strong support.

Make sure you've addressed every part of the prompt before you move on.

Step 3: Create an Outline

Decide how best to present your ideas in about four or five paragraphs. Note the main idea of each paragraph and where you'll include specific examples. *Do not write out the essay yet*—just outline.

Remember that *you only have **one** page on which to write your response.* Four or five solid paragraphs will easily fill that space (besides, you won't really have time to write much more). If you find you're outlining six or seven paragraphs, take a good look at your notes. Which ideas are the *most* important or *most* relevant? Save the less powerful or relevant ideas for another essay.

Before you begin to write, make sure your outline is logical. Once you've written the essay, you won't be able to go back and switch paragraphs or move ideas around. So check that you've organised your ideas effectively. And check for unity and development. Do any paragraphs contain too many ideas? Do any need more support? Adjust your outline accordingly before you begin to write.

Step 4: Write

Now it's time to put your ideas together in a coherent essay. Follow your outline. Write with clarity as your main goal; don't worry about trying to sound sophisticated. Simple = clear, and clarity is essential. So is neatness. Like it or not, this is a handwritten test—so your handwriting *must be legible*.

Before you begin writing, take a moment (but just a moment!) to think about how you'll introduce your essay. Getting started is often the most difficult part for writers, especially when they're under time pressure. Remember that you can always begin with a paraphrase or explanation of the proposition. However, if you can think of an introduction that will capture the reader's attention, that's even better. Think about how many essays the UCLES readers will review—a catchy introduction will help yours stand out from the masses. But don't get hung up trying to think of a great opener! A catchy introduction will do little to help your score if you don't have time to finish your essay.

Now, the question you've been waiting for: how much should you write? Your response must fit on the single answer sheet provided. But depending upon your script size, you could fill that page with 50 words or 500.

Obviously it would be difficult to complete the tasks in the prompt in 50 words. About 350-400, though, is a good number to have in mind. That should get you about four or five solid paragraphs that address all aspects of the prompt and keep you within the confines of a single page.

SPACE IS LIMITED!

Your entire essay must fit on one lined sheet of paper, so you need to be extra sure to organise your ideas effectively and only include what is directly relevant to your topic. Part of what readers are looking for is your ability to be clear and concise even in a pressure situation.

Having to fit everything on one page also means you must write neatly and in a relatively small script. If you tend to write sloppily (especially when you hurry) or write in a large hand, practise writing under timed conditions to improve your script size and legibility.

Step 5: Review

If you've paced yourself effectively, you should have a few minutes left to review what you've written and make some corrections and improvements. Read what you've written with an eye for "quick fixes"—simple steps that can significantly improve your score (see below).

TIME MANAGEMENT

On a timed writing exam, the general rule of thumb is to divide your time as follows:

- ¼ time planning
- ½ time writing
- ¼ time revising/editing

On the BMAT, however, we like to place extra emphasis on the planning stage so there will be less need for revising and editing. Here's what that means for you:

- Step 1: 1 minute
- Step 2: 3–4 minutes
- Step 3: 4–5 minutes
- Step 4: 15–20 minutes
- Step 5: 5–7 minutes

Remember that these time allotments are suggested and approximate. If you are particularly good at brainstorming and planning, for example, you may move through Steps 1–3 more quickly and have more time to write and revise.

Revising: Five Quick Fixes

Revising differs from proofreading or editing in that it involves the "big picture"—matters of structure and style rather than grammar or mechanics. Here are five quick big picture fixes you can make in the few minutes before time is called.

1. **Add an example or specific detail**. Are any of your paragraphs underdeveloped? Is one much shorter than the others? Balance it out by adding another example. Use a caret [^] to insert text above a sentence or add your example in the margin if necessary.

2. **Add transitions**. Do you have smooth transitions between paragraphs? Within paragraphs? Make sure your ideas are logically connected with transitions that show the relationship between ideas.

3. **Eliminate tangents.** Did you include anything that is irrelevant or inappropriate? Cross out or erase that idea or find a way to make it relevant.

4. **Eliminate wordiness**. Show readers that you value their time and that you know the elements of effective style by eliminating unnecessary wordiness or repetition.

   Wordy: Because of the fact that you can only write on one page, it is important and essential to organize your ideas carefully. (22 words)

   Concise: Because you can only write on one page, it is essential to organise your ideas carefully. (16 words)

MOST UNWANTED: TOP WORDINESS OFFENDERS

Here's a list of some of the most common wordy constructions and their concise counterparts:

Wordy	Concise	Wordy	Concise
in the event that	if	for the purpose of	for
in spite of the fact that	although	due to the fact that	because
because of the fact that	because	for the reason that	because
at that point in time	then	at this point in time	now
at the present time	now	has the appearance of	looks like, seems like
in the proximity of	near	until such time as	until
in the neighbourhood of	about		

5. **Improve vocabulary**. Change an ordinary word to one that is more compelling or sophisticated, or find a synonym for a word that you repeat several times in the text. (But be careful not to go overboard; being pretentious is *worse* than being unsophisticated.) Eliminate any slang or overly casual language as well; this is a formal essay.

Unsophisticated: We have to take real steps to slow down global warming, or else our planet may be in big trouble.

Sophisticated: We must implement effective measures to curb global warming; otherwise, our planet may be headed for disaster.

Repetitive: Without a doubt, a good "bedside manner" is as important a factor as clinical knowledge and experience. In fact, it may even be the most important factor. There's nothing more important in human relationships than compassion.

Varied: Without a doubt, a good "bedside manner" is as essential a factor as clinical knowledge and experience. In fact, it may even be the most significant quality. There's nothing more important in human relationships than compassion.

Can't remember the rules for comma use? Notorious for writing fragments or run-ons? Tend to write long-winded and repetitive sentences? Then spend a few weeks with Kaplan's *Grammar Source: The Smarter Way to Learn Grammar*. We'll highlight relevant chapters in the rest of this section.

Proofreading: Five More Quick Fixes

This isn't the place for an exhaustive grammar review, but it is a good place to remind you of some of the most common grammar mistakes in student writing. Keep an eye out for these errors as you review.

1. **Correct run-on sentences.** Probably the most common error in student writing is the run-on sentence: two or more complete thoughts without proper punctuation or conjunctions between them. Remember, we separate ideas in sentences so that they're easily distinguished from one another. With run-ons, ideas are easily tangled and confused. (See Kaplan's *Grammar Source* Chapter 8.)

   Run-on: Sentences need boundaries they should not just run together.

   Correct: Sentences need boundaries; they should not just run together.

   Correct: Sentences need boundaries. They should not just run together.

   Run-on: Run-ons are very common however they are also easy to fix.

   Correct: Run-ons are very common; however, they are also easy to fix.

2. **Correct fragments.** Fragments are incomplete sentences. Correct them by adding the missing subject or verb or connecting them to other sentences. (See Kaplan's *Grammar Source* Chapter 8.)

   Fragment: Don't leave a fragment standing alone. When it should be part of another sentence.

   Correct: Don't leave a fragment standing alone when it should be part of another sentence.

   Fragment: Fragments can be fixed in many ways. Such as combining sentences. Or adding a missing subject or verb.

   Correct: Fragments can be fixed in many ways, such as combining sentences or adding a missing subject or verb.

3. **Correct errors in agreement.** Subjects and verbs must agree in number and person. A first-person plural subject (*we*) needs a first-person plural verb (*digress*). Likewise, pronouns must agree in number and person with their antecedents (the words they replace). (See *Grammar Source* Chapter 5.)

   Incorrect: Audrey, like many students, are more comfortable composing on a keyboard than with pen and paper.

   Correct: Audrey, like many students, is more comfortable composing on a keyboard than with pen and paper.

   Incorrect: Someone left their wallet on the counter.

   Correct: Someone left his or her wallet on the counter. *or* Someone's wallet has been left on the counter. (to avoid the bulky his/her construction)

4. **Correct shifts in tense or person.** Verb tenses and pronouns should be consistent. For example, if you're describing an event that took place last month, all of the verbs describing that event should be in the past tense. (It's easy to get caught up in narrating and shift into the present.) Similarly, if you start using the third person (*he, she, it, they*), don't suddenly switch to the second *you*. Be consistent. (See *Grammar Source* Chapters 3 and 6.)

   Tense shift: I didn't know what to do. Then I realised I have only one real option, and I will go and tell Hani the truth.

   Correct: I didn't know what to do. Then I realised I had only one real option, and I would go and tell Hani the truth.

   Pronoun shift: Students should make sure they write legibly. You want your readers to understand your essay.

   Correct: You should make sure you write legibly. You want your readers to understand your essay.

5. **Correct spelling errors.** Because you're in a hurry, you're liable to make more spelling mistakes than usual. Pay particular attention to homophone and contraction errors such as *there* when you mean *they're* or *cite* when you mean *site*. (See *Grammar Source* Chapter 18.)

SAMPLE ESSAY

Now here's a sample essay from start to finish using the five steps we've outlined above.

Step 1: Identify the Task

Art is I; science is we.
(Claude Bernard)

Explain what you believe the author means by this statement. Are there any ways in which art can be a communal act and science an individual act? How might we reconcile this apparent difference between these two disciplines?

1. explain proposition
2. give examples of communal art and individual science
3. show how to reconcile individual/community, art/sci

Step 2: Brainstorm

Notice that the writing in this brainstorm is not always coherent or polished, and that's quite all right. The key is to get ideas down on paper. You can write in sentences or lists, whatever works best for you.

Prop means a work of art is individual expression, one person's vision while science is people working together for a common vision or goal. Also art interpreted individually (we all experience art indiv) and scientific findings are facts shared by everyone in the same way.

Art can be communal—working together on a mural for ex. or experiencing art together (motion picture or play). In research, questions and goals individual, personal interests and reasons for pursuing XYZ.

Artists and scientists more alike—both often do much work in isolation but get feedback and affirmation from others, community of critics and work must past muster.

Both begin with the vision of the "I" and end with the gift to the "we". In art, however, goal is expression of idea, not proof of idea, so results are unique; in science, results have to be duplicatable and impersonal.

Step 3: Outline

P1: explain proposition

    A.   how art is individual (personal vision, individual interpretation)

    B.   how science is communal (shared vision, shared interpretation)

P2: art can be "we" too

    A.   creating art together (motion picture, murals)

    B.   experiencing art together (plays, museums)

P3: science can be personal

    A.   individual research

    B.   individual inspiration and vision

P4: different goals, same goals

    A.   art's goal is expression of emotional truths

    B.   science's goal discovery of physical truths

    C.   both aim to expand understanding

P5: artists and scientists therefore more alike—both "I" and both "we"

Step 4: Write

Claude Bernard has it right when he says "Art is I; science is we". But only half right. Art is a very individual pursuit. Each artist has their personal vision that they want to convey through their art and they typically work alone to create their art. Although art is viewed by the public, each persons interpretation is unique. So the creation and the interpretation of art are both the experience of the "I". Science, on the other hand, is a more communal pursuit. Typically a community of scientists work on similar questions and seek similar answers. When those answers are found, they are presented to the community, which interprets those answers in much the same way. Scientists, after all, present facts, while artists present vision.

But of course it's not so simple. Because art can also be a communal experience. Throughout history artists have worked together to create great works of art. A motion picture, for example, requires the cooperation and input of many artists. A dozen artists may work together to create a mural or mosaic. Viewing or experiencing art can be a communal process. Whether we come away from a work of art with different opinions or not, we can experience it together. Whether it be a motion picture, a play, or a trip to the museum.

Science can be "I" as well as "we". Many scientists spend a lifetime pursuing individual research questions. They have their own individual inspiration and vision. Many scientists also have their own individual interpretations of theories and facts before them.

While on the surface it seems that artists and scientists have different goals, in reality, they are much the same. Both art and science aim to discover and express truths: truths about human nature (art) and truths about the natural world (science). Both aim to expand our understanding of ourselves and our world.

So to say "art is I; science is we" is only partly right. Science is also personal, art is also communal. Both begin with the vision and passion of the "I" and end with a gift to the "we".

Step 5: Revise

Claude Bernard has it right when he says "Art is I; science is we"—but only half right. Art is a very individual pursuit. Artists have their personal vision that they want to convey through their art, and similarly, they typically work alone to create their art. Although art is viewed by the public, each person's interpretation is unique. So the creation and the interpretation of art are both the experience of the "I". Science, on the other hand, is a more communal pursuit. Typically a community of scientists work on similar questions and seek similar answers. When those answers are found, they are presented to the community, which interprets those answers in much the same way. Scientists, after all, present facts, while artists present vision.

But of course it's not so simple, because art can also be a communal experience. Throughout history artists have worked together to create great works of art. A motion picture, for example, requires the cooperation and input of many artists from the screenwriter to actors to the director and cinematographer. A dozen artists may work together to create a mural or mosaic. Viewing or experiencing art can also be a communal process. Whether we come away from a work of art with different opinions or not, we can still experience it together, whether it be a motion picture, a play, or a trip to the museum.

Likewise, science can be "I" as well as "we". Many scientists spend a lifetime pursuing individual research questions. They have their own individual inspiration and vision. Many scientists also have their own personal interpretations of theories and facts before them.

Thus, while on the surface it seems that artists and scientists have different goals, in reality, they are much the same. Both art and science aim to discover and express truths: truths about human nature (art) and truths about the natural world (science). Both aim to expand our understanding of ourselves and our world.

Therefore, to say "Art is I; science is we" is only partly right. Science is also personal, art is also communal. Both begin with the vision and passion of the "I" and end with a gift to the "we".

This essay now has the marks of a 15 score. It fulfills each task in the prompt in an insightful manner. The writing flows smoothly, and the argument is logical and supported with specific examples. The style is engaging and occasionally sophisticated, and the essay is error-free.

Writing Task Practice Sets

To help you practise for the BMAT Writing Task, we present two complete model writing tasks. Do as many of the prompts as you can—all six if you know timed writing is not one of your strengths. The more you practise, the more quickly ideas will come and the more effective your writing will be on test day.

For each practice essay, set a timer for 30 minutes and have a piece of scrap paper ready for your brainstorming and outline. Use only **one** sheet of lined paper for your answer. Follow the Kaplan five-step Writing Task plan and write well. Stop when time is up, whether you've finished or not. If you weren't able to complete your essay, evaluate your performance. What kept you from finishing? Identify the hold-up(s) and work to eliminate them the next time.

After each essay, carefully evaluate your work. Compare it to the BMAT Writing Task scale and the list of what essay readers are looking for on page 390. How would you rate your performance? Why? What strengths and weaknesses can you identify? Feel good about your strengths; develop a plan to address your weaknesses.

Ask others to criticise your essay, too. If possible, have an instructor or tutor mark your essay.

Don't forget to check for legibility. Your hard work will be for nothing if readers can't read what you've written.

At the end of the chapter, we provide sample score 6, 9 and 12 essays for one topic from each practice Writing Task to help you better judge your score.

Writing Task Practice Set I

Below are three writing tasks. Choose only **one** and write your response on the single page answer sheet provided. You may make any preliminary notes on the back of this page or a separate sheet of paper. You have 30 minutes to choose your tasks and complete your essay.

The tasks give you the chance to demonstrate how well you can select, develop and organise ideas and how effectively you can communicate them in writing. Before you begin, think carefully about what you want to say in response to the prompt. Consider how you will organise your response to most effectively convey your message. You may use diagrams or other graphic forms if they enhance the communication of your ideas.

Use this opportunity to demonstrate how well you can write. Your essay must be confined to the single answer sheet, so be clear and concise. Be sure to write legibly.

You may **not** use a dictionary or thesaurus.

There will always be another reality to make fiction of the truth we think we've arrived at.
(Christopher Fry)

What do you understand the above statement to mean? How does this idea contrast with the notion that science uncovers truths about the natural world? What are the implications of this statement for scientists?

It is not every question that deserves an answer.
(Publilius Syrus)

What does the author mean by the above statement? Can you give examples of questions that some may believe do not deserve to be answered but that you believe should? What criteria would you use to determine which questions should be answered?

While becoming nuclear giants, we have remained ethical infants.
(Clifford McEntarfer)

What do you understand by the statement above? Can you provide examples of ways that we have grown morally as we have progressed scientifically? What are the implications of a lack of ethics in the nuclear age?

Writing Task Practice Set II

Below are three writing tasks. Choose only **one** and write your response on the single page answer sheet provided. You may make any preliminary notes on the back of this page or a separate sheet of paper. You have 30 minutes to choose your tasks and complete your essay.

The tasks give you the chance to demonstrate how well you can select, develop and organise ideas and how effectively you can communicate them in writing. Before you begin, think carefully about what you want to say in response to the prompt. Consider how you will organise your response to most effectively convey your message. You may use diagrams or other graphic forms if they enhance the communication of your ideas.

Use this opportunity to demonstrate how well you can write. Your essay must be confined to the single answer sheet, so be clear and concise. Be sure to write legibly.

You may **not** use a dictionary or thesaurus.

The only possible interpretation of any research whatever in the 'social sciences' is: some do, some don't.
(Ernest Rutherford)

What does the above statement imply? Advance an argument against the statement above, i.e., in support of the argument that research in the social sciences offers real, tangible results. What can we realistically hope to learn from research in the social sciences?

While the State exists, there can be no freedom. When there is freedom there will be no State.
(Lenin)

What do you think the author means by the statement above? Can you think of examples of freedom within the confines of the State (government)? Can freedom and government co-exist? How might you reconcile this apparent contradiction?

The price of progress is trouble.
(Charles F. Kettering)

What do you believe the author means by this statement? Are there situations in which you believe progress is worth that price, and others in which it is not? What criteria do you use to make the distinction?

Answers

The following sample score 6, 9 and 12 essays are in response to the following prompt from Writing Task Practice I:

> It is not every question that deserves an answer.
> (Publilius Syrus)
>
> What does the author mean by the above statement? Can you give examples of questions that some may believe do not deserve to be answered but that you believe should? What criteria would you use to determine which questions should be answered?

Sample Score 6

Publilius Syrus said "It's not every question that deserves an answer". I agree. There are some things we just shouldn't ask about.

For example, some questions don't deserve to be answered because they're rude or ignorant. For example, if you ask me the same question 10 times, I don't need to answer it 10 times. Or if it's a question about none of your business, something personal, you shouldn't ask and I don't need to answer you. It's none of your business. We need to respect the privacy of others.

If you have any questions about your health, they deserve to be answered. Your doctor should always be truthful and tell you the truth about as much as he knows. Questions about feelings do not always deserve to be answered because you may want to share those feelings.

In conclusion, not all questions deserve answers. Ask smart questions with answers that matter.

Comments:

This response fulfills most of the task but in a rather simplistic way that is short on scope; it doesn't go beyond the personal. The ideas and language are somewhat repetitive and there are several significant errors. It is also very underdeveloped, and notice the tangent ("We need to respect the privacy of others").

Sample Score 9

Publilius Syrus said "It is not every question that deserves an answer". In other words, their are some questions we should not ask. Sometimes we shouldn't ask as a matter of decency, other times we shouldn't ask because we don't deserve an answer, that is, we're not able to handle it.

For example, as a matter of privacy. There are some things you can ask me that I don't need to tell you. Your questions about my personal life are not questions that deserve to be answered unless you are a close friend. The person being asked needs to decide on a case by case basis whether the person asking deserves an answer.

Scientists and philosophers sometimes want answers to questions that some people don't think should be answered. These are the big questions, such as, What is the meaning of life. What is the secret of life? Is another, and this is one that is really debatable. Is this something we deserve to know? What happens if we find the answer? Who will control the secret of life? What will we do with that knowledge? Because knowledge, after all, is power. Therefore, that's another reason some questions should not be answered.

Comments:

This essay offers a reasonable argument and counter-argument but lacks sophistication in development of ideas and in style. Ideas come across clearly but there are errors in grammar and mechanics.

Sample Score 12

A wise man once said, "There's no such thing as a stupid question". But does that mean that all questions, no matter how stupid, deserve to be answered? No. I agree with Publilius Syrus that not every question deserves an answer. As much as I value curiosity, and as much as I believe in questioning the world around me, there are some lines that should not be crossed.

On a practical or every day level, what Syrus probably meant was that there are some questions that are simply nobody's business. For example, if a complete stranger asks me a question about my personal life. That question doesn't deserve an answer; he doesn't have a right to know. Similarly, if a classmate asks me the answer to a question in an exam, that doesn't deserve an answer, either. That's cheating.

But thinking about bigger things, like the meaning of life, here are questions where we can debate endlessly about whether or not we should be seeking an answer. The question is really, Do we deserve to know those answers? I think of Dr. Frankenstein as an example. He relentlessly pursued the secret of life, and found it, then he created a deadly monster. He asked a question that should not be answered, because he could not handle it. I do not think human beings are capable yet of knowing the answers to fundamental questions about our life and existence, because we don't know what to do with the power that would then be granted to us.

Imagine if someone really did discover the secret of life. What would we do with that knowledge? I think humans are still too ethically challenged to handle the answer.

Comments:

This essay is fully developed and effectively organised. The writing is much stronger than the 9 essay and there are fewer errors, none of which interfere with comprehension. The argument is convincing and interesting and includes specific examples, though it is a little repetitive toward the end. It needs a bit more exploration of key points and elimination of the remaining errors to be a 15 essay.

The following sample score 6, 9 and 12 essays are in response to the following prompt from Writing Task Practice II:

The only possible interpretation of any research whatever in the 'social sciences' is: some do, some don't.
(Ernest Rutherford)

What does the above statement imply? Advance an argument against the statement above, e.g., in support of the argument that research in the social sciences offers real, tangible results. What can we realistically hope to learn from research in the social sciences?

Score 6

The social sciences are sometimes called "soft" sciences unlike the "hard" sciences because they don't have "hard" results like real numbers and laws that we always follow. Ernest Rutherford doesn't think the social sciences are worth much, he seems to really think we don't have anything to learn from social sciences, the research tells us some people do some things, others don't do those things.

I like the hard sciences better too but I don't think he should down the social sciences this way, they have more to offer than that. There are some things we can learn, like what people will usually do, even if they don't do it all the time. That can be helpful in some way. We can sometimes be surprised to learn how people behave.

Maybe better experiments can be designed to really look at why people do what they do. I think in the future we'll see more experiments that are both hard and soft sciences like looking at brain chemistry combined with behaviour.

Comments:

The essay attempts to tackle the issues in the prompt but is significantly underdeveloped and sticks to a simplistic view. Notice that there is a lack of specific examples and a number of errors, particularly run-on sentences. The writing is clear, but it lacks sophistication and style.

Score 9

Ernest Rutherford doesn't seem to think much of the social sciences. He even puts the words in quotes, like it's not a real science. On one level, he's right. The social sciences aren't like physics because you don't have experiments that you can do with precise measuring instruments. Its about studying human behaviour which is more variable and unpredictable than the weather. But we can still learn alot from social science experiments.

For example, put ten hungry people in a room with nine sandwiches. If you do this experiment over and over, your going to see some patterns. Like women will be more likely to share there food or men will take food first. Or you can watch how people behave in public places and notice patterns there, too. Then you can ask questions about why people behave that way and design new experiments to dig deeper into that behaviour.

Some of this will translate into useful knowledge and applications, some won't, the point is there is more to social science research then the binary do or don't. Humans are not perfect and any science of human behaviour isn't going to be perfect either, but it's definitely better than nothing.

Comments:

This response is clear and assertive in its answers to the questions in the prompt. It is more developed and sophisticated than the score 6 essay with specific examples and more complex sentences and vocabulary. However, it could still use improvement in all the major areas, including correctness.

Score 12

Humans are not atoms, and we can't expect them to behave according to specific laws and patterns. Or can we? Research in the social sciences can give us far more insight into human behaviour than Ernest Rutherford allows. He seems to believe that the only thing we can get out of social science research is the fact that some people will do X (whatever is under observation) and some people won't. But a well-designed experiment can show us *why* some people do and others don't. It can also show us patterns of behaviour that we can use to better understand human behaviour.

It is true that humans are highly unpredictable creatures, and we will behave different according to different circumstances. That's why we can't establish true "laws" about human behaviour like we can about elements in the natural world. Additionally that's why it's hard to do experiments that are repeatable and will give us the same results over and over.

Still by observing human behaviour we can begin to understand why people do what they do. For example, let's set up an experiment where we tell people we have two new soft drinks, please try and see which one you like best. We fill both glasses with the same drink but make one glass more full than the other. Let's say more people choose the drink in the glass that's more full, they think it actually tastes better. Then we can conclude that people feel more positively about something when there is more of it.

That may not be an earth-shattering revolution but it does make the point, that we can learn about human behaviour, much more than "do" or "don't". Experiments like this offer starting points for new research. Why do we think the fuller glass tastes better? The social sciences are still young and there is much to learn about our behaviour.

Comments:

The essay is very solid and does a good job addressing the tasks laid out in the prompt. It is more sophisticated and developed than the score 9 essay with fewer errors and more eloquent prose. With a few minor corrections and a little more development (e.g., going farther with examples or exploring implications further), it would be a score 15 essay.

PART IX

Practice Test

Practice Test

SECTION 1: APTITUDE AND SKILLS

Time: 1 hour

Directions: Answer every question. Points are assigned for correct answers only. There are no penalties for incorrect answers.

All questions are worth 1 mark.

Indicate your answers in pencil on the answer sheet provided for this section. For multiple-choice questions, fill in the bubble(s) completely. For short-answer questions, write clearly and neatly in the space provided. If you make a mistake, erase it as completely as possible. Calculators are not permitted during any portion of the test.

1. The number of butterflies in Gloria's garden varies directly with the number of flowers that are in bloom. On Monday, when 50 flowers were in bloom, 10 butterflies visited the garden. By Friday, 30 more flowers had bloomed. How many butterflies visited the garden on Friday?

2. An assortment of sweets consists of x chocolates and y caramels. If 2 chocolates are added and 3 caramels are removed, what fraction of the remaining sweets, in terms of x and y, are chocolates?

    (A) $x + \dfrac{2}{y}$

    (B) $\dfrac{x}{y-1+2}$

    (C) $\dfrac{x-1}{x+y+2}$

    (D) $\dfrac{x+2}{x+y-1}$

    (E) $\dfrac{x+3}{x+y}$

3. Every human is a vertebrate and every vertebrate is a chordate. No mollusc is a vertebrate. Which **two** of the following must be true?

    (A) Only vertebrates are human.

    (B) Molluscs could be chordates.

    (C) Chordates are always human.

    (D) Every human is a chordate.

4. If Ms. Lewis travels to country A to purchase camping equipment, she must pay the prevailing sales tax of 8 percent on what she buys. The store will ship her purchase to her home in country B without charging tax, but with a fixed shipping fee of £3.20. What is the least number of pounds she can spend, so that having the purchase shipped will not be more expensive than paying the sales tax?

5. The U.S. government tracks the number of employees in 22 different mining sectors, ranging from anthracite to uranium. The following histogram displays the number of employees in each of the 22 sectors.

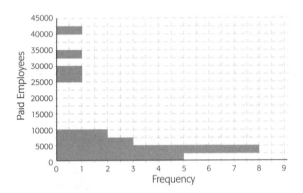

What percentage of mining sectors has 7,500 or fewer paid employees?

(A) 73%

(B) 59%

(C) 27%

(D) 16%

(E) 6%

6. The table shows how much food each animal type needs each day if it is fed a combination of three different kinds of food.

Pounds of food eaten each day			
	Hay	Clover	Fresh Grass
Zebra	8	6	6
Zebu	12	11	10

Which one of the following shows the percentage of each type of food eaten each day?

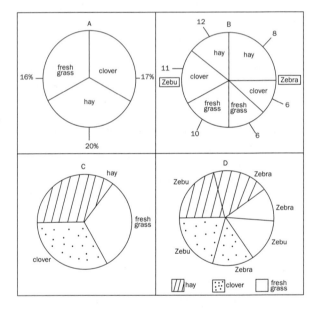

GO ON TO THE NEXT PAGE ▷

x%	on time
43%	up to 15 minutes delayed
17%	15–30 minutes delayed
12%	30–60 minutes delayed
3%	more than 60 minutes delayed

7. The chart above describes departures from a certain airport on a certain day. If 1,200 flights were delayed, how many flights departed on time?

    (A) 250
    (B) 300
    (C) 350
    (D) 400

8. Although temporary and contract employees can play an important role in completing projects and adjusting to seasonal work flow, they are not an adequate substitute for a full-time, permanent staff. In order to thrive, the company needs workers who are not just skilled and efficient but who have a personal connection to their work and a dedication to the company. A staff made up of contract or temporary employees is incomplete at best.

    Which **one** of the following is an underlying assumption of the above argument?

    (A) temporary employees are detrimental to a company's success
    (B) companies should encourage temporary employees to feel dedicated to their employers
    (C) seasonal work flow is not an important factor in assessing an employee's suitability for work
    (D) temporary employees lack connection and commitment to the companies that hire them
    (E) permanent employees are more skilled and efficient than are temporary employees

9. Ranjit was extremely upset when he received a failing grade in his engineering course because he had attended every class, participated in course discussions, and handed in every project except for the 3-D modeling project. He concluded that the grade was unfair since other students who had not turned in the 3-D project had passed the course.

    Which **one** of the following, if true, would most strengthen the above argument?

    (A) Ranjit has never failed a course before.
    (B) Ranjit received a failing grade primarily because he didn't hand in the 3-D project.
    (C) Ranjit received above-average scores on all of his assignments except the 3-D modeling project.
    (D) The 3-D project was worth 30% of the course grade.
    (E) Ranjit's performance was above average in comparison to students in other engineering courses.

10. **Advertisement:** Savvy shoppers know that the Autumn Sale at Thompson's gives you great savings on clothes for the whole family. When you make at least one purchase in each of the Men's, Women's, and Children's departments during the sale, you'll receive a voucher for 50% off any purchase in the Household department. If you're looking to clothe the family on a budget, don't miss the Autumn Sale at Thompson's!

    Which **one** of the following is the best statement of the flaw in the above argument?

    (A) Many shoppers may not make a purchase in each department during September.
    (B) The savings advertised are for household goods, not clothing.
    (C) The length of the sale is not specified in the advertisement.
    (D) A purchase in the Household department is much more expensive than a purchase in the Women's department.
    (E) The sale does not take into account other discounts that customers may redeem.

GO ON TO THE NEXT PAGE

KAPLAN

11. During the summer season, there is always a surge in the population of Oceanville. Therefore, residents of the town will want to be especially careful to keep their doors and windows securely locked.

Which **one** of the following is an underlying assumption of the above argument?

(A) Most burglaries in the United States occur during the summer months.

(B) A surge in the town's population is likely to result in a higher incidence of home burglaries.

(C) The arrival of the summer season leads burglars to start working outdoors.

(D) The beginning of the summer season inevitably leads to an increase in crime.

(E) A higher percentage of homes being occupied leads to an increase in the number of residential burglaries in any given area.

12. A code is created by pairing digits (0–9) with letters. A particular code has 5 alphanumeric pairs. The first and final pairs cannot contain any multiples of 2, and the third pair cannot contain a vowel. Finally, the fourth pair cannot contain a prime number. Every pair must use a different letter of the alphabet that comes after but not including G and a different digit.

Which **one** of the following correctly shows the possible order of pairs of the code?

(A) 1F, 6J, 7K, 9R, 0S

(B) 5M, 8Z, 1Q, 2P, 3Y

(C) 0O, 2I, 9X, 8P, 7W

(D) 1J, 0H, 7I, 3Q, 5T

13. In a class of 27 students, the average (arithmetic mean) score of the male students on the final exam was 83. If the average score of the 15 female students in the class was 92, what was the average of the whole class?

(A) 87.0

(B) 87.5

(C) 88.0

(D) 88.2

14. Josephine is having 5 friends over for tea and makes a seating arrangement for her rectangular dining table. She wants her guests to have a view of her garden, so she assigns herself the seat facing away from the window. On her right she places Audrey, to her left, Briony. Clea will be diagonally across from Briony and Desiree will be directly across from Clea. Ellen will face Josephine. Briony, Clea and Desiree arrive and take their seats. Audrey calls to cancel just before the party starts and Ellen arrives last. Ellen sits in an empty chair.

Which of the following could show the seating arrangement once the tea party begins?
(NOTE: An "X" represents a still empty seat)

(A) Figure 1 only

(B) Figure 2 only

(C) Figure 3 only

(D) Figures 1 and 2 only

(E) Figures 1 and 3 only

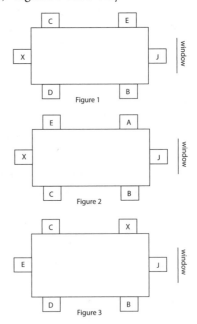

15. A garden measuring 40 meters by 50 metres is to be surrounded by a flagstone walkway 5 metres wide. If each stone is rectangular and has the dimensions 2 metres by 1 metre, how many stones will be needed to cover the walkway?

GO ON TO THE NEXT PAGE ▷

Questions 16–19 refer to the following information.

DISTRIBUTION OF AGES OF AMERICANS 55 YEARS OF AGE AND OLDER

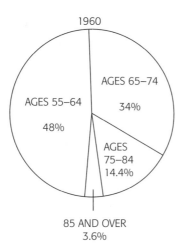

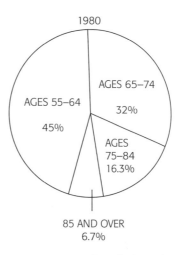

1960 Population of U.S.:   179,323,000
Total Number 55 or older: 32,134,000

1980 Population of U.S.:   226,505,000
Total Number 55 or older: 47,247,000

16. Which of the following statements must be true based on the information given?

1) You can calculate how many of the Americans who were between the ages of 55 and 64 inclusive in 1960 were still alive in 1980.

2) The percentage of Americans aged 55 or older in 1960 was greater than the percentage of Americans aged 55 or older in 1980.

3) In 1960, there were approximately 6.3 million more Americans between the ages of 65 and 74 (inclusive) than between the ages of 75 and 84 (inclusive).

(A) 3 only

(B) 1 and 2 only

(C) 2 and 3 only

(D) 1 and 3 only

17. In 1960, how many Americans were there between the ages of 55 and 64 inclusive?

_____

18. In 1980, approximately what percent of the total population of the United States was between the ages of 65 and 74 inclusive?

(A) 4%

(B) 7%

(C) 9%

(D) 16%

(E) 32%

19. How many of the given categories saw an increase in their number in 1980 over 1960?

(A) 1

(B) 2

(C) 3

(D) 4

GO ON TO THE NEXT PAGE

KAPLAN

20. A scientist added different quantities of auxin to a number of plant seedlings and observed their growth. This chart summarizes the findings.

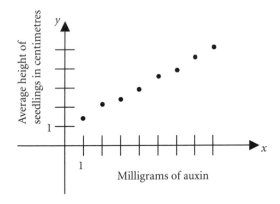

Which of the following statements must be true based on the information given?

1) There is always a positive constant correlation between the amount of auxin added and the average height of the seedlings.

2) The height of the seedlings is affected by the amount of time they grow.

3) The increase in growth from 1 mg of auxin to 2 mg of auxin was less than the increase of growth from 5 mg of auxin and 6 mg of auxin.

(A) 1 only

(B) 1 and 2 only

(C) 2 and 3 only

(D) All of the above

(E) None of the above

21. We must increase funding for nursery school programmes so that students will begin reading earlier. That's the only way to raise test scores in the area.

Which **one** of the following is the best statement of the flaw in the above argument?

(A) It assumes that funding for nursery school programmes is available.

(B) It does not consider other factors that may be causing low test scores.

(C) Strong reading skills does not guarantee a high test score.

(D) It does not consider that tests include maths and science.

(E) It compares nursery schoolers to primary students.

22. This editorial cannot be a good argument because it is barely literate. Run-on sentences, slang, and perfectly dreadful grammar appear regularly throughout. Anything that poorly written cannot make much sense.

Which **one** of the following is an underlying assumption in the above argument?

(A) This editorial was written by someone other than the usual editor.

(B) Generally speaking, few editorials are poor in style or grammar.

(C) The language of an argument is indicative of its validity.

(D) Generally speaking, the majority of editorials are poor in style and grammar.

(E) The author of the editorial purposely uses poor grammar to disguise what he knows is a bad argument.

(F) The author of the editorial purposely uses poor grammar to mimic the writing of an uneducated person.

GO ON TO THE NEXT PAGE

23. According to a recent study, a diet that is free of meat and dairy products greatly reduces the risk of suffering a heart attack. The study cites the fact that only 10% of those who consume such a diet suffer a heart attack at some point in their lives.

    Which **one** of the following would most seriously weaken the above argument?

    (A) 2% of all people who have a heart attack have more than one in their lifetime.

    (B) Those who consume only dairy but not meat are twice as likely to suffer a heart attack as those who consume neither meat nor dairy.

    (C) Some people who consume neither dairy nor meat suffer two or more heart attacks over the course of a lifetime.

    (D) Meat and dairy products are high in low-density cholesterol, which is known to harden arteries and cause other heart problems.

    (E) 7% of those who consume dairy and meat regularly suffer heart attacks over the course of their lifetime.

24. A chemical company recently introduced a new type of foam spray that it claims will reduce the rate of erosion from the walls of road cuts. A study by the company showed that the rate of erosion was low on a road cut where the foam was applied.

    Which **one** of the following, if true, most **weakens** the above argument?

    (A) Road cuts similar to the one studied typically show low rates of erosion without the foam.

    (B) Because the foam itself weathers, the foam would have to be reapplied every four years to maintain protection against erosion.

    (C) Studies by the company that produces the material are sometimes unreliable because of conflicts of interest.

    (D) The rate of erosion from the road cut in the study was greater than expected based on computer simulation models.

    (E) Other foams made from similar materials have failed to halt erosion from certain types of road cuts.

25. Kaliyani always wears skirts. Rhonda wears skirts during the week, but trousers at the weekend. Lenore wears trousers unless it is very warm and then she wears skirts.

    One of the three sees the other two women each wearing the same article of clothing.

    Which **one** of the following **cannot** be true?

    (A) It's the weekend.

    (B) It's a weekday.

    (C) It's a cold day and one of the two women is Lenore.

    (D) It's hot Saturday and one of the two women is Rhonda.

    (E) It's a very cold Tuesday.

26. If a rectangle with width 49.872 centimetres and length 30.64 centimetres has an area that is 15 times the area of a certain square, which of the following is the closest approximation to the length, in centimetres, of a side of that square?

    (A) 5

    (B) 10

    (C) 15

    (D) 20

27. Hollings is north of Derby, which is north of Jessup. Leyton is south of Derby and north of Ipswich.

    Ipswich must be south of:

    (A) Derby, but not necessarily south of Hollings or Jessup;

    (B) Jessup, but not necessarily south of Derby or Hollings;

    (C) Derby and Hollings, but not necessarily south of Jessup;

    (D) Hollings and Jessup, but not necessarily south of Derby;

    (E) Derby, Hollings, and Jessup.

GO ON TO THE NEXT PAGE

28. A computer is programmed to generate two numbers according to the following scheme: the first number is to be a randomly selected integer from 0 to 99; the second number is to be an integer which is less than the square of the units digit of the first number. Which of the following pairs of numbers could NOT have been generated by this program?

    (A) 99, 10
    (B) 60, –10
    (C) 58, 63
    (D) 13, 11

29. A magazine's survey of its subscribers finds that 20 percent are male. If 70 percent of the subscribers are married, and 10 percent of these are male, what percentage of the male subscribers are not married?

30. Time and time again, it has been shown that students who attend universities with low faculty/student ratios get the most well-rounded education. As a result, when my children are ready for university, I'll make sure they attend one with a very small student population.

    Which **one** of the following is the best statement of the flaw in the above argument?

    (A) A low faculty/student ratio is the effect of a well-rounded education, not its source.
    (B) Intelligence should be considered the result of childhood environment, not advanced education.
    (C) A very small student population does not, by itself, ensure a low faculty/student ratio.
    (D) Parental desires and preferences rarely determine a child's choice of a college or university.
    (E) Students must take advantage of the low faculty/student ratio by intentionally choosing a small university.

31. A brochure for City X highlights the reasons why residents should move there rather than to other cities in the region. One reason the brochure mentions is the relative ease of finding a job in City X, where the unemployment rate is 4.7%.

    Which of the following are underlying assumptions of the above argument?

    I. Most people find jobs easily.
    II. Unemployment is higher than 4.7% in other cities in the region.
    III. 4.7% is a record low unemployment rate.

    (A) I only.
    (B) I and II only.
    (C) II only.
    (D) III only.
    (E) I, II and III.

32. A recently published article on human physiology claims that enzyme K contributes to improved performance in strenuous activities such as weightlifting and sprinting. The article cites evidence of above-average levels of enzyme K in Olympic weightlifters and sprinters.

    Which **one** of the following, if true, most **strengthens** the above argument?

    (A) Enzyme K levels are the most important factor affecting the performance of strenuous activities.
    (B) Enzyme K has no other function in the human body.
    (C) Enzyme K is required for the performance of strenuous activities.
    (D) Enzyme K helps weightlifters more than it helps sprinters.
    (E) Strenuous activities do not cause the human body to produce unusually high levels of Enzyme K.

GO ON TO THE NEXT PAGE ⇨

Mercury in Vaccines: More Harm than Good?

Are childhood vaccines dangerous? A few years ago, that question might have seemed absurd. But with the recent publication of journalist David Kirby's book *Evidence of Harm: Mercury in Vaccines and the Autism Epidemic: A Medical Controversy*, vaccine manufacturers and the Centers for Disease Control and Prevention (CDC) are in the hot seat, accused of poisoning America's children with toxic doses of mercury. While mercury has been phased out of most vaccinations over the last six years, some, and most notably the latest flu vaccine, still contain what some believe to be dangerous amounts of the poisonous metal. And for many children who were vaccinated before mercury was removed, the damage ostensibly caused by the vaccines has already been done.

Mercury in vaccines comes in the form of thimerosal, a compound consisting of 49% ethylmercury. Thimerosal is a preservative and has been used in some vaccines since the 1930s to help prevent bacterial contamination. It is only used in multi-dose vaccination vials.

Critics point out that the level of mercury infants receive in the American childhood vaccination programme exceeds the level set as safe by the Environmental Protection Agency (EPA). Notably, the amount does *not* exceed the safety guidelines set by the Food and Drug Administration (FDA), the Agency for Toxic Substances and Disease Registry (ATSDR), or the World Health Organisation (WHO). It is also important to note that these safety standards are for *methyl*mercury, not ethylmercury, which has not been sufficiently researched to establish intake guidelines.

The CDC claims that there is no evidence of harm to infants receiving vaccines with thimerosal because the amount of thimerosal is minute and far below the FDA's safe level, an amount 10 times lower than the level at which mercury begins to cause neurological damage. But do ethylmercury and methylmercury have the same level of toxicity? This is an important unknown.

The EPA standard for mercury safety (methylmercury) is .1 micrograms per kilogram per day.[1] Kirby claims that by the end of a child's first year, he or she can receive up to 212.5 micrograms of mercury through vaccines—well above the EPA daily exposure level.[2] Worse, those 212.5 micrograms are not spread out in daily doses but administered in a handful of highly concentrated doses at two months, four months, six months and one year.[2]

Because these mercury doses are so high, Kirby and others believe that the American childhood vaccination programme may be responsible for the dramatic rise in autism, ADD, and other behavioural disorders. The sharp rise in these disorders, they argue, corresponds with the early 1990s addition of several vaccines containing thimerosal to the immunisation calendar. Statistics seem to support their case: In the 1980s, autism affected only 1–2 children in 10,000.[3] By 2004, that number skyrocketed to 1 in 166 (60 per 10,000).[3] In addition, the list of symptoms of mercury poisoning and autism are nearly identical.

But the CDC argues that there is no epidemic of autism—that we are simply getting better at diagnosing children with autism and similar disorders and that there are many other sources of mercury in the environment, including fish, pesticides, PCBs, and flame retardants. It also points out that there has been a significant rise in autism in Great Britain, yet only one vaccine in Great Britain's childhood immunisation programme contains thimerosal.[4] If thimerosal levels in vaccines increases the risk for autism, then there should not be a corresponding rise in autism in Great Britain.

The CDC admits that prior to 1999 and the thimerosal-reduction initiative, children could have received up to 187.5 micrograms of mercury during the first six months of life from routine childhood vaccinations.[4] Now, however, with many newly formulated thimerosal-free vaccines, the maximum cumulative exposure during the first six months should be less than three micrograms—a reduction of 98%[4] and far short of Kirby's 212.5 figure. But children are heavily immunised until

GO ON TO THE NEXT PAGE ➤

age four, and vaccines are always given in highly concentrated doses at annual and bi-annual doctor visits. In addition, the new flu injection—which is being marketed to the public unlike any other vaccine in the past and encouraged even for infants—contains thimerosal*.

Whether a direct link between thimerosal and autism is found remains to be seen. One thing, however, seems certain: there is a definite *potential* for harm, and the impact of concentrated doses of thimerosal and the cumulative effect of repeated thimerosal injections must be investigated.

*A thimerosal-free version of the vaccine is being produced but is more expensive and less available.

Sources [1] "Human Exposure", *Mercury Home*, US Environmental Protection Agency. 27 July 2005. http://www.epa.gov/mercury/exposure.htm.

[2] Kirby, David. *Evidence of Harm* Powerpoint Presentation. 11 January 2005. http://www.evidenceofharm.com/ppp/1–11.ppt#11.

[3] Ibid. http://www.evidenceofharm.com/ppp/1–11.ppt#5.

[4] "Thimerosal and Vaccines: Q&A", 18 May 2004. Department of Health and Human Services, Centers for Disease Control and Prevention. http://www.cdc.gov/nip/vacsafe/concerns/thimerosal/faqs-thimerosal.htm#9.

Answer the following questions, based on the information given above:

33. Which of the following statements can we safely conclude to be accurate?

    (A) Safe levels of ethylmercury have recently been established.

    (B) The flu vaccine has safe levels of thimerosal.

    (C) The EPA's safe level for mercury is lower than the FDA's.

    (D) David Kirby's children suffer from autism.

34. The author seems concerned that:

    (A) even if individual vaccines contain safe levels of thimerosal, the practice of multiple vaccinations at set intervals during infancy still puts children at risk.

    (B) the epidemic of autism will only worsen in the next decade.

    (C) the CDC is not being honest with the public about levels of mercury in vaccines.

    (D) Kirby's book will prompt many parents to stop vaccinating their children, resulting in outbreaks of previously eradicated diseases such as polio.

35. Which of the following are reasons for a suspected link between thimerosal and autism?

    I. symptoms of autism mimic those of mercury poisoning

    II. a British study found evidence of mercury poisoning in autistic children

    III. the rise in autism in the US corresponds with the 1990s expansion of its vaccination programme

    (A) I only

    (B) I and II

    (C) II and III

    (D) I and III

GO ON TO THE NEXT PAGE ⟹

KAPLAN

SECTION 2: APTITUDE AND SKILLS

Time: 30 minutes

Directions: Answer every question. Points are assigned for correct answers only. There are no penalties for incorrect answers.

All questions are worth 1 mark.

Indicate your answers in pencil on the answer sheet provided for this section. For multiple-choice questions, fill in the bubble(s) completely. For short-answer or calculation questions, write clearly and neatly in the space provided. If you make a mistake, erase it as completely as possible.

Calculators are not permitted.

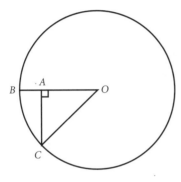

1. If the area of the circle with centre O above is 100π and AC has a length of 6, what is the length of AB?

2. What is the remainder when $5x^3 - 2x^2 + x + 1$ is divided by $x - 3$?

3. Which of the following structures is present in the nucleus of a cell?

   (A) mitochondrion
   (B) ribosome
   (C) endoplasmic reticulum
   (D) chromatin
   (E) centriole

4. Fermentation may result in the production of:

   I. Oxygen
   II. Carbon dioxide
   III. Lactate
   IV. Ethanol

   (A) I only
   (B) II only
   (C) II and IV only
   (D) III and IV only
   (E) II, III, and IV

5. A drug called Brefeldin A blocks transport from the endoplasmic reticulum to the Golgi apparatus. If a cell that typically secretes enzyme X is treated with Brefeldin A, what effect will be observed on the secretion of enzyme X?

   (A) There will be no effect on secretion.
   (B) Secretion of enzyme X will increase.
   (C) Secretion of enzyme X will decrease.
   (D) Enzyme X will accumulate in the plasma membrane.
   (E) Enzyme X will accumulate in the nuclear membrane.

GO ON TO THE NEXT PAGE

KAPLAN

6. The transport of which ions across the plasma membrane is important for the transmission of nerve impulses?

(A) Na^+, K^+
(B) Na^+, Cl^-
(C) Mg^{2+}, K^+
(D) Ca^{2+}, Cl^-
(E) H^+, K^+

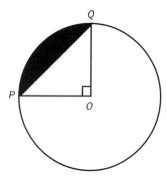

7. In circle O above, if $\triangle POQ$ is a right triangle and radius $OP = 2$, what is the area of the shaded region?

(A) $4\pi - 2$
(B) $4\pi - 4$
(C) $2\pi - 2$
(D) $2\pi - 4$
(E) $\pi - 2$

8. Which of the following elements is classified as a metalloid?

(A) As
(B) Be
(C) Cl
(D) Hg
(E) Sn

9. Brass is an alloy of copper and zinc. If a brass coin has a mass of 12.3 grams and has a mass percent of 70% copper, what is the mass of zinc in the coin?

(A) 3.0 g
(B) 3.7 g
(C) 7.0 g
(D) 8.6 g
(E) 70 g

10. The radioactive isotope chromium-57 has a half-life of 21 sec. If a sample has 10.0 grams of chromium-57, how much chromium-57 would it have in 1.4 minutes?

(A) 0.625 grams
(B) 1.25 grams
(C) 2.50 grams
(D) 5.00 grams
(E) 10.0 grams

11. A 50-pound child and a 200-pound adult are at a park swinging on two swings of identical length. In the time it takes the adult to make a complete oscillation, the child can make

(A) one quarter of an oscillation
(B) half of an oscillation
(C) one oscillation
(D) two oscillations
(E) four oscillations

12. We are given a fixed length of a heating wire with a known resistance, which we connect across a 120-V line. If we cut the wire in half and connect each half across the 120-V line, how will the total power output change?

(A) It will double
(B) It will be half as large
(C) Total power output will not change
(D) It will increase by a factor of four
(E) Not enough information is provided

GO ON TO THE NEXT PAGE

13. If $8<\sqrt{(n+6)(n+1)}<9$, then n could equal

    (A) 5
    (B) 6
    (C) 7
    (D) 8

14. $\dfrac{3^5+\dfrac{1}{3^5}}{3^5}=$ _____

_____

15. Rearrange $x=\dfrac{x+y}{y}$ to make z the subject.

    (A) $z=\dfrac{x}{y}+x$

    (B) $z=\dfrac{x}{y}+1$

    (C) $z=\dfrac{y}{x}+y$

    (D) $z=\dfrac{y}{x}+x$

    (E) $z=\dfrac{y}{x}+1$

16. Which of the following statements regarding evolution is true?

    (A) Certain phenotypes are more fit in certain environments than others.
    (B) Natural selection creates new alleles.
    (C) Genotype, not phenotype, influences fitness.
    (D) Mutations always affect the fitness of an organism.
    (E) all of the above

17. A culture of algae is inoculated with small numbers of two different species of protozoan ciliates, Protozoans A and C, that feed on the algae. Protozoan A replicates asexually once every hour and Protozoan C replicates asexually once every 1.5 hours under these conditions, as long as the algae is not limiting. Which of the following is most likely to be observed?

    (A) The protozoans will evolve to have a mutualistic relationship.
    (B) Both populations of protozoans will increase in size initially, but then Protozoan C will die off from the culture.
    (C) The algae will rapidly evolve to avoid predation.
    (D) The algae will die off from the culture due to overfeeding.
    (E) Protozoan C will evolve to replicate more rapidly.

18. A black male mouse (I) is crossed with a black female mouse, and they produce 15 black and 5 white offspring. A different black male mouse (II) is crossed with the same female, and the offspring from this mating are 30 black mice. Which of the following must be true?

    (A) The female mouse is homozygous.
    (B) Male mouse II is heterozygous.
    (C) Two of the mice are heterozygous.
    (D) All the progeny of mouse II are homozygous.
    (E) All three mice are homozygous.

GO ON TO THE NEXT PAGE

KAPLAN

19. Which of the following pairs of substances will react to produce H_2 (g)?

    (A) HCl (aq) and $NaHCO_3$ (aq)

    (B) HCl (aq) and Cu (s)

    (C) HNO_3 (aq) and Cu (s)

    (D) H_2O (l) and Na (s)

    (E) NaOH (aq) and NH_4Cl (aq)

20. A certain elemental substance is a gas at room temperature and atmospheric pressure. It is most likely a

    (A) metal.

    (B) metalloid.

    (C) nonmetal.

    (D) halogen.

    (E) transition element.

21. Using a sensitive laboratory balance, a chemist determines the mass of a ball-point pen to be 11.1064 g. He or she uses the pen to record an experiment in a lab notebook, and then finds that the mass of the pen is 11.0344 g. How can the mass of ink used be most appropriately represented?

    (A) 720 mg

    (B) 0.072 g

    (C) 0.0720 g

    (D) 7.2×10^{-2} g

    (E) 7.20000×10^{-2} g

22. Which of the following particles will feel the greatest force due to a magnetic field?

    (A) An electron moving perpendicular to the magnetic field lines

    (B) A neutron moving perpendicular to the magnetic field lines

    (C) An electron moving parallel to the magnetic field lines

    (D) A neutron moving parallel to the magnetic field lines

    (E) An electron at rest

23. An $8 \times 10{-}4$ C charge and a $2 \times 10{-}4$ C charge are 2 m apart. Which of the following is closest to the force between them?

    (A) 360 N

    (B) 720 N

    (C) 3.6×106 N

    (D) 7.2×106 N

    (E) 3.6×1010 N

24. In a laboratory, you connect two identical small light bulbs in a series circuit with a battery. Which of the following best describes what happens and gives the correct explanation?

    (A) The brightness of both bulbs is the same because the bulbs are the same size.

    (B) The first bulb in the circuit is brighter because it uses the current first.

    (C) The brightness of both bulbs is the same because current is the same throughout a series circuit and there is the same potential difference across the bulbs.

    (D) The first bulb in the circuit is brighter because the current and potential difference are both higher in this bulb.

    (E) The second bulb in the circuit is brighter because the current and potential difference are both higher in this bulb.

25. Which of the following elements would be the least electronegative?

    (A) Al

    (B) Cs

    (C) F

    (D) I

    (E) Li

GO ON TO THE NEXT PAGE

26. Which of the following statements is true?

    (A) The liquid phase of a substance cannot exist above its critical temperature.

    (B) Above the critical pressure, only the liquid phase of a pure substance can exist.

    (C) At the critical point, all phases of a pure substance can exist simultaneously.

    (D) The critical temperature and pressure cannot be produced simultaneously.

    (E) All of the above statements are true.

27. An electron is moving in a straight line through a region of space in which no forces act on the electron. A uniform magnetic field is suddenly turned on in this region of space, such that the magnetic field lines are not parallel (or anti-parallel) or perpendicular to the electron's velocity. Which of the following best describes the path the electron will take after the magnetic field is turned on?

    (A) It will continue to move at the same speed and direction.

    (B) It will move in a circular path, with the plane of the circle perpendicular to the magnetic field lines.

    (C) It will move in a circular path, with the plane of the circle parallel to the magnetic field lines.

    (D) It will move in a helical (spiral) path around the magnetic field lines.

    (E) It will come to a complete stop.

GO ON TO THE NEXT PAGE

KAPLAN

SECTION 3: WRITING TASK

Time: 30 minutes

Directions: Below are three writing tasks. Choose only one and write your response on the single page answer sheet provided. You may make any preliminary notes on the following page or a separate sheet of paper. You have 30 minutes to choose your tasks and complete your essay.

The tasks give you the chance to demonstrate how well you can select, develop, and organise ideas and how effectively you can communicate them in writing. Before you begin, think carefully about what you want to say in response to the prompt. Consider how you will organise your response to most effectively convey your message. You may use diagrams or other graphic forms if they enhance the communication of your ideas.

Use this opportunity to demonstrate how well you can write. Your essay must be contained to the single answer sheet, so be clear and concise. Be sure to write legibly.

You may **not** use a dictionary or thesaurus.

Technological progress is like an axe in the hands of a pathological criminal.
(Albert Einstein)

Explain what you believe the author means by this statement. Provide examples of how technological progress can be dangerous and how it can be beneficial. Can you reconcile the rapid pace of technological progress with its purported dangers?

What we see depends mainly on what we look for.
(John Lubbock)

What does the above statement imply? Can you provide examples that support this statement and contradict it? What are the implications of this statement for scientists?

Knowledge is more valuable than morals.
(Maxim Gorky)

What do you think the author means by this statement? Do you agree? Advance an argument in support of this statement or against it. Provide specific examples of how knowledge is more valuable than morals or how morals are more valuable than knowledge.

GO ON TO THE NEXT PAGE

Use this page for notes.

GO ON TO THE NEXT PAGE

Practice Test
Answer Sheet

Section 1: Aptitude and Skills

1

2 (A) (B) (C) (D) (E)

3 (A) (B) (C) (D)

4

5 (A) (B) (C) (D) (E)

6 (A) (B) (C) (D)

7 (A) (B) (C) (D)

8 (A) (B) (C) (D) (E)

9 (A) (B) (C) (D) (E)

10 (A) (B) (C) (D) (E)

11 (A) (B) (C) (D) (E)

12 (A) (B) (C) (D)

13 (A) (B) (C) (D)

14 (A) (B) (C) (D) (E)

15

16 (A) (B) (C) (D)

17

18 (A) (B) (C) (D) (E)

19 (A) (B) (C) (D)

20 (A) (B) (C) (D) (E)

21 (A) (B) (C) (D) (E)

22 (A) (B) (C) (D) (E) (F)

23 (A) (B) (C) (D) (E)

24 (A) (B) (C) (D) (E)

25 (A) (B) (C) (D) (E)

26 (A) (B) (C) (D)

27 (A) (B) (C) (D) (E)

28 (A) (B) (C) (D)

29

30 (A) (B) (C) (D) (E)

31 (A) (B) (C) (D) (E)

32 (A) (B) (C) (D) (E)

33 (A) (B) (C) (D)

34 (A) (B) (C) (D)

35 (A) (B) (C) (D)

Section 2: Aptitude and Skills

1

2

3 (A) (B) (C) (D) (E)

4 (A) (B) (C) (D) (E)

5 (A) (B) (C) (D) (E)

6 (A) (B) (C) (D) (E)

7 (A) (B) (C) (D) (E)

8 (A) (B) (C) (D) (E)

9 (A) (B) (C) (D) (E)

10 (A) (B) (C) (D) (E)

11 (A) (B) (C) (D) (E)

12 (A) (B) (C) (D) (E)

13 (A) (B) (C) (D)

14

15 (A) (B) (C) (D) (E)

16 (A) (B) (C) (D) (E)

17 (A) (B) (C) (D) (E)

18 (A) (B) (C) (D) (E)

19 (A) (B) (C) (D) (E)

20 (A) (B) (C) (D) (E)

21 (A) (B) (C) (D) (E)

22 (A) (B) (C) (D) (E)

23 (A) (B) (C) (D) (E)

24 (A) (B) (C) (D) (E)

25 (A) (B) (C) (D) (E)

26 (A) (B) (C) (D) (E)

27 (A) (B) (C) (D) (E)

ANSWERS AND EXPLANATIONS

Section 1: Aptitude and Skills

1. 16

If a quantity b varies directly as another quantity f, the relation between them can be expressed as $\frac{b}{f} = k$, where k is a constant. In this case, b and f represent the number of butterflies and the number of flowers in the garden. You can use the given values of b and f to find k.

$$\frac{10}{50} = k$$

$$0.2 = k$$

So $\frac{b}{f} = 0.2$

Now find b when $f = 50 + 30 = 80$.

$$\frac{b}{80} = 0.2$$

$$b = 16$$

2. D

You are asked to find what fraction of all the sweets will be chocolates after the total has been adjusted. This fraction is simply the number of chocolates over the total number of sweets after the change has been made. Find the number of chocolates and caramels by translating the question. Then divide the number of chocolates by the total number of chocolates and caramels. Alternatively, since all the answer choices contain variables, you could try picking numbers.

You initially had x chocolates, but now have two more, or $x + 2$. The original number of caramels was y, and 3 were removed, so the number of caramels is $y - 3$.

So the fraction of sweets which are chocolates =

$$\frac{\text{number of chocolates}}{\text{number of sweets}} = \frac{x+2}{x+2+y-3} = \frac{x+2}{x+y-1}$$

If translating this problem was difficult—many people have trouble sorting out parts and totals—you should have tried plugging in numbers. For instance, say there are initially 5 chocolates and 5 caramels—10 sweets total. After the 2 chocolates are added and the 3 caramels are removed, there are 7 chocolates and 9 sweets in total. Plugging in 5 and 5 for x and y in the answer choices, only choice **(D)** works out to $\frac{7}{9}$. This question illustrates that picking numbers can be a useful strategy for some problems.

3. B, D

Choice **(B)** is true because if you are a mollusc, you are not a vertebrate. The first statement notes that all vertebrates are chordates, but it does not say that all chordates must be vertebrates. Therefore, it is possible to be a mollusc (non-vertebrate) and a chordate and this choice must be true. Choice **(D)** is true because if every human is a vertebrate and every vertebrate is a chordate, then every human is a chordate. Choice **(A)** and choice **(C)** do not have to be true, therefore they are incorrect.

4. £40

The sales tax on her purchase must equal the fixed shipping fee of £3.20. Let $x =$ the purchase amount, in pounds. Find the smallest number of pounds that can be spent so that the cost of having the purchase shipped will not be more expensive than paying the sales tax. In other words, find the smallest number of pounds that can be spent so that the cost of having the purchase shipped will be less than or equal to the sales tax. So $3.20 \le 0.08x$. Then $\frac{3.20}{0.08} \le x$.

Now $\frac{3.20}{0.08} = \frac{3.20 \times 100}{0.08 \times 100} = \frac{320}{8} = 40$. So $40 \le x$. That is $x \ge 40$. The smallest possible values of x is 40.

5. A

The histogram shows 16 of the 22 mining sectors have 7,500 or fewer paid employees, for 73% of the mining sectors, so **(A)** is correct. If you misread the table and only consider the sectors employing 5,000 or fewer people, you get choice **(B)**. If you work with the sectors employing more than 7,500 you get 27%. The table shows frequency, but if you misread it and believe it shows percentage instead, you will get choice **(D)**. If you combine the mistakes of **(C)** and **(D)**, you get **(E)**.

6. C

The question does not require that the chart show the percentage of food eaten each day by each animal type, therefore choices **(B)** and **(D)** should be eliminated. Choice **(A)** shows the numerical values of the number of kilograms of food eaten each day, but has incorrectly converted the amount to a percentage. Only choice **(C)** shows the correct percentage of hay (approximately 37%), clover (approximately 32%) and fresh grass (approximately 30%).

7. D

The chart shows what percentage of the flights were late, and the text states what number of flights were late (the number of flights that the percentage represents). You have to figure out the number of flights that were *not* late (that were on time). 43% + 17% + 12% + 3% = 75% of the flights were late. That is a nice, neat percentage, representing $\frac{3}{4}$. So $\frac{3}{4}$ of the flights were late, which means $\frac{1}{4}$ of the flights were on time. That makes the calculation very easy: 1,200 flights were late, which is equal to $\frac{3}{4}$ of all the flights. Call the total number of flights F. Then, since 1,200 flights is equal to $\frac{3}{4}$ of all the flights, write the equation $\frac{3}{4} F = 1,200$. Solve for F.

Thus:

$$\frac{3}{4} F = 1,200$$

$$3F = 1,200(4)$$

$$3F = 4,800$$

$$F = \frac{4800}{3} = 1,600$$

The total number of flights is 1,600. You know that of all the flights were on time. So the number of flights that were on time is $\frac{1}{4} F = \frac{1}{4} (1,600) = 400$.

8. D

The author concludes that a staff made up of contract or temporary employees is "incomplete at best". Why? The evidence says it's because a company needs workers who have a personal connection to their work and a dedication to the company. We're looking for the assumption that ties the idea that we need dedicated, connected workers to the idea that temporary workers aren't enough. Otherwise, temporary workers would indeed be an acceptable substitute for permanent staff. (D) sums this assumption up nicely. (A) distorts the point; the author states only that temporary staff by themselves are inadequate, not that they cause the company any harm. (B) might be tempting because it suggests a possible remedy for the problem the author raises, but that's not what we've been asked for. We're looking for the missing piece that leads to the conclusion that temporary workers are *not enough*. The idea that they could be encouraged to develop that dedication actually weakens the conclusion. (C) directly contradicts the author's statement that temporary and contract workers can play an important role with regard to

seasonal work flow. (E) is another distortion: the passage mentions that skilled and efficient employees are important to a company, but it doesn't attribute those qualities to either group.

9. C

Ranjit thinks it was unfair that he failed the course because other students who neglected to hand in the same project he failed to turn in had passed the course. To strengthen the argument, we need information that would show how Ranjit performed in the rest of his work in comparison to the other students. If, for example, he did poorly in other classwork, a failing grade might not be unfair. But if he did well in all of his other work, and other students who did not hand in the project passed, then it seems that something would be amiss in the calculation of his grade. (C) tells us that Ranjit received above-average scores in all of his other coursework. That means excepting the 3-D project, he certainly should have passed the course. And since other students passed the course without the 3-D project, it's unlikely that the project was worth a high enough percentage to have Ranjit fail despite good scores on all his other work. Thus (C) is the best answer. (A) is irrelevant; he might be extra upset because he'd never failed before, but that fact has nothing to do with the fairness of his failing the engineering course. (B), if true, would actually weaken the argument as the failure to turn in the 3-D project would be the main reason for his failing grade. (D) likewise undermines the argument: if the 3-D project were worth such a significant portion of the grade, Ranjit would have to have earned top scores in all of his other coursework to pass the course. Finally, (E) compares apples to oranges. The issue isn't how Ranjit compares to students in *other* engineering courses; it's how he fared in this one.

10. B

This question asks us to find the flaw in the logic of an advertisement. We are told that the Autumn Sale offers savings on clothing. The supporting evidence is that if you purchase clothing in three different departments, you receive a discount off of a purchase in the Household department. (B) points out that, although the sale is advertised as offering "great savings on clothes for the whole family," the only discount available is in Household. (A) isn't a criticism of the argument because it focuses on people who are outside the scope of the offer (those who won't make the purchases required to get the coupon). As for (C), the length of the sale doesn't affect whether shoppers are saving money on clothes. The comparison in

(D) is irrelevant; it may speak to whether or not shoppers save money overall, but it does not address the claim that consumers will save money *on clothing*. It's certainly possible that the coupon will help some shoppers save some money, but not, contrary to the advert's claims, on clothing. Similarly, other discounts, **(E)**, don't have any impact on the validity of the claim that this sale will save shoppers money on clothing.

11. B.

This argument concludes that the residents of Oceanville should be extra careful to keep their homes locked. The evidence? Summer has arrived and, as a result, the town's population has increased. The only way for the author to get from evidence about the increased population to a conclusion about the need to secure one's home is by assuming **(B)**: an increase in population causes a higher incidence of burglaries, warranting the advice to lock the doors. **(A)** is outside the scope of the argument; the stimulus focuses on Oceanville and not the United States. **(C)** implies that the change in the weather raises the risk of burglary, but we're told it's an increase in population that we should be worried about. **(C)** also introduces an irrelevant element, "working outdoors". **(D)** is too broad; we're not concerned with, nor do we know anything about, crime statistics overall. It's residential burglaries we're concerned with here. Finally, **(E)** confuses the causation (percentage of homes occupied versus rise in population) and extends beyond the scope of the argument by its application to "any given area" rather than Oceanville itself.

12. C

Choice **(A)** is incorrect because in the first pair, 1 is paired with F and the rules state that every pair must use a different letter of the alphabet *after* G. Choice **(B)** is incorrect because 2 is a prime number and the rules state that the fourth pair cannot contain a prime number. Choice **(D)** is incorrect because the third pair cannot contain a vowel and the letter *I* is a vowel.

13. C

If 15 of the 27 students are girls, the remaining 12 must be boys. You cannot simply add 83 to 92 and divide by two. In this class, there are more girls than boys, and therefore, the girls' test scores are "weighted" more—they contribute more to the class average. So the answer must be either **(C)** or **(D)**.

To find each sum, multiply each average by the number of terms it represents. After you have found the sums of the different terms, find the combined average by plugging them into the average formula.

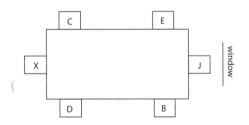

$$\text{Total class average} = \frac{\text{Some of girls' scores} + \text{sum of boys' scores}}{\text{Total number of students}}$$

$$= \frac{(\text{\# of girls} \times \text{girls' average score}) + (\text{\# of boys} \times \text{boys' average score})}{\text{Total \# of students}}$$

$$= \frac{15(92) + 12(83)}{27} = \frac{1{,}380 + 996}{27} = 88$$

So the class average is 88, answer choice **(C)**.

14. E

If you want to test the figures against the rules, you may need to reorient the diagrams first. You might also find drawing your own blank diagram helpful. Do whatever is most comfortable for you.

If you draw your own blank diagram, you should draw two of them. Careful reading of the question shows that after Audrey's cancellation, there are two empty seats available when Ellen arrives. Ellen can be at the opposite end of the table as Josephine:

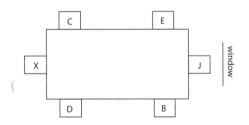

Ellen can also be in the empty seat to the right of Josephine where Audrey was originally assigned to sit:

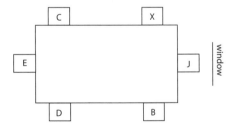

If you compared the given figures to the rules, you should have been able to eliminate choices **(B)** and **(D)** because Figure 2 shows Audrey in attendance (she cancelled) and Desiree is not shown (she was seated across from Clea when the party began). Remember, just because Figure 1 matched the rules and you were able to eliminate Figure 2 does not mean you do not have to test Figure 3. This figure also shows a possible seating assignment, which makes choice **(E)** the correct answer.

15. 500

There are two rectangles: one with dimensions 40 metres by 50 metres (the lawn); one with dimensions 50 metres by 60 metres (the lawn and the walk). The area of the walk alone is the difference between the two rectangular areas, or $(50 \times 60) - (40 \times 50) = 3,000 - 2,000 = 1,000$ square metres. Since each stone has area $2 \times 1 = 2$ square metres, you would need 500 stones for the whole walk.

16. A

Because statement 3 is found in three of the answer choices, you should test it first.

The pie chart shows that 34% of all Americans 55 or over fell into the 65 to 74 age group in 1960, and 14.4% fell into the 75 to 84 age group. That means the difference in their number will be 34 percent—14.4 percent or just under 20 percent of the total number. Just under 20 percent of 32 million means just under 32 million or a little more than 6 million. This means statement 3 is true and you can eliminate choice **(B)**.

Statement 1 is impossible to prove true. More information would be required to calculate how many Americans from the 1960 information were still alive in 1980. You can also eliminate choice **(D)**.

To test statement 2, you have to calculate the percentages and compare. In 1960, approximately 18% of the population was aged 55 or older. In 1980, approximately 20% of the population was aged 55 or older. Therefore, statement 2 is not true and only choice **(A)** is correct.

17. 15.4 million

Under the 1960 pie chart it is stated that there were 32,134,000 Americans 55 or older during that year; the pie chart shows that of these, 48 percent were between the ages of 55–64 inclusive. That must be just a little less than one-half of the total figure; 15.4 million is the only answer less than one-half of 32 million.

18. B

Find approximately how many Americans were between 65 and 74 (inclusive), then find what percentage this is of the entire population. You know from the pie chart that 32 percent or just under a third of all Americans 55 or older fell into the 65 to 74 age group. The information beneath the graph states that 47,247,000 Americans were 55 or over; a third of this will be a bit less than 16 million. The total population of the United States at this time is given as around 226 million. What percentage of 226 is 16? Well, obviously, it is less than 10%, which would be 22.6 million; and it is also greater than 5%, which would be 11.3 million. So it is either 7%, or 9%. At this point, it is simplest to multiply:

7% of 226 is $0.07 \times 226 = 15.82$.

This is close to 16; choice **(B)** is the correct answer.

19. D

In 1980 there were about 47 million Americans 55 or older, while in 1960 there were only about 32 million; these figures are found under the charts. The proportions of some of the categories decreased from 1960 to 1980 (for example, the 55–64 group decreases from 48% to 45%), but given that the whole is so much bigger in 1980 than in 1960, it is pretty clear that the number of people must increase in each category, too. This is the kind of question where you should not do any calculations; since the whole is almost 50 percent more in 1980, you would need a much more dramatic decrease in any one category to get a decrease in number. All four categories increase; the answer is choice **(D)**.

20. E

Based only on the information given, you cannot assume that statements 1, 2 and 3 must be true.

For statement 1, the given information shows a positive correlation between the amount of auxin added and the average height of the seedling, but it is not constant. Eliminate choices **(A)** and **(B)** since they have statement 1 as answers.

Statement 2 mentions information (height over time) that is not included in this chart. The chart shows only the relationship between milligrams of auxin added and the average height of the seedlings. You can now eliminate choice **(C)**.

Because **(A)**, **(B)**, and **(C)** have been eliminated, you can also eliminate choice **(D)**, but it is wise to check statement 3, just in case.

Statement 3 is also untrue. There is a greater increase between 1 and 2 milligrams of auxin added than the increase between 5 and 6 milligrams of auxin added. Choice **(E)** is correct.

21. B

The author presents a chain of cause and effect here: increase funding for nursery school programmes, and students will begin to read earlier. Get students to read earlier, and it'll raise test scores in the area. Sounds logical enough. But the conclusion goes farther by saying that this is the *only* way to raise test scores. Clearly there are *many* factors that can affect an area's scores; the age at which students begin to read is just one of them. The argument would be much stronger if the author stated "That's the *best* way to raise test scores". or "That's *one of the best ways* to raise test scores." While the argument is based on two unstated assumptions—that increased funding for nursery school will result in students reading at an earlier age and that earlier reading will result in higher test scores—there's no discussion of availability of funding, so **(A)** is outside the scope. **(C)** and **(D)** may be true, but they do not directly address the conclusion of the argument (the issue of funding being the *only* way to raise test scores). **(E)**, of course, is incorrect—there's no comparison being made in the argument—and therefore irrelevant.

22. C

The author's claim that the editorial's argument is no good because it is poorly written depends on the assumption that an argument's validity is related to its use of language. After all, if an argument's language didn't indicate its validity, the author's argument wouldn't make any sense at all. **(A)** is not assumed because the main argument doesn't concern who's to blame for the poorly written editorial. **(B)** and **(D)** fail because the argument addresses this editorial only and therefore does not make any assumptions about what happens generally. And **(E)** goes too far: the author needn't assume that the writer deliberately wrote badly to hide a bad argument, just that, as **(C)** says, the poor writing indicates a poor argument.

23. E

The conclusion here is that a diet free of meat and dairy products greatly reduces the risk of heart attack, based on the evidence that only 10% of those who omit meat and dairy from their diets suffer heart attacks. The assumption is that more that 10% of those who do eat dairy and meat suffer from heart attacks. If we knew that those who eat meat and dairy are *less* likely to suffer heart attacks **(E)**, the assumption would be contradicted and the argument weakened. **(A)** is out of scope. The issue isn't how many heart attacks a person has in a lifetime but how diet affects the likelihood of a heart attack. **(B)** comes closer to

strengthening the argument than weakening it by providing evidence that people who eat meat are more likely to have heart attacks. But it is still out of scope, since the passage doesn't mention people who eat meat but not dairy. **(C)** tells us that some of the people who eat neither meat nor dairy have more than one heart attack. Because we do not have a parallel statistic telling us how many dairy- and meat-eating heart attack sufferers experience more than one heart attack, this information does little to affect the argument in either direction. **(D)** strengthens the argument because it explains in more detail exactly how meat and dairy consumption is responsible for heart disease. **(E)** matches our prediction exactly. If we knew that only 7% of those who consume meat and dairy suffer heart attacks, then the fact that 10% of those who *don't* consume such foods suffer heart attacks is not evidence that a diet free of meat and dairy reduces the risk of heart attacks.

24. A

According to this argument, the new foam will reduce erosion from road cuts. The evidence? On a particular road cut to which the foam was applied, the erosion rate was low. The critical assumption is that the erosion rate on the road that was studied is lower than it would have been *without* the foam. If that's not true, then the effectiveness of the foam is in doubt. By pointing out that road cuts similar to the one tested typically have low erosion rates without the foam, **(A)** considerably weakens the argument. **(B)** is concerned with the long-term use of the foam and its maintenance; even if true, it doesn't contradict the conclusion that the foam will lower erosion at the time that it is applied. **(C)** doesn't indicate whether *this* study is unreliable, so it is irrelevant. **(D)** is concerned with an erosion prediction model made by a computer simulation; the fact that the foam is less effective than predicted doesn't mean it's not effective at all. **(E)** is concerned with other foams, not the one under study.

25. D

The most effective way to solve this is to test each choice methodically.

(A) It's the weekend.
This could be Kaliyani seeing Rhonda and Lenore in trousers. Since the temperature is not specified, Lenore could be wearing trousers.

(B) It's a weekday.
This could be Lenore seeing Kaliyani and Rhonda in skirts.

(C) It's a cold day and one of the two women is Lenore.

This could be Kaliyani seeing Rhonda and Lenore in trousers. Even though it is not specified that it is a weekend, it is possible for Kaliyani to see Rhonda and Lenore in trousers on a cold weekend day.

(D) It's a hot Saturday and one of the two women is Rhonda.

This could be Rhonda seeing Kaliyani and Lenore in skirts. However, the choice says that one of the two women being seen is Rhonda and she wears trousers, not skirts, on Saturdays. This cannot be true.

(E) It's a very cold Tuesday.

This could be Lenore seeing Kaliyani and Rhonda in skirts.

26. B

Follow the question carefully. Ultimately you are interested in the length of a side of "a certain square". You have been given a clue: the square's area is $\frac{1}{15}$ the area of a rectangle measuring 49.872 by 30.64. Fortunately, you have been told you need only the "approximate" length of a side, so you can work with approximates throughout. The area of the rectangle, then, is approximately 50 × 30, or 1,500. The area of the square will be approximately $\frac{1}{15}$ of that, or 100. The length of the side of a square is always the positive square root of the area (side × side = area), so this square has sides of approximately 10 centimetres.

27. C

As you learned in the problem solving lesson, draw a diagram to depict what the question is stating.

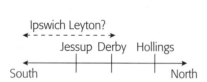

Ipswich must be south of Derby and Hollings, but there is no way to know whether it is south of Jessup. For example, Ipswich and Leyton could be south of Derby and north of Jessup. Choice **(C)** is the correct answer.

28. D

Do not get caught up in abstractly pondering the question's special instructions; turn to the answer choices and start testing the given pairs of numbers. **(A)**, **(B)**, and **(C)** do not work.

For **(D)**: The units' digit of 13 is 3, and $3^2 = 9$; $9 < 11$, so this pair does not meet the conditions, making **(D)** correct. The technique of Backsolving helps you ignore all of the strangeness and focus on exactly what the question is asking.

29. 65%

Pick a number to represent magazine subscribers. Pick 100 because it is easy to find percentages of 100. 70% of the magazine subscribers are married, so there are 70 married subscribers. 10% of the married subscribers are male, so there are 10% × 70 = 7 married male subscribers. 20% of all the subscribers are male, so 20 of them are males.

If 7 of the 20 males are married, 20 − 7 = 13 of them are not married. So the percentage of male subscribers who are not married is given by $\frac{\text{part}}{\text{whole}} \times 100\%$, which is $\frac{13}{20} \times 100\% = 65\%$.

30. C

The evidence says that students who attend universities with low faculty/student ratios get well-rounded educations, but the conclusion is that the author will send his kids to universities with small student populations. Since universities can have the second without necessarily having the first, **(C)** is correct. **(A)** claims that the author confuses cause and effect, but how could getting a well-rounded education cause a low student/faculty ratio? Anyway, the real problem is the scope shift from faculty/student ratios to student populations. As for **(B)**, the author never mentions intelligence at all, so this is out of scope as well. **(D)** fails because it doesn't point to a problem in the reasoning, just in implementing it. And **(E)** claims that students must do something extra to take advantage of the low faculty/student ratio. Since the author never claimed the benefits would be conferred automatically, this isn't a flaw; more importantly, **(E)** misses the real flaw, which we find in **(C)**.

31. C

The conclusion is that people should move to City X rather than other cities in the region in part because City X has a 4.7% unemployment rate, and that makes it relatively easy to find a job there. This is only true if unemployment rates are higher elsewhere. In other words, the assumption is that 4.7% is a low unemployment rate relative to other cities in the region. The argument states that this low rate enhances the ability to find a job, but it does not state that most people find jobs easily (choice I); in any case, this is outside the scope, because the argument only makes a claim about finding jobs in City X, not finding jobs in general. Likewise, though the argument assumes 4.7% is a low unemployment rate, there's no claim in the argument to suggest that 4.7% is a record low (choice III).

32. E

Because the article claims that enzyme K caused better performance, this is an example of a causality argument – an "X causes Y" situation. The evidence is that Olympic weightlifters and sprinters have above-average levels of enzyme K. To strengthen it, we need to find a choice confirming that X (high levels of enzyme K) does in fact cause Y (better performance). **(A)** is out of scope; the article is only concerned with enzyme K, not other factors affecting performance. **(B)** is irrelevant and uses extreme language. **(C)** distorts what the article claims; the article says only that enzyme K improves performance, not that it is required. **(D)** is an irrelevant comparison; both weightlifters and sprinters are presented as equal evidence. **(E)** states that increased levels of enzyme K are not the result of strenuous activity; this strengthens the conclusion that enzyme K contributes to better performance because the enzyme is found in people who excel at strenuous activities but is not produced by the strenuous activity. Its presence must therefore help performance. If **(E)** were not true, strenuous activity could actually be causing the increased enzyme levels, and the argument would be weakened because it reversed cause and effect.

33. C

Paragraph 3 states that the safety level for mercury is based on methylmercury, not ethylmercury, and that the latter "has not been sufficiently researched to establish intake guidelines". Thus choice **(A)** is incorrect. The exact amount of thimerosal in the flu vaccine is not stated, so we do not know if it is at a safe level (choice **(B)**); further, the article points out that the level of safety itself is debatable. Choice **(B)** therefore cannot be correct. Paragraph 3 clearly states that while mercury in vaccines exceeds the safe level established by the EPA, it does not exceed those set by other organisations, including the FDA. Therefore it is logical to conclude that the EPA's safe level is lower than

the FDA's—choice **(C)**. Choice **(D)** is a wild assumption. Just because David Kirby has investigated and written about the possible connection between thimerosal and autism does not mean that he has children who suffer from autism.

34. A

The author's concern with concentrated doses of thimerosal through multiple vaccines is expressed in paragraph 5, and especially in the last sentence in that paragraph: "Worse, those 212.5 micrograms are not spread out in daily doses but administered in a handful of highly concentrated doses at two months, four months, six months and one year". This concern is repeated in paragraphs 8 ("and vaccines are always given in highly concentrated doses") and 9 ("the impact of concentrated doses of thimerosal…must be investigated"). Thus **(A)** is the correct answer. If thimerosal is in fact responsible for the rise in autism, it is unlikely that the epidemic will worsen in the years ahead because thimerosal has been removed from most vaccines, so **(B)** is incorrect. There is no indication that the author mistrusts the CDC (choice **(C)**); in fact, the author seems to take pains to point out that both sides have evidence for their conflicting claims. Finally, it is possible that Kirby's book will prompt some parents to stop vaccinating their children, but there is no evidence that this is the author's concern, and there is no evidence that this would lead to new outbreaks of old diseases. Thus choice **(D)** is incorrect.

35. D

Paragraph 6 points out that the number of cases of autism rose in correspondence with the increase in the number of thimerosal-laden vaccinations in the 1990s and states that "the list of symptoms of mercury poisoning and autism are nearly identical", so I and III are reasons for the suspected link between thimerosal and autism. II is not; there is no mention of a British study in the passage. Thus **(D)** is the correct answer.

Section 2: Scientific Knowledge and Applications

1. 2

Since you know the area of the circle, you can find the length of radii *OB* and *OC*. You cannot find *AB* directly, but if you can find the length of *OA*, then *AB* is just the difference between *OB* and *OA*.

The circle's area, πr^2, is 100π, so its radius is $\sqrt{100}$ or 10. So *OC* is 10 and, as the question states, *AC* is 6. $\triangle AOC$ is a right triangle, so use the Pythagorean theorem to find *OA*. Ideally, you should recognize that $\triangle AOC$ is a 3-4-5 right triangle; *OC* is twice 5, *AC* is twice 3, so *OA* must be twice 4, or 8. (If you did not see this: $(OA)^2 + 6^2 = 10^2$, $(OA)^2 + 36 = 100$, $(OA)^2 = 64$, and $OA = 8$.) *AB* is the difference between the radius *OB* and segment *OA*, so its length is $10 - 8$, or 2.

2. 121

$$\begin{array}{r} 5x^2 + 13x + 40 \\ x - 3 \overline{) 5 x^3 - 2x^2 + x + 1} \\ \underline{-5x^3 - 15x^2} \\ 13x^2 + x \\ \underline{-13x^2 - 39x} \\ 40x + 1 \\ \underline{40x - 120} \\ 121 \end{array}$$

3. D

Mitochondria, ribosomes, endoplasmic reticulum, and centrioles are all organelles found in the cytoplasm of the cell. Mitochondria are surrounded by double membranes and are involved in energy production for the cell. Ribosomes synthesise proteins, and the endoplasmic reticulum sorts and transports many of those proteins. Centrioles organise microtubules in the cell and are important for cell division. Chromatin is uncondensed chromosomal material, composed of DNA and protein, and is found in the nucleus of the cell.

4. E

Fermentation is the process of energy production that occurs in the absence of oxygen. In the presence of oxygen, pyruvate produced by glycolysis can enter the citric acid (or Krebs) cycle. However, in the absence of oxygen, this pathway is not used, and fermentation is instead employed to degrade the pyruvate and generate energy. This process can produce ethanol (alcoholic fermentation, such as is performed by yeast), lactate (lactic fermentation, as occurs in muscle), and carbon dioxide.

5. C

Transport from the endoplasmic reticulum to the Golgi apparatus is required for secretion of proteins from cells. When transport is disrupted by Brefeldin A, the cell will be unable to secrete enzyme X. In addition, transport is necessary to direct proteins to the plasma membrane, so enzyme X would not accumulate in that location. Finally, sorting of proteins to the nucleus or nuclear membranes does not require either the endoplasmic reticulum or the Golgi apparatus, so it would be unaffected. Since enzyme X does not typically accumulate in the nuclear membrane and localisation to this membrane would be unaffected, enzyme X would not appear in the nuclear membrane following treatment.

6. A

Nerve impulses, also known as action potentials, are propagated by the opening of voltage-gated Na^+ channels. Because the concentration of Na^+ ions outside the cell is much higher than inside the cell, the opening of these channels allows Na^+ ions to flow into the cell. This flow of ions changes the voltage potential between the exterior and interior of the cell—thereby, the nerve impulse is generated. The voltage potential is restored to its original value by the opening of K^+ channels. K^+ concentration is higher inside the cell than outside the cell, so when these channels are opened, K^+ ions flow out of the cell, counteracting the electrical change caused by the influx of Na^+ ions.

7. E

The area of the shaded region is the area of sector *OPQ* minus the area of $\square POQ$. Since $\square POQ$ is 90°, sector *OPQ* is a quarter-circle. The circle's radius, *OP*, is 2, so the area of the circle is $\Pi (2^2) = 4\Pi$. Therefore, the quarter-circle's area is Π.

$\square POQ$'s area is $\frac{1}{2} (b \times h) = \frac{1}{2} (2 \times 2) = 2$. So, the area of the shaded region is $\Pi - 2$.

8. A

A metalloid is an element that has some typical properties of metals as well as non-metals. They are found on the periodic table between the metals and non-metals. Arsenic is a metalloid.

9. B

Percent mass is the mass of one component divided by total mass. For brass, the mass percent must be 30% (100%-70% = 30%), so 30% = (m_{Zn}/12.3 grams) (100). The m_{Zn} is 3.7 grams.

10. A

In 1.4 minutes the sample would have undergone 4 half-lives. After the first 21 seconds, the chromium would have 5.00 grams. After another 21 seconds or a total of 42 seconds, the chromium sample would have 2.5 grams and then after the third 21 seconds or a total of 63 seconds the sample would have 1.25. Then after a total of 1.4 minutes, it would have completed its fourth half-life and have 0.625 grams.

11. C

The swings act as pendulums. The period of a pendulum depends on the length of the pendulum and the local acceleration of gravity, not the mass on the end of the pendulum. If the swings both have the same length, they will swing back and forth in the same amount of time, i.e., they will have the same period, regardless of the weight of the person on the swing. Both the child and the adult take the same amount of time to make a complete oscillation.

12. D

The total power for the wire(s) is given by $P = V/R^2$, where $V = 120$ for both situations. When we cut the wire in two, the resistance of each new wire is half the original. Therefore, the power output of each wire is double the original. Adding the effects of both wires, the power output quadruples.

13. A

When solving an inequality like this one, treat it like an equation, that is, by doing the same thing to all its parts. There are two important things to remember when dealing with inequalities: (1) multiplying or dividing an inequality by a negative number reverses the sign, and (2) you are solving for a range of values rather than a single value.

To begin, you can get rid of the radical sign by squaring all the elements in the inequality $8 < \sqrt{(n+6)(n+1)} < 9$. The direction of the signs will not change since all the elements are greater than 0.

So $64 < (n+6)(n+1) < 81$. Now you could try Backsolving; the answer choice for which this relationship is true will be correct.

Start with choice (**C**): $(n+6)(n+1) = (7+6)(7+1) = 104$. This is greater than 81, so discard and move onto a smaller answer choice. (**B**) $(n+6)(n+1) = (6+6)(6+1) = 84$. This is still greater than 81, so the correct answer choice must be smaller still, which only leaves (**A**).

14. $3^{10} + \dfrac{1}{3^5}$

$$\frac{5\sqrt{14}}{2\sqrt{2}} \times \frac{4\sqrt{2}}{3\sqrt{7}} = \frac{5\sqrt{14} \times 4\sqrt{2}}{}$$

$$= \frac{5 \times 4 \times \sqrt{14} \times \sqrt{2}}{}$$

$$= \frac{10 \times \sqrt{14}}{}$$

$$= \frac{10}{3} \times \sqrt{2}$$

$$= \frac{10\sqrt{2}}{3}$$

15. E

You must solve for z here, so begin by taking z out of the denominator by multiplying both sides by z:

$x = \dfrac{x+y}{z}$, so $zx = x + y$. Now you can divide both sides by x:

$z = \dfrac{x+y}{z}$. Next distribute out the denominator on the right side of the equation:

$$z = \frac{x}{x} + \frac{y}{x} = 1 + \frac{y}{x} = \frac{y}{x} + 1.$$

16. A

In Darwin's theory of natural selection, some organisms in a species have variations in traits that give them an advantage over other members of the species. These adaptations enable these organisms and their offspring to survive in greater numbers than organisms that lack them, giving them greater fitness.

17. B

When two populations are in direct competition for the same resource, one population will compete more effectively and will, with time, force out the other population. This is particularly true with the relatively short time spans and restricted conditions in laboratory experiments. This means that (**B**) is the best answer. While resources are not limiting, both populations will grow.

When they compete, the protozoan that reproduces faster, Protozoan A, will out-compete Protozoan C and cause Protozoan C to die out. **(A)** is wrong–the relationship between these populations is a competitive one, and there is no reason to believe that this relationship will reverse itself to one in which both populations benefit. There is little an algae can do to escape predation (**(C)** is not the best choice). The populations of predator and prey are likely to reach an equilibrium state which is more or less stable. If the predator population increases and eats more of the prey, as the prey population decreases, the predator will decrease as well. Predators rarely hunt a prey to extinction (**(D)** is wrong). It is also unlikely that protozoans will be able to evolve so rapidly as to change a fundamental property in a few generations (**(E)** is wrong).

18. C

In the cross of Mouse I with the female, the ratio of the offspring phenotypes is 3:1, indicating a Bb ✕ Bb cross with BB and Bb animals black and bb animals white. Therefore, mouse I is Bb, while the female is Bb. In the second cross of mouse II and the female mouse, 100 percent of the offspring are black. Hence Mouse II must be homozygously dominant.

19. D

The alkali metals react with water to produce H_2 (g) and OH^- ions. The substances in **(A)** would react to produce CO_2 (g); **(B)** would give no reaction (though HCl does react with active metals such as Mg and Zn to produce H_2); **(C)** would react to produce NO gas, which would be converted to brown NO_2 on contact with air; **(E)** would produce NH_3 (aq) and NaCl (aq).

20. C

Only the nonmetal elements are gases under these conditions. Don't be fooled by **(D)**; while some of the halogens are gases, there are also many non-halogen elements that occur as gases—oxygen, nitrogen, and the entire group of noble gases.

21. C

When adding or subtracting numbers, keep the same number of decimal places; in this case, four decimal places means keeping one zero at the end of the number. The significant digits are 7, 2, and the final 0.

22. A

The magnetic force, F_B, on a particle with a charge, q, moving in a magnetic field, B, with a speed, v, is given by

$$F_B = qvB\sin\theta$$

where θ is the angle between the magnetic field and the velocity. A neutron has no charge, so it can have no magnetic force acting on it. A charged particle at rest also has no magnetic force acting on it because its speed is zero. A charged particle moving parallel to the magnetic field also experiences no force because $\sin\theta = 0$. The electron moving perpendicular to the magnetic field has none of the quantities in the above equation equal to zero, so it can have a magnetic force acting on it.

23. A

To answer this question, find the force, F, between two charges from Coulomb's law

$$F = \left(\frac{1}{4}\pi\varepsilon_o\right)\frac{q_1 q_2}{r^2}$$

where q_1 and q_2 are the charges and r is the distance between them. From the question stem, $q_1 = 8 \times 10^{-4}$ C, $q_2 = 2 \times 10^{-4}$ C, and $r = 2$ m. Plugging these values into the equation for Coulomb's law gives us

$$F = 9 \times 10^9 \text{ N} \times \text{m}^2 / \text{C}^2 \frac{(8 \times 10^{-4} \text{ C})(2 \times 10^{-4} \text{C})}{(2 \text{ m})^2}$$

$$F = 360 \text{ N}$$

So, the force between the charges is 360 N.

24. C

The brightness of the bulb will be determined by the electrical power the bulb uses. The power is the current passing through the bulb multiplied by the potential difference across the bulb. In a series circuit, the current is the same everywhere in the circuit. The potential difference across each bulb will be half the potential difference across the battery, because the bulbs both have the same resistance. Thus, the bulbs will be equally bright because they have the same current passing through them and the same potential difference across them.

25. B

Electronegativity is a measure of the attraction of the electron in a bond. The electronegativity decreases down a group and increases across a period. Therefore, caesium is the least electronegative.

26. C

This is the definition of **normal** boiling point; it's the boiling point of a substance at sea level, where atmospheric pressure is 1 atm. **(A)** and **(C)** are describe the boiling point, but not specifically normal boiling point. **(D)** is the value of the normal boiling point of water (the problem doesn't specify what liquid).

27. D

The electron's velocity will have components parallel and perpendicular to the magnetic field lines. If the electron's velocity were completely parallel to the magnetic field, there would be no force on the electron and its velocity would not change. If the electron's velocity were completely perpendicular to the magnetic field, the force would be continuously perpendicular to the velocity, resulting in circular motion around the magnetic field lines. The result when the electron's velocity has components both perpendicular and parallel to the magnetic field lines is that the electron has a helical or spiral path around the magnetic field lines.

Section 3: Writing Task
Sample Score 15 Essays

Technological progress is like an axe in the hands of a pathological criminal.

Albert Einstein was perhaps one of the greatest thinkers of the 20th century, both as a physicist and as a visionary observer of events (subatomic, atomic, cultural, historical and political). He also had a way with words. For such a gifted scientist to clearly paint such a picture of gloom regarding modern "technological progress" is frightening – for an axe in the hands of a pathological criminal is, well, *deadly!*

Clearly Einstein had a deep belief that the state of modern technological progress through the early-to-mid 20th century was headed toward imminent death and destruction. Perhaps the combination of his proximity to leading scientific research, his own pursuit of the theory of relativity, and the impending "atomic revolution" (he was aware of early studies in nuclear fission – the splitting of atoms that releases a devastating burst of energy in the form of a cataclysmic explosion), mixed with the cultural and political climate of his age (a world economy based on global scale wars with hundreds of millions of casualties and rapidly advancing means to kill people) resulted in his imaginative brain foreseeing a future without one.

During Einstein's lifetime, much of technological advancement was achieved through government funding (either directly or indirectly) and through commercial interests in the expanding military machine -- the industrial military complex became the largest segment of world gross production during the first half of the 20th century. Einstein clearly felt that this was a dangerous proposition: focusing scientists around the globe on the goal of splitting atoms to achieve maximum devastation of a foe.

While ultimately, and in everyday life, it could be argued that technological progress saves lives (vaccines, safety equipment, drugs etc.). But when this "tool" (read 'axe') is put in the hands of a body (the world's political leaders and industrialists) that is willing to use – no, *preconditioned* to use – violence and crime as a means to an end, then you simply cannot reconcile the dangers with any potential benefits.

What we see depends mainly on what we look for.

We all know someone who always seems to be looking for trouble – and finding it. We also know people who always seem to be on the lookout for exciting opportunities – and finding them. As John Lubbock said, "What we see depends mainly on what we look for." That seems to be true of every aspect of our lives, from the personal to the professional to the spiritual.

Let's consider a concrete example. Hypochondriacs are people who are always looking for, and finding, symptoms of some horrible ailment. They are always watching for signs that something (else) is wrong – a new disease has entered the body or an old one flared up again. A backache is the sign of cancer in the spine; an itchy rash evidence of a rare disease. If you seek negative, you will find negative. Likewise, if you seek positive, you will find positive – though not necessarily in the form you imagined. Think of the person who's always able to find the good in a situation. It's not just positive thinking; it's a way of *seeing*.

When it comes to perception and desires, one particular area of concern is science. How much does what we want to see impact what we actually see when we conduct scientific investigations?

Scientists are supposed to be objective, but of course they aren't, at least not entirely. That's because as hard as they try, their desires and hypotheses influence their findings.

It's not that scientists manufacture results (though certainly there have been some guilty of doctoring data), but it is possible to "see" something that simply isn't there or to misinterpret results. It's also possible to be so busy looking for X that you neglect to see Y and Z, which might disprove or at least overshadow X. And it's certainly possible to be so certain a hypothesis is true, that you ignore evidence that it is false.

A good scientist, of course, cannot deny facts, especially if the same facts come up over and over again after repeated experiments. No matter how much you want a red dot to turn green, it's not going to do so. But after a while, it may start to take on shades of celery or sage. When we are actively seeking something, it's easy to develop blinders to all else around us. That's why replication and peer review are so essential to good science. These are the checks and balances that help us ensure what we see really is there.

Knowledge is more valuable than morals.

I sincerely hope Maxim Gorky was being facetious when he said "Knowledge is more valuable than morals". If he wasn't, then that helps explain why Albert Einstein would say something like "Technological progress is like an axe in the hands of a pathological criminal". If we place knowledge above morality, we may indeed be headed for disaster.

I do not mean to say that knowledge isn't important, but it cannot supersede morality if we are to remain a *civilised* people. Morals guide our actions; they tell us what to do with our knowledge. Without moral guidelines, knowledge too easily becomes a weapon, not a tool for advancement.

Some examples are in order, and nuclear weapons come first to mind. One of the most frightening prospects of our time is the possibility that we might suddenly cease to exist because someone lacking moral restraint decided to annihilate us with nuclear weapons. All the knowledge required to create this great weapon becomes nothing in an instant.

On a more practical level, morality keeps us from using everyday knowledge to harm others. I might know how to hack into your computer, for example, but my morality will prevent me from violating you in that way. Similarly, you might know a secret about my past, but your morality will keep you from hurting me by telling others that secret.

I don't mean to imply that knowledge isn't important. Most certainly we should always strive to learn. I believe that knowledge is power – and it is precisely for this reason that we must value morality at least as much as we value knowledge. Without moral guidelines keeping us in check, that power can simply be too dangerous.